RESOLVING
OCD

RESOLVING OCD

Understanding Your Obsessional Experience

Volume 1

Frederick Aardema, PhD

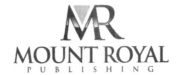

MOUNT ROYAL
PUBLISHING

Library and Archives Canada Cataloguing in Publication

Title: Resolving OCD / Frederick Aardema, PhD.
Other titles: Resolving obsessive-compulsive disorder
Names: Aardema, Frederick, author.
Identifiers: Canadiana 20240495837 | ISBN 9780987911940 (set) | ISBN 9780987911926 (v.1 : softcover)
Subjects: LCSH: Obsessive-compulsive disorder—Popular works. | LCSH: Obsessive-compulsive
disorder— Treatment—Popular works.
Classification: LCC RC533 .A27 2025 | DDC 616.85/227—dc23

Dedicated to the love of my life, Moni,
without whom this book would not
have been possible, let alone
probable.

Acknowledgements

First and foremost, I would like to express my deepest gratitude to the patients who have shared their stories and struggles with me over the years. Your courage, perseverance, and willingness to embrace new ways of thinking have been a profound source of inspiration, fueling much of the research and practical work behind this approach. It is through your dedication to understanding and managing OCD that this book has become possible.

To the practitioners who have taken this approach into their work with clients, thank you for your commitment to making a difference in the lives of those struggling with OCD. Your dedication to applying these methods with care and expertise has been essential in helping individuals break free from OCD. Your openness to exploring new methods and your passion for improving lives have made a significant impact. Without your belief in this approach, we wouldn't be where we are today.

I am also immensely grateful to the wider academic community, including students, researchers, and scholars. Your collaboration, feedback, and insights have enriched this field and contributed profoundly to our shared mission. Together, we strive for a deeper understanding of OCD, and your dedication has been instrumental in guiding this work.

And finally, to my wife. This book, and much of my life's work, is dedicated to you. From the very beginning, you have been by my side—attending conferences, reviewing grant proposals, and helping navigate the many challenges along the way. Your unwavering belief in this project and your support through the ups and downs made this book a reality. You were alongside me throughout the writing process, always gently encouraging me to achieve the best. Your patience, your wisdom, and your editorial eye have shaped this book into what it is today. For all of this and more, I am endlessly thankful. This book exists because of you.

DISCLAIMER

The information in this self-help manual and workbook is not intended as a substitute for consultation with healthcare professionals, nor is it meant to diagnose or assess your individual situation. Neither author or publisher warrants that the information contained in this book is in every respect accurate or complete and they bear no responsibility for any errors or omissions, or for any outcomes resulting from the use of the information presented herein. While this guide is designed to empower you, it may not fully address all your needs and is not intended to replace the expertise of a healthcare professional. If you experience any mental health concerns, you are advised to seek the help of a licensed mental health professional for assessment and treatment.

CONFIDENTIALITY

To maintain confidentiality, none of the vignettes or obsessional stories in this book represent real clients or individuals. Instead, they are fictionalized amalgamations inspired by insights from a broad range of clients and sources, and do not represent any specific individual or real-life client.

Volume 1

Table of Contents

PART 1 - FUNDAMENTALS OF OCD

PART 2 - THE OUTER WHEEL

PART 3 - THE INNER WHEEL

List of Downloadable Materials

Chapter 3: The Obsessional Sequence

Chapter 4: Everyday and Obsessional Doubt

Chapter 5: The Obsessional Narrative

Introduction

This fully interactive official guide is the first to bring *Inference-based Cognitive-Behavioral Therapy* (I-CBT) directly to individuals struggling with OCD in a comprehensive, self-help format. I-CBT represents a fresh perspective in OCD treatment, departing from the traditional focus on behavioral techniques that, while effective, have largely remained rooted in their original framework over the past six decades. Unlike existing self-help resources, this manual offers a truly innovative approach, providing a new lens through which to understand and overcome OCD symptoms.

I-CBT has already made a far-reaching and powerful impact on OCD treatment, with a growing number of mental health professionals incorporating it into their practices. This widespread adoption is not the result of mere hype; rather, it stems from the resonance of I-CBT principles among individuals with OCD, including therapists with lived experience. Their testimonials have been instrumental in advancing and disseminating I-CBT, serving as powerful endorsements.

Furthermore, I-CBT stands as an evidence-based intervention rooted in scientific principles. Extensive research has bolstered its theoretical foundations and demonstrated its efficacy in multicenter randomized trials conducted by independent scientific laboratories. With such robust support, I have every confidence that the number of professionals offering I-CBT will continue to rise.

This first volume of the *Resolving OCD Series* endeavors to make I-CBT readily accessible to those dealing with OCD, with the sincere hope that it will serve as a valuable tool on your journey toward liberation from OCD. By the end of this volume, you will have a clear understanding of the many manifestations of OCD and your personal patterns, including your obsessional narrative. The focus of this volume is to help you build a foundational awareness of your own OCD, setting the stage for advanced techniques covered in Volume Two.

Who am I?

I am the co-creator of I-CBT, the psychological treatment framework underpinning this self-help guide. My journey with OCD began during my studies at the University of Groningen in the Netherlands in the mid-1990s, under the esteemed guidance of Professor Paul Emmelkamp. It was during this formative period that I delved into the intricacies of OCD and its treatment, particularly through exposure and response prevention (ERP), still widely viewed as a fundamental approach in OCD therapy. However, despite its reputation as an effective treatment modality, ERP doesn't universally achieve success, often leaving lingering symptoms in its wake. Furthermore, the requirement to directly confront fears can pose a formidable challenge for many individuals.

In my quest for alternative approaches, I found myself drawn to cognitive models of OCD. These models focus on the impact of thoughts and beliefs on behavior, pinpointing specific cognitive patterns underlying OCD symptoms. However, cognitive interventions were typically only used to supplement ERP rather than standalone treatments, leaving a gap in addressing OCD comprehensively through cognitive means.

In 1996, while researching for my Master's thesis, I stumbled upon a novel cognitive approach proposed by psychologists Kieron O'Connor and Sophie Robillard. This approach offered a fresh perspective on OCD, emphasizing unusual reasoning processes and suggesting a treatment avenue that bypassed the need for ERP. Intrigued, I embarked on validating this cognitive model empirically, confirming its efficacy in predicting OCD symptoms.

Driven by this discovery, I pursued a doctoral degree focused on further exploring reasoning processes in OCD, collaborating closely with Professors Paul Emmelkamp and Kieron O'Connor. Expanding the model to encompass all forms of OCD, not just contamination and checking, marked a significant milestone in my research journey. During this foundational period, I also developed the first treatment manual to support therapists and clients in our treatment trials, which was later published in *Beyond Reasonable Doubt: Reasoning Processes in Obsessive Compulsive Disorder and Related Disorders*. This work laid the groundwork for a new, reasoning-focused approach to OCD treatment.

In 2009, following my postdoctoral studies, I joined the University of Montreal as a professor and researcher at the Montreal Mental Health University Institute Research Center. Subsequent awards, including scholarships and research funding, have bolstered my commitment to advancing OCD research and treatment.

My dedication remains unwavering in providing effective treatment options for individuals suffering from OCD, particularly those unresponsive to standard interventions. I am indebted to the insights gathered from clients and collaborators, which have shaped my mission to alleviate the burden of OCD. This self-help book is a tangible manifestation of that mission, offering hope and guidance to those navigating the complexities of OCD.

Who is This Book For?

This book is primarily intended for individuals with OCD. Regardless of the specific manifestation of your OCD, whether it's contamination fears, unwanted thoughts, or compulsive behaviors, they all stem from the same core: unnecessary doubt. This doubt can permeate any aspect of life, regardless of its subject matter.

While this resource is designed for individual use, it's important to emphasize that it's not a substitute for professional treatment. If your symptoms are severe, or if you find yourself struggling with feelings of depression or suicidal thoughts, seeking the guidance of a qualified mental health professional is imperative.

Mental health professionals will also find this book an invaluable resource. Whether you're a seasoned therapist or new to the field, this guide serves as a comprehensive companion for I-CBT. Packed with handouts, exercises, and diagrams, it is designed to complement therapy sessions with clients, making it a practical and interactive tool. Even therapists who are well-versed in I-CBT will benefit from the latest strategies, insights, and therapeutic frameworks presented in this manual. It can enhance your practice, offering a structured yet flexible approach to help clients break free from OCD through cognitive and inferential reasoning techniques.

Finally, if you're someone who simply wants to deepen your understanding of OCD, perhaps because you have a loved one battling the condition, this book offers a comprehensive exploration. By gaining insight into the intricacies of OCD, you can offer meaningful support and compassion. However, it's essential to respect individuals' autonomy and readiness for help; forcing this resource upon someone who isn't receptive may be counterproductive.

How Can This Book Help You?

Building on the principles of I-CBT, this book aims to address OCD at its core by targeting the unique reasoning styles that fuel obsessive-compulsive symptoms. I-CBT has proven its effectiveness in helping individuals with OCD, as evidenced by randomized controlled trials across multiple research centers. These studies consistently demonstrate that I-CBT achieves significant symptom improvement for most individuals, with a considerable number reaching full remission.

What sets I-CBT apart is its acceptability and tolerability. In contrast to treatments heavily reliant on exposure, I-CBT doesn't demand confronting fears or enduring uncertainty. Instead, it targets the underlying dysfunctional reasoning to eradicate obsessional doubt without the need for ERP. At its core, I-CBT teaches that obsessions lack inherent validity, thus eliminating the need for direct confrontation of fears.

> In I-CBT, you don't confront fears; you overcome them by realizing there's nothing to fear in the first place.

While proven to be effective, it's important to acknowledge that I-CBT isn't a one-size-fits-all solution. If previous treatments have been successful for you, that's fantastic. This book doesn't discredit your achievements. However, if you're still struggling, it might be time to explore alternative approaches. Different treatments can yield different outcomes for different individuals, and failure to respond to one doesn't equate to personal failure. This self-help manual aims to provide you with the support and tools you need for a different approach, recognizing that everyone's journey to overcoming OCD is unique.

How do I Use this Book?

Try approaching this book with a relaxed mindset, allowing it to unfold naturally without jumping to conclusions or dismissing it prematurely. Maintaining an open and curious attitude will enable you to derive the most benefit from this self-help guide and workbook. I-CBT requires some work and persistence, but it is primarily a therapy of insight, rather than one of exhaustive effort. Its essence lies in understanding how obsessional doubts arise and recognizing their falsehood.

It's also crucial to understand that the approach outlined in this manual isn't purely intellectual, despite its focus on cognition and reasoning. I-CBT aims to reduce *unnecessary* thought and reasoning, a common feature in OCD, guiding you back to your true self and a life free from pointless obsessions.

In contrast to psychodynamic or psychoanalytical therapies, I-CBT doesn't delve into the depths of the unconscious or trace symptoms back to childhood. Instead, it focuses on observable elements in the present, including the narrative and reasoning behind your obsessional doubts, which are often readily accessible with the right questions.

The book is structured logically to aid in overcoming OCD, with each chapter and exercise building upon the previous. Skipping ahead or rushing through may impede progress rather than accelerate it. Merely reading the exercises isn't sufficient; active participation is essential, often over extended periods. Remember, resolving OCD requires more than just thinking about it — it involves thinking differently.

What is Inside?

This first volume of the series, *Resolving OCD: Understanding Your Obsessional Experience,* is structured into three main parts, designed to provide a foundational understanding of OCD while building a deep awareness of how it manifests in your life. Through a comprehensive and practical approach, this book delves into the nature of OCD and helps you identify and understand your own obsessional patterns. It lays the groundwork for more advanced work in the next installment of the series, *Resolving OCD: Advanced Strategies for Overcoming Obsessional Doubts,* equipping you with the tools to take your journey toward freedom to the next level.

Part 1 focuses on the *Fundamentals of OCD and its Treatment.* It begins with an in-depth exploration of the different forms of OCD and the wide range of symptoms that accompany it. In *Chapter 1,* you'll receive a broad overview of how OCD manifests in various forms and you'll be encouraged to reflect on how these manifestations apply to your personal experience. By recognizing your own symptoms, you'll begin the process of identifying the specific ways in which OCD influences your thinking and behavior.

Moving into *Chapter 2,* the focus shifts to understanding how different cognitive-behavioral theories have evolved in the treatment of OCD. This chapter delves into the key models to treating OCD, including the limitations and benefits of these models. You'll explore why some traditional methods have been successful for some but challenging or incomplete for others. Crucially, this chapter introduces you to an inference-based approach to OCD, which offers a fresh and innovative lens through which to understand OCD. The groundwork laid here forms the foundation of the manual, helping you understand how I-CBT specifically targets the underlying reasoning that drives obsessional doubt.

Part 2 shifts the focus to what I-CBT describes as *The Outer Wheel of OCD.* This part explores the visible and most recognizable symptoms of OCD, such as compulsions, triggers, and emotional reactions to obsessional doubt. *Chapter 3* introduces the concept of the obsessional sequence, helping you to trace how OCD operates in a step-by-step manner in your mind. By understanding how obsessional doubts emerge, escalate, and lead to compulsive actions, you'll gain a clearer picture of how OCD takes hold of your thought processes. This chapter will guide you in mapping out your personal obsessional sequence—a critical exercise in identifying the patterns of thought and behavior that keep you trapped in the cycle of OCD.

In *Chapter 4,* we dive deeper into the nature of obsessional doubt, uncovering what sets it apart from the everyday doubts that everyone encounters. This chapter highlights the unique nature of obsessional doubt, which persists without resolution, thrives in the absence of concrete evidence, and leaves you trapped in a cycle of perpetual uncertainty—questioning your actions, thoughts, or intentions. By clearly distinguishing between everyday doubt and obsessional doubt, you will gain the insight needed to confront the reasoning driving obsessional doubt and take the first steps toward breaking its hold on your thinking.

The final section of Volume One, introduces *Part 3: The Inner Wheel of OCD*, which delves into the deeper cognitive processes that drive OCD from within. *Chapter 5*, which concludes this volume, focuses on one of the central elements of the Inner Wheel—the obsessional narrative. The obsessional narrative is the story that OCD creates around your doubts, making them feel more real and convincing. In this chapter, you'll explore how OCD builds an elaborate story around your fears, often convincing you that your worst-case scenarios are plausible or even inevitable. By identifying this false narrative, you'll learn to question its validity and begin crafting an alternative, non-obsessional narrative. Chapter 5 provides you with the tools to turn away from the stories that OCD tells you and start shifting your thinking toward a different, more balanced perspectives.

While *Volume One* introduces you to Part 3, which focuses on the obsessional narrative, the work in this section will continue in *Volume Two* of the series, *Resolving OCD: Advanced Strategies for Overcoming and Breaking Free from OCD*. In *Volume Two*, you'll dive deeper into the remaining elements of the Inner Wheel of the OCD, starting with *Chapter 1*, which explores the confusion between imagination and reality in OCD during reasoning. This chapter explains how OCD blurs the line between what is real and what is imagined, leading you to distrust your senses and common sense. You'll learn how to identify and dismantle the tricks of the OCD, allowing you to regain trust in your own reasoning and judgments.

Following this, Volume Two continues with *Chapter 2*, which examines the feared possible self—a distorted version of yourself that OCD convinces you is real or could become real. This chapter will guide you in disengaging from the obsessive fears that cause you to doubt your identity and capabilities, helping you realize that you are not, and will not become, the person you fear.

Finally, Volume Two transitions into *Part 4: The Doing*, where you'll begin applying the knowledge you have gained in real-world cognitive and behavioral exercises. In *Chapters 3 through 5*, you will learn practical strategies to break free from OCD's grasp, including exercises like reality sensing and techniques to stay out of the OCD bubble—a metaphor for the alternate reality OCD creates when you're trapped in obsessive thinking. These exercises will guide you in re-engaging with the real world and building lasting change as you move forward in your recovery.

In summary, *Volume One* sets the stage for understanding the nature of OCD and its obsessional patterns, particularly through exploring the obsessional narrative. *Volume Two* will build on this foundation by guiding you through deeper cognitive work and practical exercises, equipping you with the tools to fully overcome OCD.

Downloadable Exercises, Handouts, and Diagrams

To support your journey with this self-help guide, a selection of key materials—including highlights, diagrams, tables, and forms—are available for download and printing. These resources are thoughtfully designed to enhance your learning and can be accessed online in various formats. If you have purchased this book, you're welcome to download these resources for personal use or, if you're a practitioner, to utilize them in supporting your work with clients. You can find them at www.icbt.online. Please note that reproducing these materials for anything other than personal or client use, whether for commercial or non-commercial purposes, is prohibited (refer to the copyright page for details). Additionally, please be aware that all other content in this book is protected by copyright, with all rights reserved.

How to Start?

Begin by avoiding the temptation to start randomly or rush through this book. Rushing can lead to setbacks or frequent backtracking, ultimately slowing your progress. Taking your time allows for deeper understanding, reflection, and integration. It gives your mind the chance to process new information, connect it to existing knowledge, and form meaningful insights, leading to more effective learning.

To get ahead is to start with where you are.

Starting at the beginning helps establish context, build a solid foundation of understanding, and progress systematically towards your goals. This approach provides clarity, structure, and often highlights key elements necessary for success. With that being said, the best way to get ahead is still to just get started. So, let's get going.

Frederick Aardema, Ph.D., Clinical Psychologist.
Full Professor, Department of Psychiatry and Addiction, University of Montreal
Clinical Researcher, Montreal Mental Health University Institute Research Center
Director, Obsessive-Compulsive Disorders Study Center
Montreal, November, 2024

PART 1

Fundamentals of OCD and its Treatment

Chapter 1

Obsessive-Compulsive Disorder

Obsessive-Compulsive Disorder (OCD) is a complex mental health condition that still affects millions of people worldwide. Early on in 1926, Sigmund Freud referred to it as "...unquestionably the most interesting and repaying subject of analytic research. But as a problem, it has not yet been mastered." Nearly a century later, while much has been learned, OCD remains one of the most intriguing yet challenging disorders to understand.

OCD comprises two primary elements: obsessions and compulsions. Obsessions are persistent, unwanted, and repetitive thoughts, images, or urges that intrude into an individual's consciousness and are difficult to control. These obsessions often center around fears related to contamination, harm, taboo thoughts, symmetry, and order. Compulsions, on the other hand, are repetitive behaviors or mental acts performed in response to obsessions, aimed at reducing the anxiety they cause. Examples include checking, washing, counting, arranging objects, or seeking reassurance.

Compulsions always arise from obsessions; without the thoughts triggering anxiety or discomfort, there would be no compulsion to act. Obsessions create the foundation for compulsions, driving repetitive behaviors or mental rituals aimed at alleviating the distress they provoke. Regrettably, these actions seldom provide lasting relief; instead, they reinforce the obsession, increasing its frequency and intensity.

For instance, if you have the thought that one might have left the stove on: the obsession with its feared potential consequences, like a fire or harm to others, induces anxiety. Consequently, you may compulsively check the stove to ease your fears, inadvertently reinforcing the obsession. Understanding this intricate interplay between your obsessions and compulsions is vital for grasping OCD dynamics.

But that's just the start — OCD is way more complicated than just reacting to thoughts. It's not merely a response problem; it's about the nature of the thoughts themselves. An obsession isn't just a passing worry. It manifests as a relentless presence in the individual's mind, often alien and at odds with their true desires and values. Unlike typical concerns, obsessions are persistent, intense, and seemingly immune to rational dismissal.

Many individuals with OCD are acutely aware that their obsessions are irrational or improbable. They often express sentiments like, "I know it's irrational, but I can't shake the thought," or, "It seems unrealistic, but I can't help performing the [ritual]." This recognition reflects the ego-dystonic nature of OCD, where the obsessions feel intrusive and inconsistent with their sense of self. Yet, despite this awareness, the obsessions continue to exert control, compelling compulsive behaviors in a desperate attempt to alleviate the distress they generate.

For others, obsessions may feel plausible or connected to genuine concerns, making the drive to act even more compelling. In such cases, the obsessions are not necessarily perceived as ego-dystonic, but rather as valid and reasonable, demanding immediate attention. Regardless of whether obsessions are experienced as irrational or credible, they consume time and energy, disrupting daily life in a relentless cycle of distress and attempted resolution.

OCD's complexity lies in its ability to adapt to personal fears and concerns, shaping a unique but equally disruptive experience for each individual. Recognizing this complexity is essential for understanding its challenges and addressing the misconceptions that surround it. By demystifying OCD, we can break down the stigma that hinders understanding, support, and access to effective treatment.

Highlight 1.1
Key Learning Points

- The principal components of OCD are obsessions and compulsions.
- Without the obsession, there is no compulsion to act.
- Obsessions are relentless thoughts that may feel senseless or entirely realistic, yet they demand action to alleviate distress.
- OCD adapts to personal fears, creating unique yet equally disruptive experiences for each individual.

OCD Myths and What it is Not

There are many misconceptions about OCD, often fueled by misinformation disseminated through various media channels. These myths not only perpetuate stigma but also hinder understanding and support for those affected by the condition. The following sections address some of the more common misconceptions and clarify what OCD truly entails.

"It's all in the brain…"

The idea that OCD is solely the result of brain abnormalities can feel disempowering, suggesting a fixed and unchangeable condition. However, this view overlooks the transformative potential of psychological intervention. While it's true that the brain plays a key role in shaping thoughts and emotions, OCD is not a hard-wired or permanent affliction. Psychological treatments have been proven effective in managing OCD symptoms and can even lead to measurable changes in brain activity, challenging the notion that OCD is immutable. Instead of viewing OCD as a lifelong sentence, it is more helpful to see it as a condition made up of persistent thoughts, feelings, and behaviors—elements that are, crucially, open to change.

Psychological approaches reveal that obsessional doubts stem from distorted reasoning rather than objective reality. These doubts may feel urgent and compelling, but they arise from flawed mental processes rather than actual evidence. By addressing the reasoning errors that fuel these doubts, psychological strategies can diminish their influence over time. In fact, changing the way you think can literally reshape your brain, demonstrating the profound power of the mind to influence brain function.

Although it can be daunting to realize that OCD originates within your own mind, this understanding is also a source of hope. Recognizing your role in generating symptoms puts the power for change in your hands. By exploring psychological strategies, you can learn to challenge obsessional thinking, reframe unhelpful patterns, and ultimately regain control over your thoughts and behaviors—reshaping your brain pathways in the process.

"You're obsessed..."

In more superstitious eras, tracing back to the mid-16th century, the term "obsession" directly implicated the hostile actions of the devil or malevolent spirits. It was closely associated with the idea of being haunted or possessed, believed to necessitate prayer, confession or exorcism rather than psychotherapy for treatment.

Thankfully, contemporary understanding acknowledges that the obsessions experienced by those with OCD originate internally, devoid of external or malevolent influences. Yet, traces of these historical beliefs persist, subtly skewing our perceptions of OCD. That is, over time, the meaning of the term obsession evolved from the influence of an evil spirit, to that of voluntary pursuits that bring pleasure.

For example, colloquial usage of the term "being obsessed" commonly denotes an excessive preoccupation that the person takes pleasure in, such as being "obsessed with sports," "obsessed with work," or "obsessed with sex." While innocuous in everyday conversation, it's crucial not to confuse it with the obsessions experienced in OCD.

Individuals with OCD derive no pleasure from their obsessions, especially those revolving around harm. They dread the intrusive thoughts, images, and urges that afflict them. This starkly contrasts with mental disorders where individuals take pleasure in these thoughts and are actually a danger to others.

Misunderstandings about the nature of obsessions and their conflation with other meanings can lead to profound misconceptions. Even healthcare professionals lacking experience with OCD may misinterpret the aversive thoughts and urges experienced by individuals with OCD as genuine threats, potentially resulting in misdiagnosis with adverse consequences.

Similarly, individuals with OCD, overwhelmed by their obsessions, might erroneously believe that turning themselves in to authorities is the "right" thing to do. However, this action stems from confusion and distress, rather than any genuine threat they pose to others. It's essential to understand that those with OCD merely fear they "might be" a danger, but in reality, they are not.

"It's your personality and values..."

People with OCD are frequently stereotyped as rigid, perfectionistic, meticulous, stubborn, intolerant, dogmatic, controlling, argumentative, or difficult to engage with. These stereotypes are commonly reinforced in media and films. However, personality traits are unrelated to OCD. In reality, none of these characteristics define individuals with OCD any more than they might apply to the general population. So, why do these stereotypes persist to the extent they do?

The notion that OCD is directly linked to personality likely originates from early psychodynamic theories. These theories suggested that OCD arises from issues with control and personality development. Specifically, OCD was believed to be closely associated with what was then termed "obsessional character," now recognized as Obsessive-Compulsive Personality Disorder (OCPD).

Individuals with OCPD often display traits and behaviors such as rigidity in routines, perfectionism, inflexibility, stubbornness, and a strong need for control. However, it's important to note that OCPD is a distinct disorder from OCD. Unlike OCD, OCPD lacks the hallmark features of true obsessions and compulsions.

While both disorders may coexist, with estimates suggesting a co-occurrence rate of around 17%, this does not imply they are identical or share common origins. In fact, given the ongoing tendency to mix-up OCD with OCPD, it's reasonable to scrutinize whether the reported co-occurrence rate accurately reflects the distinct nature of these conditions.

Consider someone with OCD who compulsively washes their hands to achieve maximum cleanliness. This behavior might appear to stem from meticulousness or rigid standards regarding hygiene. However, Individuals with OCD don't wash their hands repeatedly for these reasons; rather, they do so because they obsess over the idea of their hands being unclean. It's a fixation that isn't rooted in any inherent personality trait or characteristic.

The idea that individuals with OCD are inherently rigid, overcontrolling, or intolerant of uncertainty is also misguided. Their attempts to control their environment stem from relentless obsessions that convince them something is seriously wrong, rather than from an inherent tendency to be more rigid or controlling than others.

For instance, when someone with OCD experiences the obsession that they might pose a danger to their loved ones, they will naturally feel compelled to seek certainty and control their thoughts and to ensure that they are not a threat. This need for certainty and control arises from the distressing nature of their obsessions, rather than from a personality trait.

Misinterpretations of OCD go beyond the general public and media; individuals with OCD and their therapists can also misinterpret its nature, often confusing symptoms with personality traits. For instance, a client might attribute their compulsions to a need for things to be well-done or even perfect. Consequently, they might receive advice to be more flexible in their thinking, tolerate uncertainty, or be less perfectionistic. Yet, once more, this overlooks the fact that compulsions stem from obsessions, not inherent traits.

Much like how OCD can sometimes be mistaken for aspects of one's personality, it can also be confused with personal values. For instance, you may think that your symptoms are the result of religious devotion, industriousness, honesty, or responsibility. However, there is no evidence that these attributes directly cause OCD behaviors. You do not have to change your personality, standards or values to overcome OCD.

"To be compelled..."

Like the expression "to be obsessed", the phrase "to be compelled" also encompasses a wide range of experiences that go beyond OCD. We all encounter moments where we feel driven to take action, yet not every instance qualifies as a compulsion. While individuals with OCD often experience strong urges in response to their obsession, experiencing such urges doesn't inherently imply the presence of OCD. Indeed, an intense urge to act can emerge in completely ordinary scenarios, such as when ensuring the safety of one's child.

Furthermore, several other mental health conditions are characterized by repetitive and compulsive behaviors, potentially leading to confusion with OCD. For instance, habit and tic disorders, like nail biting, eye blinking, or sudden muscle movements, may resemble OCD due to the presence of a strong urge to act. However, in habit and tic disorders, the compulsion is typically driven by a sensory sensation aimed at alleviating physical discomfort rather than neutralizing obsessions and associated anxiety.

Compulsive-like behaviors may also be observable in autistic individuals, occasionally causing confusion. However, autism and OCD are distinct conditions, though they can co-exist. In such cases, it's important to differentiate between the repetitive behaviors often associated with autism and those stemming directly from OCD. For autistic individuals, repetitive behaviors and routines often serve a soothing or regulatory purpose, helping to manage sensory overload or underload.

Compulsive behavior also manifests prominently in substance use disorders, and behavioral addictions. For example, in substance use disorders, compulsive drug-seeking and drug-taking behaviors become central despite adverse consequences, driven by an overwhelming urge to alleviate cravings or withdrawal symptoms. Similarly, in behavioral addictions like gambling disorder, compulsive shopping, individuals experience irresistible urges to engage in repetitive behaviors despite negative consequences. However, unlike OCD, these behaviors aren't driven by the need to alleviate obsessions or perceived threats. They are driven by an overwhelming urge to satisfy cravings.

In OCD, compulsions always aim to resolve a problem posed by the obsession. They are goal-directed strategies with a discernible logic or purpose behind them, despite their inability to truly resolve the underlying issue. The themes of these obsessions are vast and deeply personal, reflecting the unique concerns of each individual. However, before delving into the various manifestations of OCD, let's first briefly explore some of different types of compulsive strategies individuals with OCD use to manage their obsessions.

Highlight 1.2.
Key Learning Points

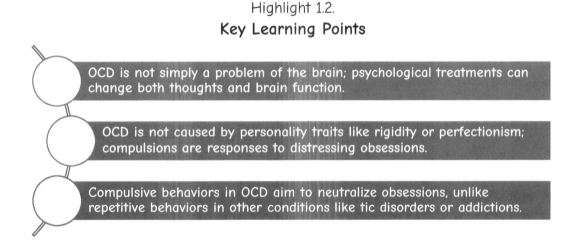

OCD is not simply a problem of the brain; psychological treatments can change both thoughts and brain function.

OCD is not caused by personality traits like rigidity or perfectionism; compulsions are responses to distressing obsessions.

Compulsive behaviors in OCD aim to neutralize obsessions, unlike repetitive behaviors in other conditions like tic disorders or addictions.

Compulsive Strategies

Compulsive strategies in OCD are varied, and although they provide temporary relief from distress, they ultimately perpetuate the cycle of obsessions and compulsions. Overt compulsions are visible actions that are often performed to neutralize a perceived threat. These include behaviors such as washing hands repeatedly to avoid contamination, checking the stove multiple times to prevent a fire, or rearranging objects until they feel "just right." For example, someone afraid of illness might spend hours cleaning their home, scrubbing every surface until their hands are raw, even when there is no evidence of contamination. Similarly, a person worried about accidentally hitting someone with their car might retrace their driving route repeatedly to ensure no harm was done, leading to significant time loss and disruption of daily activities.

On the other hand, covert compulsions, which are more subtle and often unnoticed by others, include mental rituals such as repeating phrases in one's head, counting, or mentally reviewing past events to seek reassurance. For instance, someone afraid of unintentionally offending others might replay a conversation in their mind over and over, searching for signs that their words were misunderstood. Another example is a person worried about moral wrongdoing, who might mentally list reasons why their actions were justified or acceptable. Although they are not visible, covert compulsions serve the same function as overt behaviors: to neutralize or undo the anxiety triggered by the obsession. These internal actions may provide a temporary sense of control, but much like overt compulsions, they strengthen the obsession in the long run. Because covert compulsions are not outwardly visible, they can be particularly challenging to identify and address, even for the person experiencing them.

Reassurance-seeking is another commonly used compulsive strategy, where individuals seek external validation from others or conduct exhaustive research in an effort to negate their obsessions. Whether it's repeatedly asking a loved one for reassurance or compulsively searching the internet for answers, the short-term relief these actions provide reinforces the obsession. Despite the temporary sense of security, reassurance-seeking keeps individuals reliant on external sources for comfort, which only strengthens the obsessive thought and ensures its recurrence. For instance, a person obsessing over their health might repeatedly ask a doctor if they are "truly fine" or seek out forums and articles online. Each new reassurance temporarily quiets their fear but ultimately feeds the obsession.

Safety behaviors is another type compulsive strategy. These behaviors involve subtle precautions intended to prevent feared outcomes from occurring. For example, someone with OCD centered on fears of harm might consistently keep their hands in their pockets to avoid accidentally touching or harming someone. A person with contamination fears might wear gloves or sanitize excessively to avoid perceived contamination. Although these actions may seem protective, they inadvertently reinforce the belief that the feared situations or objects are dangerous, perpetuating the anxiety they were intended to reduce.

Avoidance strategies, often intertwined with safety behaviors, involve actively steering clear of situations that might trigger obsessions or compulsions. These strategies can range from avoiding specific places, like kitchens where knives are present for someone afraid of accidentally harming others, to avoiding people or events that might increase anxiety. Over time, avoidance can limit the individual's ability to live freely, as they feel compelled to avoid an increasing number of situations. For example, someone afraid of contamination might avoid public spaces altogether, resulting in isolation and a diminished quality of life. elf-testing, a unique compulsive strategy, differs from avoidance in that it involves approaching obsessional situations in an attempt to disprove the doubts.

Finally, people engaging in self-testing confront their fears head-on, but not to overcome them; instead, they are trying to confirm that the feared scenario won't happen. Examples of self-testing include touching potentially contaminated surfaces to "test" whether they will feel dirty, or handling sharp objects to see if they can control themselves. Another example would be someone concerned about radiation standing close to a microwave to see if harmful rays are emitted. Similarly, a person doubting their sexual orientation may look at same-sex imagery to check for any physiological or emotional reaction. While the person hopes to find clarity, self-testing often amplifies doubt because OCD twists the results, leaving the person more confused than before.

Table 1.1.
Types of Compulsive Strategies in OCD

Compulsive Strategy	Examples
Overt Compulsions Repetitive behaviors or actions that are observable and visible to others.	Ordering, checking, washing, tapping, touching, aligning, repeating, counting out loud.
Covert Compulsions Mental rituals or internalized behaviors not readily observable to others.	Repeating mantras, mental counting, mental neutralizing, self-analysis, praying, reviewing, ruminating, monitoring.
Reassurance seeking The act of repeatedly seeking validation, confirmation or comfort from outside sources.	Consulting with authorities, doctors, family members, friends, therapists, internet searches, researching.
Safety Behaviors Subtle avoidance behaviors to prevent or reduce the likelihood of obsessions and distress	Using gloves, masks, protective gear, driving slowly, distracting oneself, paying too much attention.
Avoidance Evading stimuli that trigger distressing obsessive thoughts and anxiety.	Avoiding places, people, objects, items, topics of conversation, news, media, activities, decisions.
Self-Testing Purposely engaging with situations that provoke obsessions to reassure oneself.	Purposely thinking blasphemous thoughts to test if you feel guilty or anxious enough, looking at individuals to test for sexual attraction.

Compulsive strategies—whether overt or covert, active or avoidant—ultimately reinforce the cycle of OCD by validating the false belief that the obsession holds some truth. These behaviors provide temporary relief but strengthen the conviction that the obsessional doubts are worth acting upon. To truly alleviate the distress caused by OCD, individuals must learn to disengage from these compulsive behaviors, but for the person with OCD, this is not as simple as it sounds.

When you have OCD, the doubts and fears can feel intensely real and compelling, making it incredibly difficult to resist acting on them. The obsessive thoughts are often accompanied by a powerful sense of urgency or dread, leading to a near-automatic response to perform a compulsion. This makes breaking free from the cycle of compulsions extremely challenging, even when there is a desire to stop. Thus, while disengaging from compulsions is critical, it requires more than willpower.

Ultimately, any action that reinforces your obsession is a compulsion. The key is to recognize when you're engaging in these behaviors, rather than over-analyzing different types of strategies. While these actions may not explain the origins of your obsessions, they do play a major role in keeping them alive. Compulsions are something you'll want to let go of. They don't offer a path to resolution; they only sustain the cycle.

> Compulsive actions are failing strategies to resolve an obsession.

The OCD Kaleidoscope

No manifestation of OCD is ever entirely alike. Every person has their own story, with distinct thoughts, emotions and coping mechanisms. Despite this diversity, certain recurring themes tend to emerge around which obsessions and compulsions cluster. Among the most prevalent are: 1) disturbing thoughts, 2) contamination-related OCD, 3) concerns about negligence and mistakes, and 4) a preoccupation with symmetry, ordering, and arranging.

However, the spectrum of OCD is vast, encompassing many other variations beyond these categories. The manifestation of symptoms varies widely among individuals, defying neat categorization into subtypes. Labeling them as such can be misleading, as many individuals experience symptoms in more than one theme, and these can evolve over time. A more accurate depiction acknowledges these varied experiences as symptom dimensions of OCD, rather than distinct types, recognizing their intersection and fluidity.

In the following sections, we delve into some of the more prevalent symptom dimensions within the intricate tapestry of OCD, including several lesser-known forms as well. However, it is important to acknowledge that obsessions can manifest in virtually limitless ways, rendering any list inherently incomplete. Therefore, if your experience doesn't neatly align with the descriptions provided, there's no cause for concern or feeling of being outside the realm of help. Your unique manifestation simply reflects a less common facet of OCD.

> Trying to classify OCD into fixed subtypes is as futile as trying to encapsulate the vastness of human imagination.

Disturbing Thoughts

Obsessions centered around disturbing thoughts represent one of the most prevalent forms of OCD. These obsessions often conflict with societal norms and the individual's personal values, leading to significant distress. It is estimated that around 20-30% of those with OCD consider them to be their primary problem. Frequently, these obsessions involve taboo and forbidden thoughts deemed unacceptable or immoral by personal or societal standards.

Obsessions revolving around disturbing thoughts can be further delineated into several subcategories, although substantial overlap between them is common:

1) **Aggression** (e.g., fear of smothering one's infant, hitting an elderly person, stabbing or torturing your loved one; hurting oneself).
2) **Sexuality** (e.g., intrusive images of sexual assault or molestation; thoughts about engaging in taboo sexual acts such as necrophilia or bestiality; fears of committing incest).
3) **Religion** (e.g., blasphemous thoughts or images, fears of having committed a religious sin; fear of not believing in God).
4) **Morality** (e.g., fears of engaging in immoral behavior, being deceitful or causing offense).

Not everyone experiences obsessions in these categories in the same manner. While they often seem to appear as sudden intrusive thoughts, they can also manifest in other ways, such as vivid mental imagery or sudden, compelling impulses. For some, these obsessions might involve recurrent thoughts of accidentally harming a loved one or committing a morally reprehensible act. Others may be plagued by distressing images of violence or overwhelmed by seemingly real urges to engage in harmful behaviors.

Regardless of the form they take, the core fear remains consistent: the concern of having or engaging with a prohibited thought, image, or action, even though the individual's actual intention and moral compass are different. This fear of wrongdoing, despite one's best intentions, challenges one's sense of identity and integrity. It creates a persistent state of anxiety and self-doubt, making it difficult for the individual to trust their own mind and intentions.

Table 1.2.

Disturbing Thoughts
Aggression
Fear of stabbing someone, fear of hurting oneself, images of murders or accidents or other gory images, fear of violent words, fear of driving a car into a tree, fear of being a psychopath, fear of shouting obscenities, fear of hurting one's baby, fear of running someone over on impulse, fear of hitting random strangers, fear of harming vulnerable groups.
Sexuality
Unwanted sexual thoughts about strangers, family, or friends; fear of being a pedophile, unwanted thoughts or images about sexual assault and molestation, images committing incest, fear of being sexually perverted, fears that one may commit rape or may cheat on their partner.
Religion and Spirituality
Saying evil things, fear of being a blasphemer, fear of making mistakes that go against religious or metaphysical higher authorities, a fear of shouting obscenities, fear of going to hell, fear of desecrating holy places, fear of offending the dead, fear of not being religious or spiritual enough.
Morality
Worries about having told a lie or having cheated someone, fear of thinking or saying something offensive, inappropriate or disrespectful, fear being dishonest, inauthentic, fake or unreal, worries about always doing things in the morally correct way, fear of being judged for wrong doing.

Obsessions revolving around disturbing thoughts, images and impulses often trigger covert compulsions, primarily in the form of mental rituals. For instance, a person might try hard not to think about certain things, or they might replace negative thoughts with positive ones or repeat a specific phrase to ease the anxiety. This often leads to a cycle where the more one tries to counteract the disturbing thoughts, the more intrusive they become, reinforcing the obsession. Additionally, it becomes more difficult to identify these rituals because they are internal, giving the illusion that no active behavior is occurring. These mental rituals can sometimes be disguised as helpful coping strategies, but they are, in fact, just another way OCD perpetuates itself.

Religious obsessions can trigger compulsive praying, which can in turn breed new doubts of wrongdoing, like whether prayers were done correctly or if impure thoughts intruded during prayer. Other mental compulsions include repeatedly reviewing situations in one's mind or deliberately focusing on thoughts opposite to the ones causing distress. This constant analysis can consume a significant amount of time each day. The preoccupation with moral correctness or the fear of divine punishment often makes these religious compulsions particularly distressing.

Various subtle strategies are also often employed by individuals with disturbing thoughts to alleviate their distress, some of which may go unnoticed even by the person themselves, such as tensing a small part of their body or instinctively shaking one's head to dispel the thoughts.

While overt compulsions are less prevalent among those with disturbing thoughts as compared to other forms of OCD, they are not entirely absent. For instance, individuals with sexual obsessions may engage in frequent bodily checks, such as monitoring oneself for signs of arousal. Similarly, physical actions like touching or arranging objects perceived as "safe" are used to neutralize the obsession, such as touching a religious object in response to blasphemous thoughts or images.

Reassurance seeking manifests in various ways with disturbing thoughts. For instance, individuals with religious obsessions might repeatedly seek guidance from clergy to determine if they've committed any sins. Similarly, those with moral obsessions may constantly seek validation from their spouse regarding their behavior. Apart from seeking validation from others, reassurance seeking can also manifest through excessive online research. For instance, a person with obsessions about harm and wrong doing might endlessly peruse religious texts on whether one has broken the rules or do extensive research on psychopaths or pedophiles to determine whether one shares similarities with them.

Safety behaviors typically aim to prevent the obsession from occurring, or to mitigate the distress caused by it. For instance, someone with aggressive obsessions may rely on the use of plastic knives to feel secure. Similarly, someone with religious obsessions might avoid saying anything at all when in a place of worship for fear of saying something inappropriate.

Avoidance takes safety behaviors a step further by steering clear of potential triggers, like completely avoiding children, or places of worship. While this might offer temporary relief, it's not a long-term solution. New triggers can easily emerge, worsening symptoms over time. Ultimately, avoidance always fails and perpetuates the cycle of OCD.

Self-testing behaviors are also quite common among those with disturbing thoughts, more so than in many other forms of OCD. For instance, an individual worried about shouting obscenities in public might softly whisper them to assess their capability to do so. Alternatively, a person with sexual obsessions might test themselves during sex whether or not they think or feel anything inappropriate. Needless to say, this approach never resolves the issue; instead, it exacerbates it.

Case Vignette 1.1.
Aggressive Theme
Jack

Jack, a 28-year-old graphic designer, had always been a calm and composed individual, known for his creativity and meticulous attention to detail at work. He enjoyed peaceful activities like reading, spending time outdoors, and relaxing with friends, which always helped him maintain a sense of calm and balance. However, about six months ago, while using a large kitchen knife to prepare dinner, he found himself suddenly reminded of a horror movie he had recently watched. Out of nowhere, an unsettling thought struck him: "What if I do something violent?" or worse, "Maybe I'm a violent person without knowing it?" Almost immediately, these thoughts triggered a barrage of horrific mental images—vivid scenes of him stabbing his family. The intensity of these images consumed him instantly, making it impossible to dismiss or rationalize.

As time passed, these disturbing thoughts expanded beyond the kitchen. Jack started to experience terrifying mental images of attacking his friends with sharp objects, pushing strangers into oncoming traffic, or even suffocating someone while they slept. He'd once read about a person who seemed perfectly normal until they suddenly lashed out violently, and it terrified him to think that anyone might have such hidden tendencies. These thoughts were deeply frightening and completely out of character, but no matter how hard he tried to rid himself of them, they persisted. Jack felt consumed by guilt and fear, horrified by the possibility that he might lose control and harm someone.

Jack's anxiety about these thoughts grew so overwhelming that he began questioning his own sanity. He wondered, "What if I actually do something violent?" or "Could I be a dangerous person without realizing it?" These doubts tormented him, and he became terrified that he might unknowingly hurt someone. He even worried, "I might have already harmed someone and just forgot about it." He knew that everyone was capable of anger and impulsivity under certain circumstances, and that thought made him question how much control he actually had over his actions. To avoid even the smallest possibility of losing control, Jack began avoiding situations where he might be tempted to act violently. He stopped using knives in the kitchen and declined invitations to social gatherings, terrified of being near others in case something went wrong.

The worry of hurting someone became Jack's all-encompassing fear, filling him with dread and unbearable guilt. He couldn't shake the vivid images of the emotional trauma he could cause—picturing the pain and suffering of his imagined victims and their devastated families. The thought of being responsible for such harm was too much to bear. Once, he'd read an article that stated some people carry subconscious tendencies for years without realizing it, and the possibility of this only increased his sense of guilt and self-doubt. Beyond this, Jack became consumed with fears of legal and social consequences. He imagined being arrested, tried, and imprisoned for a crime he might commit. The idea of losing his freedom and living out the rest of his life in prison haunted him. He also feared that he might suddenly snap, like the people he read about in the news who seemed normal until they committed horrific acts. Jack started to think, "I might be capable of doing something terrible."

The fear of losing control took over Jack's entire life. He mentally reviewed his past actions again and again, desperately trying to assure himself that he hadn't hurt anyone. He obsessively replayed his thoughts, checking for signs of violent intent, and even engaged in silent prayers or rituals in an attempt to counteract the disturbing images. At work, Jack avoided using sharp tools like scissors, fearing that the smallest mistake could lead to disaster. Even mundane tasks—such as holding a pen or using a simple tool—could trigger distressing thoughts of harm. His productivity plummeted as he constantly left his desk to perform cleansing rituals, such as washing his hands, in a futile attempt to rid himself of the violent thoughts. His frequent absences and strange behavior raised concerns among his colleagues.

Socially, Jack withdrew from everyone he cared about. He turned down invitations to parties and gatherings, worried that being around others might cause him to lose control. His mind constantly reminded him, "If you think you could be a threat, it's only responsible to take precautions." On the rare occasions he did attend, Jack kept his distance, constantly monitoring himself to ensure he didn't act out. His friends noticed his absence and strange behavior, but Jack was too ashamed to explain the true nature of his fears.

At home, Jack's compulsions became even more pronounced. He insisted on using only plastic utensils, fearing that metal ones could be used as weapons. He would repeatedly check and recheck that all knives and dangerous objects were securely locked away. When friends or family visited, he asked them to handle cooking tasks involving sharp tools, which sometimes led to tension or misunderstandings. They, unaware of the severity of his fears, grew frustrated with what they saw as irrational and unreasonable demands.

Jack's obsessive thoughts and compulsive behaviors took an enormous toll on his mental health. He was overwhelmed with shame and guilt, convinced that having such thoughts made him a terrible person. Sometimes, when he thought about it, he even questioned why he would be having these thoughts if he wasn't somehow dangerous. The relentless anxiety and fear of losing control left him feeling hopeless and deeply depressed. He even began to doubt his own memory and perception, questioning whether he might have already harmed someone and simply forgotten about it. This led Jack to compulsively seek reassurance from friends and family, repeatedly asking them to confirm that he hadn't done anything wrong.

Jack's pain and desperation were palpable. He felt trapped in a relentless cycle of fear, self-doubt, and confusion, unable to shake the haunting question: "Am I truly capable of something terrible?" He knew he couldn't continue living this way. Jack needed help.

Case Vignette 1.2.
Sexual Theme
Rachel

Rachel, a 32-year-old kindergarten teacher, had always taken pride in her compassionate and nurturing nature. She found joy in guiding and teaching young children, and her colleagues often commented on how patient and attentive she was. However, about a year ago, during an ordinary day at school, an unsettling and distressing thought suddenly crossed her mind: "Maybe I have inappropriate feelings toward the children I work with? What if I am sexually attracted to them?"

The thought jolted her, and although it felt completely out of place, it stuck with her. At times, Rachel would experience vivid mental images or fleeting sensations that seemed to align with her worst fears, as if she had actually crossed a boundary she never intended to approach. These mental impressions felt disturbingly real, making it seem as if her mind was betraying her. At first, she tried to dismiss the doubt as a passing thought. But as the days went by, it resurfaced, each time more alarming, planting deeper uncertainty: "Could these thoughts mean something about me?" After all, some people have hidden feelings or tendencies they are unaware of until later in life. Could be the case for her as well? Though she had never questioned her intentions before, she found herself growing more anxious at work, second-guessing every touch, smile, or interaction with her students.

What had once been a source of joy—working with children—suddenly became a source of dread. She started avoiding close contact with her students. Simple gestures, like giving a hug or comforting a child, now filled her with unease. Rachel began distancing herself emotionally, too, afraid that she might *unintentionally cross a line she didn't even know existed. The warmth and connection she once cherished were now overshadowed by fear and doubt.*

The intrusive thoughts didn't stop there. Rachel soon found herself questioning her interactions outside of work, too. At family gatherings, the same sense of unease crept in when she was around younger relatives. She began avoiding physical contact with her nieces and nephews, fearing that something in her subconscious was driving her thoughts. Every innocent hug or touch now felt loaded with uncertainty, as if she could no longer trust her own instincts. These moments filled her with shame and self-recrimination: "What kind of person has these thoughts?"

"I'm a terrible person," Rachel thought repeatedly, the doubt wrapping tighter around her sense of self. "I will have to give up my job to protect the children." This fear became overwhelming, making it seem as though the only way to keep others safe was to leave the environment she once loved.

As the thoughts persisted, Rachel started to engage in subtle compulsions to reassure herself. She would mentally review her interactions from the day, checking for any signs that something had been "off" or inappropriate. At work, she became more vigilant, positioning herself in ways that minimized physical contact and interaction with the children. She made sure never to be alone with a child, always finding a way to be in a group or near other teachers, just to protect herself from her own doubts.

Rachel also began researching compulsively. She spent countless hours online, reading articles and forums about people who had inappropriate sexual thoughts. She learned that these thoughts could occur in both OCD and in cases of genuine inappropriate attraction. She wanted reassurance—proof that her fears didn't reflect reality. But the more she searched, the more confused and anxious she became. "Why would I question myself if there was not some truth to it? What if I'm actually a pedophile? What if I'm just fooling myself it is OCD only?"

At home, the impact of these doubts was even more pronounced. Her relationship with her partner, who had always been a source of comfort and stability, became strained. Rachel began to question her feelings during intimate moments, wondering if she was somehow capable of harboring inappropriate thoughts there as well. She felt compelled to test herself—analyzing her emotions and reactions—to make sure everything was "normal." This constant self-monitoring left her exhausted, and she withdrew emotionally, fearing that she couldn't trust her own responses.

The emotional toll was undeniable. Rachel, once so confident and capable, was now gripped by a paralyzing sense of shame. She started isolating herself from friends and family, too embarrassed to share the nature of her fears. How could she explain these thoughts without people judging her? How could she continue working with children when she couldn't trust herself? The thought of losing the career she loved due to thoughts she didn't even want to have was devastating. Her doubts became an endless cycle— each one reinforcing the next, leaving her trapped in fear.

The internal conflict soon became impossible to ignore. At work, she had grown so distant that her colleagues noticed her reluctance to engage with the children. She could no longer participate in activities she once loved, like reading stories to her class or playing games with the kids. Every interaction was clouded by the question: "What if I'm dangerous to them?" And at home, her relationship continued to suffer. Rachel couldn't enjoy the closeness she once shared with her partner, and the joy she used to find in simple moments had disappeared. She couldn't escape the constant mental noise of second-guessing and testing.

Desperate to make sense of it all, Rachel even wondered if she had repressed memories or was in denial about some hidden truth about herself. She felt lost, questioning her entire identity. "Am I the person I thought I was?" became the question that haunted her daily. Despite never having acted on the thoughts, Rachel was consumed with guilt, afraid that her mind had betrayed her, turning her into someone she couldn't recognize.

Case Vignette 1.3.
Religious Theme
John

John, a 40-year-old accountant, had always been deeply committed to his faith. Raised in a religious household, he found great comfort and purpose in his spirituality. He attended worship regularly, volunteered in his community, and spent time in prayer and reflection. His faith gave him meaning and direction in life. However, over the past year, things began to shift. During a spiritual gathering, an unsettling thought struck him: "Perhaps I don't believe in God anymore."

At first, John dismissed it as a passing doubt. But the thought lingered, growing louder each time he attended worship. "Maybe I've lost my faith." This thought gnawed at him, creating a cascade of doubts: "What if I'm not a true believer?" He remembered hearing that even the most faithful people could lose their faith, and this idea unsettled him deeply. The more he tried to dismiss the thought, the stronger it became. John found himself questioning whether his faith was genuine, doubting his own spiritual connection.

Over time, his doubts began to infiltrate other parts of his religious practice. During prayer, he became preoccupied with the thought: "Maybe my prayers don't mean anything." He would repeat prayers multiple times, struggling to feel sincere. John recalled moments in his past when he felt disconnected during spiritual practices, which now seemed like evidence that his faith might not be as strong as he believed. He remembered reading that doubt could indicate a lack of true belief, and it made him question whether he was truly committed. The thought followed: "What if God thinks I don't mean it?" This led John to obsess over the words he used, constantly second-guessing the sincerity of his prayer. He tried to control his thoughts, desperately avoiding blasphemous or inappropriate ideas. Yet, no matter how hard he tried, the thoughts grew more intrusive.

John also feared: "Perhaps I've committed a terrible sin." He mentally reviewed his past, searching for any disrespectful or doubtful moments in his spiritual life. He thought about stories he'd heard of people who lost their faith after a period of intense questioning and wondered if he was going down the same path. He had heard from a friend about someone they knew who lost their faith after questioning it for too long, and now that fear seemed to apply to him. "Maybe I doubted God without realizing it." These doubts *led him to feel like he was spiritually lost, creating an intense need to retrace every prayer and religious act.*

His doubts and fears began to affect his life profoundly. What was once a source of comfort—attending spiritual gatherings—became a source of dread. John began to avoid study groups and other faith-based events, fearful that others might sense his doubts. When he did attend worship, he stayed quietly in the back, afraid that his thoughts would betray him. Instead of feeling spiritually renewed, he left worship burdened with the thought: "I could be losing my faith entirely." He knew that even the most faithful people could lose their belief, and this idea haunted him, making him feel that he might be losing something essential to his identity. He feared that he might be condemned by God and face eternal punishment. The thought of being rejected by God filled him with dread, as though his life might be meaningless without his faith.

Even in everyday life, the fear followed him. John scrutinized his behavior, wondering: "What if I'm not living up to God's teachings? Maybe every small mistake I make is a sin." He feared that he could be unknowingly offending God at every turn, with each decision carrying heavy moral weight. This thought consumed him in mundane situations, making even small tasks feel loaded with consequences.

At home, his wife, Sarah, noticed a change in him. He seemed distant and withdrawn. When she asked what was wrong, John couldn't explain his mental turmoil. He was ashamed to admit his doubts to anyone, including Sarah, fearing judgment. He worried that if others discovered the extent of his doubts, they would judge or reject him, and he might lose the relationships closest to him. This shame drove him to further isolation, cutting him off from the people closest to him.

The weight of these doubts grew heavier over time. Each prayer felt like a test of faith, and every act of worship like a trial of his spiritual standing. He feared that no matter how hard he tried, he would never regain his connection to God, leaving him spiritually lost forever. The idea of living without God's grace haunted him, making it impossible to relax or find peace.

In desperation, John sought reassurance from his spiritual advisor, asking the same questions repeatedly: "Am I still in God's grace?" However, no amount of reassurance seemed to calm his mind. He feared that even his spiritual's advisor's reassurances were meaningless if he had already fallen out of favor with God. He felt trapped in an endless loop of doubt and prayer, never able to shake the fear: "Maybe I've already lost my connection to God."

Case Vignette 1.4.
Morality Theme
Laura

Laura, a 29-year-old marketing professional, had always been known for her strong moral compass and integrity. She prided herself on doing the right thing and being fair to others. Whether at work, with friends, or in her personal life, Laura held herself to a high standard of honesty and accountability. However, about six months ago, she began to experience troubling doubts that shook her sense of self. It started with a simple mistake at work, when she accidentally forgot to credit a colleague for their contribution on a project. She had heard that even small, unintentional actions could reveal deeper character flaws, and the idea began to take hold in her mind. The thought struck her suddenly: "What if I'm a liar?"

Though her colleague hadn't seemed bothered, the thought lingered. Laura couldn't shake the feeling that she had done something deeply wrong. "If my colleagues think I lied, they might stop trusting me." "Maybe I'm a dishonest person without even realizing it?" she wondered. What had been a minor oversight turned into a gnawing doubt she couldn't ignore. "If I am a dishonest person, I'd lose respect from everyone at work." She replayed the incident over and over in her mind, scrutinizing her actions and words. She'd heard that even small actions could reveal hidden flaws in character. Could that be true for her too? "Did I lie on purpose? What if I'm hiding something even from myself?"

As time went on, these doubts expanded beyond the workplace. Laura started questioning her behavior in everyday situations, constantly worried that she had said or done something wrong. During casual conversations with friends, she would suddenly wonder, "If they think I lied, they might avoid me." "Did I just tell a lie?" She would replay the conversation in her head, searching for any sign that she had exaggerated or misrepresented something. If she couldn't recall every word, she would worry that she had been dishonest without meaning to. If she did do something wrong, then it would hurt others and they'd stop trusting me.

Laura's doubts soon turned into a compulsive need to review her actions throughout the day. Each night before bed, Laura would go over every interaction, checking for any possible sign of dishonesty or wrongdoing. She would mentally replay her conversations, retrace her steps at work, and even analyze her social media posts for any inaccuracies. She remembered a news story about someone who unknowingly committed fraud, which made her question if she could also act unethically without realizing it. "If I said something misleading, even accidentally, I could damage my reputation." There were times she felt unsure if she'd been entirely truthful in her words. Could that uncertainty mean she was truly dishonest? If she couldn't find anything wrong, she would feel momentary relief—only for the doubts to resurface the next day with even more intensity.

Laura's social life began to suffer. She became overly cautious in conversations, carefully choosing her words and avoiding situations where she might be misunderstood. "Maybe it's safer to avoid people altogether than risk offending someone." Even with her closest friends, she felt a constant pressure to ensure that everything she said was 100% accurate. A casual joke or playful comment would later fill her with dread, as she questioned whether she had unintentionally lied or been deceitful. She stopped sharing opinions or engaging in debates, worried that she might accidentally mislead someone. "If I offend someone, they might cut me out of their life."

At work, her doubts became even more consuming. Laura found herself double- and triple-checking every email she sent, rereading them over and over to make sure she wasn't exaggerating or presenting information incorrectly. The fear that she might be dishonest in a report or presentation haunted her, causing her to spend excessive time perfecting even the smallest tasks. "If I make a mistake, I could lose my job or damage my career." Her productivity dropped as she became fixated on making sure everything she said or did was beyond reproach. Even minor mistakes felt catastrophic, as they triggered intense guilt and fear that she was fundamentally dishonest.

One particularly stressful moment occurred when Laura mistakenly overcharged a client for a service. Though it was quickly corrected, the thought spiraled out of control: "What if I did that on purpose? Maybe I'm the kind of person who cheats people?" "If my clients believe I'm dishonest, they'll stop working with me." She'd heard stories of people who, despite seeming honest, were later exposed for hiding something. Could she be like them without even knowing it? She became consumed with the fear that she might be secretly unethical or manipulative. She started to question every decision she had ever made in her career, wondering if she had been unintentionally deceitful.

Outside of work, these fears continued to affect her personal life. Laura found herself avoiding certain social situations, especially with people she didn't know well, out of fear that she might accidentally say something dishonest or offensive. "If I offend someone, word might spread, and my reputation could be ruined." When friends invited her to gatherings or social events, she often declined, worried that casual conversations could lead to more doubts about her character. She felt trapped, unable to trust her own words or actions, even though she knew deep down that she valued honesty above all else.

Despite her efforts to control the doubts, Laura's compulsive need to review her behavior only intensified the problem. She began to seek reassurance from friends and colleagues, asking them repeatedly if she had said or done anything wrong. While her friends initially brushed it off as unnecessary worry, they soon noticed how fixated she had become. She would ask her friends things like, "Was I honest about everything?" or "Did I say anything offensive?" The constant need for reassurance strained her relationships, as friends grew frustrated with her repeated questions and doubts.

Laura felt overwhelmed by guilt and self-doubt, consumed with the fear that she wasn't living up to her own standards of integrity. "Maybe I'm not as moral as I think I am, and people will find out." "What if I'm not as good a person as I think I am?" became the question that haunted her daily. She couldn't escape the feeling that she might be dishonest, manipulative, or even morally corrupt without knowing it.

Her once-strong sense of self was now clouded by doubt. Laura began to question whether she could continue in her job, fearing that she might unknowingly deceive a client or make an ethical mistake. "If I mess up at work, I could lose my job and career." The doubts had become a constant companion in her mind, undermining her confidence and making her feel disconnected from the person she believed herself to be. Laura was trapped in a cycle of fear, guilt, and endless questioning, unable to find relief from the persistent doubts about her integrity.

OCD Related to Negligence and Making Mistakes

Obsessions related to fears of negligence and making mistakes are commonly associated with a dimension of OCD often called "checking OCD." However, checking—the compulsive behavior—can occur across various forms of OCD. Therefore, it's more accurate to describe this symptom dimension as revolving around unintentional fears of negligence and making errors.

Concerns typically involve everyday tasks and routines, such as closing doors, turning off appliances, or locking up. Each action becomes a source of anxiety as individuals obsess over whether they've completed it correctly.

Despite appearing trivial, obsessions about negligence can trigger significant distress. Individuals often dread the potential consequences of their perceived mistakes, fearing harm to loved ones if, for example, they left the stove on. Moreover, not all concerns about negligence are confined to routine events. However, if the obsession encompasses fears of intentionally causing harm, it aligns more closely with the previously described symptom dimension of disturbing thoughts. For instance, someone might fear suddenly going crazy and driving into pedestrians.

Obsessions about negligence and their potential outcomes can trigger significant distress, prompting compulsive behaviors in response. The primary form of compulsion in this symptom dimension is checking, aimed at averting negligence or rectifying perceived mistakes. However, this isn't just a casual once-over; it involves repeated and often excessive checking,

For instance, consider someone obsessing about accidentally hitting a child while backing out of the driveway. They wouldn't be satisfied with the usual mirror and blind-spot checks; instead, they meticulously survey their surroundings before even getting into the car. Then, any slight distraction intensifies the obsession, prompting them to exit the vehicle and thoroughly inspect for any signs of impact. Even if everything appears fine, doubts persist, leading to a cycle of repeated checking.

Table 1.3.

Obsessions About Negligence and Mistakes
Worrying about making mistakes while reading, writing, or doing simple calculations, fear of losing things, worries about having left doors and windows unlocked, worries about appliances that may have been left on (stoves, toasters, coffee machines, etc.), worries about mistakes when filling in checks or forms, fears of having caused an accident, fears of being careless, fears of poisoning someone accidently, repeated checking and counting prescription pills to make sure no mistake has been made, checking related to the presence of insects or animals (without any specific contamination fears), reassurance seeking for possible mistakes or accidents one may have caused.

Covert compulsions often accompany overt checking. For example, mentally counting while checking, often for superstitious reasons, or reassuring oneself aloud during the process. Additionally, individuals may excessively focus on the checking task, imprinting it in their memory more than necessary. Reflecting on past events where negligence or mistakes occurred is another common mental ritual. Sometimes, these rituals even extend to past events believed to have happened decades ago.

Reassurance seeking often entails seeking information from others or external sources to alleviate concerns about negligence or mistakes. It may also arise from a desire to share the responsibility for imagined acts of negligence. For instance, repeatedly asking a spouse if the door has been properly closed.

Safety behaviors are typically undertaken to lessen the likelihood of making any mistake, or to reduce distress in situation where this is anticipated. For instance, a person with obsessions about hitting someone with your car might drive very slowly to be extra cautious.

Extending these behaviors can result in avoidance, like avoiding areas with many pedestrians while driving, or even quitting driving altogether. Alternatively, some may stop checking even essential tasks, fearing they'll become preoccupied for hours.

Case Vignette 1.5.
Negligence and Mistakes Theme
Ethan

Ethan, a 35-year-old IT specialist, was always in a hurry, but not because he was disorganized or running late. Every morning before he could leave his apartment, he found himself tangled in a relentless series of checks. It wasn't the typical last-minute glance around the house; it was far more exhaustive. Just as he was ready to leave, a thought would pop into his mind: Maybe I forgot to turn off the stove. After all, it's possible to overlook small details or make mistakes without realizing it. He would rush back to the kitchen, checking each burner, pressing his hands close to make sure everything was cool.

But it never stopped there. As soon as he left the kitchen, another thought would hit him: Perhaps the toaster is still on. Appliances can sometimes fail unexpectedly, even if they seem to be functioning. Back he would go, unplugging the toaster, even though he hadn't used it that morning. As he walked towards the front door, another wave of doubt would strike: Maybe the windows are left open. I've read stories about accidents caused by small oversights, like leaving something unsecured, and I don't want to take that chance. Even after a quick check, the thought gnawed at him, making him circle the apartment again. He'd read before that even small oversights, like a window left open or an appliance left on, could lead to larger issues. He didn't want to risk missing something that could be easily avoided.

The process seemed endless. Just as he reached for the door handle, his mind flooded with new worries: What if I left the light on in the bathroom? or Maybe I don't have everything I need in my wallet. He would stop, go back, and double-check his wallet—confirming that his ID, credit card, and cash were all there, even though he had checked them before. Despite everything being in order, the thoughts persisted. Ethan believed that being responsible meant making absolutely sure that things were in order, even if it took extra time. Every step out the door felt like a potential mistake waiting to happen.

At work, the doubts didn't disappear. They transformed into different worries. Ethan would be sitting at his desk, focused on a project, when a new concern interrupted his concentration: What if the refrigerator isn't cooling properly? He would picture his food spoiling and becoming unsafe, wondering if he should have checked it one more time before leaving the house. The anxiety grew as the day went on. Once, he'd thought he'd left something secure, only to find it wasn't, and that experience left him cautious ever since. He would mentally replay his morning, trying to remember if he had done everything right.

Driving home was no relief either. Ethan's worries took on a different form when he was in his car. He constantly questioned whether the handbrake was properly engaged. Even though he physically checked it, he couldn't trust that it was secure. Every stop at a red light or parking space was an opportunity for doubt: Maybe the car will roll away, he feared. He would tug on the brake again and again, even after hearing the familiar click of the mechanism engaging.

At home in the evenings, the same thoughts and routines played out over and over. Ethan would sit on the couch, ready to unwind, but before he could relax, another thought surfaced: What if the smoke detector isn't working? He would climb up on a chair, press the test button, listen for the beep, and feel a moment of relief—only for the doubt to return minutes later. He would check the smoke detector repeatedly throughout the night, worried that it might have malfunctioned in the brief time since his last test. He remembered hearing stories about house fires caused by devices that failed unexpectedly, even if they seemed fine before. The idea of missing something small that could cause a problem filled him with dread.

The doubts extended to the smallest of details. He found himself checking the temperature of his laptop to make sure it wasn't overheating, even though he hadn't run any intensive programs. He worried that leaving it on overnight would cause it to catch fire, so he would unplug it and place it on a cool surface, only to wake up in the middle of the night, wondering if he had truly unplugged it.

His weekends, once a time for relaxation, had also become an ordeal. Before going to bed, Ethan would check the doors over and over, wondering if they were really locked. He would press down on the handle, make sure the deadbolt was turned, and then return to his bedroom, only for the doubt to reappear: I might have left the door unlocked. And so he would get up, walk to the door, and repeat the process, sometimes three or four times before he felt safe enough to sleep.

The constant checking began to take a toll on his social life. He stopped going out with friends, fearing that he would leave something undone at home. He couldn't enjoy a night out without the persistent thought that something was left on or unlocked. His friends noticed that he was growing more distant, but he didn't know how to explain what was happening. The doubts seemed so trivial when he thought about them rationally—how could he tell his friends that he was afraid he hadn't turned off a light or locked a door?

Work wasn't much better. Ethan's performance began to slip because he was spending so much mental energy on whether he had done everything properly. He found it hard to focus on his tasks because of the never-ending mental replay of his morning routine: Did I close the windows before I left? What if the fridge door isn't closed all the way? He installed cameras in his apartment so he could check everything remotely, but even that didn't help. He would pull up the camera feed repeatedly during the day, scanning the images for any sign that something was wrong.

No matter how many times Ethan checked, no matter how many safety measures he put in place, the relief never lasted. The moment he convinced himself that everything was fine, a new doubt would take its place: Maybe the door was unlocked after all. What if the refrigerator door didn't seal properly this time? It was a never-ending cycle that left him feeling drained and overwhelmed.

Ethan's mind was constantly searching for errors, constantly questioning whether things were functioning the way they should. His doubts were scattered, covering every aspect of his daily life, from his home appliances to his car, to his wallet. No task seemed too small to warrant a thorough check, no process too simple to escape doubt. And the more he tried to gain control, the more his thoughts spiraled into a sea of uncertainty.

Contamination OCD

Obsessions surrounding contamination represent the most prevalent symptom dimension of OCD. Typically, these obsessions center on fears of encountering germs and viruses, though they can encompass a wide array of contaminants, including pesticides, asbestos, chemicals, radiation, plants, and animals. Individuals may even harbor apprehensions about seemingly innocuous items like cleaning products or tissue paper.

While contamination OCD is now the most common form, it is a relatively new phenomenon, emerging alongside the advent of germ theory in the 19th century. Unlike obsessions involving intrusive or disturbing thoughts, which have historical accounts dating back to the 4th century, there are no clear references to contamination-related fears before the modern era. This shift may reflect the growing societal awareness of microbial dangers, public health campaigns, and medical advancements that began emphasizing hygiene and disease prevention.

However, the concept of what constitutes a contaminant is highly individualized and personal in contamination OCD. Contrary to popular media portrayals that often depict contamination OCD as stemming from perfectionistic cleanliness standards, individuals' concerns are diverse not tied to hygiene ideals. For instance, someone might fear contracting the Hepatitis C virus while remaining unconcerned about other pathogens like HIV or E. coli. This selectivity cannot be attributed to inherent personality traits; rather, it reflects the complex nature of OCD.

Contamination obsessions can also extend to fears of *mental* contamination. Individuals with mental contamination OCD experience thoughts or feelings of being "dirty" or "contaminated" on a psychological or moral level. These thoughts can be triggered by various stimuli, such as interactions with specific individuals, exposure to certain environments, or engaging in activities that are perceived as morally wrong.

For instance, someone might feel an inner sense of contamination or "dirtiness" after interacting with a person they perceive as morally impure, touching objects they consider tainted, or being in environments that provoke feelings of guilt or shame. In this way, contamination obsessions with aversive content can lead to secondary feelings of mental contamination, where distress arises not from physical germs or dirt but from perceived moral or emotional taint.

Regardless of whether contamination obsessions stem from physical or non-physical sources, they typically elicit strong feelings of discomfort and distress. Anxiety is often heightened by concerns about the potential consequences of contamination, such as serious illness, infecting loved ones, or being held accountable for spreading disease. However, not all individuals with contamination obsessions fixate on the fear of illness; the mere notion of being contaminated can induce extreme distress in itself.

Consider the account of an individual with OCD from the 19th century:

> *"Now, I can touch nothing without feeling irresistibly compelled to wash my hands afterwards. If I am prevented from doing so, I experience the most horrible sense of fear. I am always looking at my hands to ascertain if I can see anything on them, and I have a lens which I use to aid my oversight. I have no particular apprehension of contracting small-pox or any other disease I can specify. It is an overpowering feeling that I shall be defiled in some mysterious way, that presses me with a force I cannot resist...And lately, even gloves do not seem to afford me entire protection. I know they are porous, and that therefore, the subtle influence, whatever it may be, is capable of passing through them to my hands" (From Hammond, 1863; P. 426-427).*

Additionally, obsessions frequently evoke feelings of disgust, particularly when individuals believe they have been contaminated. This reaction may be intensified in those predisposed to experiencing disgust easily, whether triggered by foul odors, certain foods, or unsanitary conditions. However, the level of disgust sensitivity varies among individuals and can significantly impact their behaviors and responses in diverse situations. Disgust sensitivity can exacerbate OCD symptoms, intensifying the emotional response to perceived contamination, but it does not fully account for the disorder. For most people, contact with something repulsive can be easily resolved through washing, but for those with OCD, this process is far more complex and prolonged.

Table 1.4.

Obsessions About Contamination
Fears about acquiring germs or viruses through common interactions, such as shaking hands, touching doorknobs, or handling surfaces in public spaces, fear potential contamination from animals and insects, including bats, lice, ticks, birds, worms, dogs, spiders, flies, and cats, apprehension about asbestos, radon exposure or other hazardous substances, fear of coming into contact with animal products like eggs or feces, fearing transmission of diseases or parasites, fear of coming into contact with animal products like eggs or feces, fearing transmission of diseases or parasites, fear of bodily fluids such as urine, feces, semen, or vaginal secretions, fear of sticky substances or objects that could trap contaminants, contracting specific diseases like HEP C, HIV, MERS, SARS, E-Coli, Botulism, or Meningitis due to contamination, fear of ingesting certain foods perceived as contaminated, fear of being exposed to chemicals such as lead, pesticides, mold, or toxic substances in cleaning products.

Compulsions in contamination OCD typically involve efforts to remove the perceived contaminant and alleviate associated anxiety and harm. These can manifest as excessive handwashing or other cleaning rituals. Ritualistic behaviors and specific rules often accompany these compulsions, such as washing in a particular sequence or for a set number of times. In many cases, individuals may feel compelled to wash until they "feel" clean, regardless of visual cues, leading to prolonged and repeated washing sessions. This can make everyday tasks feel exhausting and overwhelming, turning basic routines into time-consuming rituals.

The frequency and severity of washing can vary among individuals with contamination OCD. Some may engage in frequent and prolonged rituals multiple times daily, while others may do so less often. Excessive washing can result in skin irritation or other dermatological issues, especially when harsh cleaning products or hot water are used. Additionally, washing rituals often extend beyond handwashing alone, encompassing repetitive cleaning of surfaces such as toilets, doorknobs, faucets, kitchen counters, and tableware in an effort to ward off contamination.

Not all compulsions in contamination OCD center on washing or cleaning. Individuals with fears of radiation or toxic substances may ingest excessive amounts of charcoal or supplements to rid their bodies of contaminants. Similarly, those fearing animal or insect-related contaminants may engage in checking behaviors rather than washing. Checking compulsions may also include keeping track of individuals and their actions throughout the house to ensure they do not touch or contaminate anything.

There are numerous other strategies employed by individuals with OCD in attempts to alleviate their obsessions of contamination. Reassurance seeking may involve consulting spouses or medical professionals regarding the risk of disease. Many individuals spend significant amounts of time scouring the internet for information on potential contaminants and diseases.

Safety behaviors in contamination OCD are invariably aimed at preventing contamination. For instance, wearing gloves or protective clothing to avoid contact with perceived contaminants is a common safety measure. Additionally, individuals may implement systems, rules, and rituals, such as dividing items based on their perceived level of cleanliness, to control or prevent contamination spread.

Similarly, avoidance behaviors in contamination OCD are directed at minimizing contact with contaminants. Social events may be avoided due to the potential for physical contact, such as handshaking. Medical appointments might also be skipped out of fear of increased exposure to germs, viruses, or blood. In some cases, individuals may insist on special arrangements for medical appointments, such as being the first patient of the day when instruments are believed to be the least "infected".

Avoidance behaviors aimed at preventing the spread of contaminants can severely limit individuals with contamination OCD over time. For example, individuals may restrict themselves to only one set of "safe" or "clean" clothes, deeming all others contaminated, even newly purchased ones. This can lead to secondary worries and fears, such as being unable to leave the house or losing one's livelihood if the last set of clothing becomes contaminated. Ultimately, entire parts of an individual's living environment may be deemed unusable or uninhabitable due to fear of contamination. In extreme cases, individuals may find themselves confined to only their personal bedroom or bed only as the last perceived safe space.

Case Vignette 1.6.
Contamination Theme
Sophie

Sophie, a 29-year-old event planner, had always been careful about cleanliness, but over the past year, her concern had spiraled into an overwhelming fear of toxic exposure. It began when she read an article highlighting the dangers of household cleaning products, warning of potential long-term health risks from exposure to certain chemicals. That article planted a seed of fear: Perhaps I could be contaminated by toxic chemicals.

Everyday products Sophie once used without hesitation became sources of intense anxiety. Cleaning her apartment was no longer a routine task but a dangerous endeavor. As she sprayed cleaner on her countertops, a thought surfaced: Maybe the cleaning products I use are toxic. She remembered that experts often warn about the risks of long-term exposure to certain household chemicals, and this idea stuck with her, making her cautious of every product she used. She wore gloves and a mask every time she cleaned, convinced that even brief exposure could harm her. After each session, she opened all the windows, but the fear remained: Could the air still be filled with toxic particles?

Determined to find a solution, Sophie began experimenting with different "safe" cleaning products, hoping to eliminate her fears. She tried eco-friendly sprays, homemade vinegar solutions, and organic cleaners. But no matter how many products she switched to, the doubts persisted: Perhaps even these products aren't truly safe. Eventually, the frustration became too much, and she stopped using any cleaning products altogether, relying on water alone to wipe surfaces in an attempt to feel safe.

Her anxieties soon extended beyond her apartment. At work, Sophie handled anything made from synthetic materials with unease. Research she'd read emphasized the potential dangers of synthetic materials and chemicals in everyday items, adding to her belief that many surfaces and materials around her could be hazardous. Maybe this material contains toxic chemicals, she thought. She scrubbed her hands vigorously after touching anything she suspected might be unsafe, her skin becoming dry and irritated from the constant washing. Despite these efforts, the same doubts haunted her: Could I have spread contaminants from one item to another?

Sophie's thoughts grew darker: If I am contaminated, then I could contract a severe illness from these chemicals. The fear of personal harm now intertwined with fears for her loved ones. If I unknowingly expose my family to these substances, then they might get sick because of me. She became consumed with the idea that the chemicals she encountered throughout her day could linger on her clothing or skin, potentially contaminating everything she touched. When visiting family, Sophie would sit stiffly on the edge of the couch, afraid to spread contaminants onto furniture.

At home, Sophie's routines became more rigid. She divided her apartment into "clean" and "contaminated" zones. Simple tasks—like using the bathroom—felt like navigating a minefield. Maybe chemicals are still lingering from the last time I cleaned in here. To stay safe, she avoided certain areas of her home altogether, confining herself to a small corner of her bedroom.

If I fail to clean thoroughly, I could be responsible for someone else's illness. The thought that she might unknowingly be responsible for spreading toxic substances filled Sophie with guilt. If I spread contamination to others, then I might be responsible for someone else getting sick. She started second-guessing every action: Had she rinsed her hands well enough? Had she changed clothes after cleaning? No matter how many precautions she took, she couldn't shake the feeling that she might still pose a danger to others.

Social situations became overwhelming. Sophie avoided gatherings at friends' houses, fearful that they had recently used strong cleaners or air fresheners. Shopping for groceries turned into a stressful ordeal. She scrutinized every product, searching for "chemical-free" labels, and often left the store empty-handed when nothing met her strict criteria. Even fruits and vegetables, which should have felt safe, became a source of worry, as she remembered hearing that pesticide residues could remain on produce no matter how thoroughly she washed them.

Despite her meticulous efforts to control contamination, Sophie's world kept shrinking. She stopped cooking, afraid that packaging materials and cookware might contain toxins. She even limited her use of personal care products, abandoning lotions, makeup, and scented shampoos for fear of chemical exposure. Yet the same doubt always lingered: Could I have missed something dangerous?

The emotional toll became unbearable. Sophie felt trapped in her own mind, paralyzed by fears of contamination. What once brought her joy—organizing events and spending time with loved ones—now filled her with dread. She grew isolated, afraid to explain her fears to others for fear they would judge her. Even in moments of rest, the same thought returned: Maybe I'll never feel safe again.

Sophie's need to prevent contamination drove her to perform endless rituals, but no amount of cleaning or avoidance could bring lasting relief. Each time she thought she had done enough, a new doubt surfaced: Perhaps I didn't clean thoroughly enough. No matter how much she tried to stay ahead of her fears, the anxiety never subsided. The cycle of doubt and compulsion left her exhausted, yet the fear of toxic chemicals remained ever-present, dictating her every move.

OCD Related to Symmetry, Order and Arrangement

The fourth most common dimension of OCD revolves around obsessions with symmetry, order, and arrangement, often dubbed "just right OCD." Individuals experiencing this form of OCD feel a persistent sense of incompleteness or dissatisfaction, fixating on details like the arrangement of items on their desk or in their home. They may feel intense discomfort if things aren't arranged precisely as they feel they should be, leading to repetitive adjustments until achieving a sense of completion. Others may obsess over their writing or typing, feeling compelled to erase and retype words until satisfied. Additionally, some may focus on the preparation of their food, feeling driven to cut, chop, or arrange it in specific ways.

The level of anxiety in "just right" OCD varies depending on whether the person worries about potential consequences of things not being "just right." These consequences can range from superstitious fears, like harm coming to loved ones, to more common concerns, such as worrying that one might lose their job if things are not done "just right". However, some individuals with OCD may not fear any consequences, yet still experience discomfort or a strong sense of something being amiss, driving their compulsions. In certain cases, anxiety may seem nearly absent, adding to the challenge of distinguishing "just right" OCD from obsessive-compulsive personality disorder.

However, although individuals with "just right" OCD and those who excessive perfectionism both pursue a sense of perfection or alignment in their behaviors, their underlying motivations diverge significantly. Rather than "merely" seeking flawlessness or pursue perfection, those with "just right" OCD are driven by persistent obsessions that something is fundamentally wrong, often despite lacking tangible evidence. Consequently, they engage in compulsive ordering and arranging behaviors as a means to alleviate this sense of wrongness.

Of course, both motivations can occur in the same individual, as someone with OCD may also have perfectionistic tendencies. However, it is important to recognize that repetitive behaviors in OCD are not the same as those stemming from pathological perfectionism. The compulsive actions in OCD are rooted in distressing obsessions and an overwhelming drive to neutralize discomfort, whereas perfectionism typically reflects a deliberate pursuit of exceptionally high, often unattainable, standards.

Table 1.5.

Obsessions About Symmetry, Order and Arrangement
Worrying that calculations are done incorrectly, thinking handwriting is not good enough, stressing over the alignment of objects like papers, pens, books, or ornaments, worrying about finding the precise word or phrase to effectively convey thoughts or respond to others in conversations, presentations, or writing, concerns about not being able to articulate ideas clearly or express emotions accurately, fixating on the evenness or symmetry of sensory experiences, obsessing over maintaining symmetry in personal grooming, like ensuring haircuts are precisely balanced or clothes are symmetrically arranged, doubting the accuracy or completeness of memories, past actions, or the organization of information in one's mind, thinking one's food might not be prepared correctly unless done in a very specific way

Compulsions in "just right" OCD naturally follow from obsessions about symmetry, order and arrangement (e.g., the idea that something is "not right"). Symmetry rituals frequently involve repetitively arranging or aligning objects until they achieve a perceived state of symmetry or evenness. Ordering compulsions manifest as creating specific sequences or patterns with objects or tasks, such as arranging items numerically or alphabetically. Arranging behaviors entail organizing items in predetermined ways, like lining them up or forming geometric patterns. Individuals with this form of OCD may also feel compelled to mentally reorder or categorize memories or past events to alleviate uncertainty or distress.

Checking rituals are also common, involving frequent verification of arrangements to ensure symmetry and orderliness. Counting rituals may involve repetitive counting of objects or actions to establish a sense of completion or order. Additionally, individuals might engage in magical rituals, such as performing actions according to a favored number, silently reciting specific phrases or prayers, or tapping objects for a desired sense of correctness.

Similar to other manifestations of OCD, individuals with "just right" OCD often seek reassurance from others to validate that a task has been completed accurately or to their satisfaction. They may repeatedly ask for confirmation or feedback, hoping to alleviate their uncertainty about whether something has been done "right." Additionally, safety behaviors are prevalent, typically taking the form of compulsions aimed at correcting perceived imperfections or ensuring that everything is as "right" as possible.

These compulsions can become so consuming that individuals actively avoid situations where they fear becoming entangled in their rituals for extended periods. For instance, they may steer clear of touching or engaging with certain objects that trigger feelings of discomfort or the need for correction. Procrastination and indecision may also become coping mechanisms, as individuals attempt to evade the distressing sensation of things not being "just right." This avoidance can extend to social interactions, personal challenges, and opportunities for personal growth, as individuals may fear these situations will exacerbate their feelings of things not being right. As a result, they may withdraw from social engagements or forego chances for advancement, all in an effort to maintain a semblance of control over their obsessions.

Case Vignette 1.7.
Symmetry, Order and Arrangement Theme
Matthew

Matthew, a 27-year-old architect, had always appreciated structure and balance, but what started as an eye for detail had turned into something much more consuming over the past year. His daily life was dominated by a nagging sense that things weren't quite right. Whether he was at work or at home, he felt a constant pressure to arrange, fix, and adjust his surroundings until they felt symmetrical, even if nothing appeared out of place to others.

It began innocuously enough. Matthew would spend a few extra seconds straightening objects on his desk—pencils, papers, his computer mouse—making sure everything was aligned. But as time went on, the need for symmetry intensified. He could no longer simply place items where they belonged; they had to be arranged in a way that felt just right. If something is misaligned or out of place, then it could reflect poorly on me, making me seem careless or inattentive. Maybe the papers aren't lined up properly. He would spend minutes adjusting and readjusting them, convinced that even the slightest misalignment would bother him for the rest of the day.

He remembered hearing from colleagues that small details often leave strong impressions, which made him worry that even minor imperfections could reflect poorly on him. Once, he read an article that discussed how alignment and order are crucial for creating spaces that feel both pleasing and functional, reinforcing his need to ensure everything looked just right.

This obsession spread to other parts of his life. At work, Matthew would check his architectural drawings repeatedly, convinced that something was off. Even after verifying that his measurements were accurate, the feeling persisted: What if the lines aren't perfectly straight? What if I missed something small? If I don't repeatedly check and adjust things, then I might miss a crucial mistake, which could lead to embarrassment or failure, especially at work. His training emphasized that precision is fundamental in architecture, as even slight mistakes could compromise the integrity of a design. He found himself erasing and redrawing the same lines over and over, long past the point of necessity, unable to move on until everything looked flawless. Each revision seemed to create more uncertainty, and the more he tried to get things "right," the more out of balance everything felt.

Outside of work, these feelings followed him home. Matthew became fixated on the arrangement of objects in his apartment. He couldn't sit down to relax until he had spent time straightening the cushions on his couch, adjusting the books on his shelf so they were evenly spaced, and centering the paintings on his walls. He felt an underlying sense of responsibility for ensuring everything appeared just right, as though maintaining order would reflect his care and diligence. It wasn't enough for things to look orderly; they had to feel right. He would stand back, survey the room, and if anything seemed off, he would start the process over again.

His kitchen became another battleground for his sense of order. Whenever he prepared meals, Matthew found himself obsessing over the arrangement of ingredients. "What if I haven't chopped the vegetables evenly?" he would think, carefully inspecting each piece. He would spend time cutting and recutting the vegetables until their size and shape matched perfectly. Even after completing the meal, he would question whether the food had been arranged correctly on the plate, leading him to rearrange it several times before eating.

At work, Matthew's productivity started to decline. He would become stuck in loops of checking and rechecking his drafts, unable to submit them for fear that something was still off. His colleagues began noticing his delays, and even simple tasks took him twice as long as they used to. He spent hours arranging objects on his desk and double-checking the alignment of his computer screen, convinced that something was out of place. Even the way he typed on his keyboard became a source of stress—he would delete and retype entire sentences multiple times.

The constant need for things to feel "just right" became exhausting. Matthew started avoiding activities that might trigger his compulsions. He steered clear of certain work assignments that required precision, fearing he would get trapped in a cycle of endless adjustments. Even in social situations, he found it hard to relax. At restaurants, he couldn't help but rearrange the silverware and glasses on the table, adjusting them until they were symmetrically placed. His friends noticed his behavior and would gently tease him about it, but Matthew felt a growing sense of shame and frustration that he couldn't control it.

At home, Matthew's rituals became more elaborate. He would spend hours in the evenings straightening his apartment, ensuring that every object was perfectly aligned. Maybe the books on the shelf aren't evenly spaced, he would think, pulling them down and rearranging them until he felt satisfied. But the satisfaction never lasted long—minutes later, he would feel the need to adjust something else, leading to another round of straightening and realignment.

Even his grooming routine was affected. Matthew became preoccupied with symmetry when styling his hair and getting dressed. Perhaps my hair isn't symmetrical on both sides, he would think, spending excessive time in front of the mirror. Perhaps my shirt cuffs are uneven, he would wonder, adjusting his clothes repeatedly, trying to make sure that every part of his outfit was balanced and aligned. The feeling of imbalance would gnaw at him until he made these adjustments, but no matter how much he tried, the discomfort always returned.

Matthews concerns extended to how he interacted with others. When speaking to colleagues or friends, he would obsess over finding the exact right words. Maybe I didn't explain that clearly enough, he would think, replaying conversations in his head, trying to figure out if he had phrased things properly. He would correct himself mid-conversation, sometimes multiple times, until he felt his words were accurate. This made social interactions stressful, and he found himself withdrawing from them more and more, worried that he would say something that didn't come out perfectly.

Despite his best efforts, Matthew couldn't escape the feeling that perhaps something is still wrong with the way I've left things. He would check his work emails multiple times before sending them, reading and rereading to make sure the tone was exactly what he wanted. Even after hitting "send," he would worry that he had made a mistake, feeling compelled to check his sent folder to reassure himself that everything was as it should be.

The more Matthew tried to get things "just right," the more out of control he felt. The constant doubts that things were not done well enough had taken over nearly every aspect of his life—his work, his home, his appearance, and his interactions with others. Despite devoting countless hours each day to adjusting and perfecting, the sense of balance and satisfaction he craved always seemed just out of reach. The lingering feeling of imbalance haunted him, compelling him to repeat his rituals endlessly, trapped in a cycle he couldn't escape.

Sensorimotor OCD

Sensorimotor OCD is characterized by obsessions centered around bodily functions, movements, or bodily sensations, leading to compulsive behaviors aimed at neutralizing or alleviating associated anxiety. These obsessions typically revolve around concerns about bodily functions not performing correctly, such as heartbeat, breathing, or blinking.

For example, individuals with sensorimotor OCD may worry if their heart is beating correctly and continuously check their pulse for reassurance. Others may fear whether they are urinating correctly or question the timing of urination based on bladder pressure. Some individuals may experience anxiety about the movement of their eyes, fearing that they may involuntarily fixate on the genital area of another person. This manifestation is sometimes referred to as "Staring OCD" or "Visual Tourettic OCD," but it is essentially another form of sensorimotor OCD.

Sensorimotor OCD can also overlap significantly with other forms of OCD. For instance, individuals may worry about accidentally harming themselves or others through involuntary movements. Additionally, if there's an overlap with "just right" OCD, individuals may be concerned about the lack of alignment or asymmetry in experiencing certain bodily sensations. Similarly, individuals may worry about bodily functions in relation to contamination fears, such as accidentally ingesting harmful substances.

In sensorimotor OCD, concerns often center around fears of losing control over bodily functions like breathing, swallowing, or blinking, due to the obsession that these functions might not work correctly. There's also a persistent fear of never being able to stop thinking about these bodily functions, movements, or sensations. This arises from a fundamental doubt about trusting the body to operate automatically, alongside the worry that one may be unable to stop monitoring these functions.

Compulsions in sensorimotor OCD may include repetitive movements or behaviors aimed at correcting or controlling bodily sensations, such as repetitive swallowing, blinking, or breathing patterns, excessive checking of bodily sensations or movements, seeking reassurance from others about bodily sensations, or engaging in rituals to achieve a sense of bodily symmetry or alignment.

Avoidance is not typical in sensorimotor OCD, not because individuals are not motivated to avoid, but because we carry our bodies with us at all times. There is often significant distress about never feeling normal again.

Case Vignette 1.8.
Sensorimotor OCD
Olivia

Olivia, a 31-year-old investment manager at a prominent firm, had always been highly attuned to the needs of others, whether with her clients or her family. But lately, her attention had turned inward, fixating on her own body in ways that left her feeling trapped and anxious. It began one evening when she suddenly became aware of her own breathing. She had never paid much attention to it before, but now she couldn't stop thinking about it. Am I breathing too shallowly? she wondered. Maybe I'll forget how to breathe properly. As she tried to push the thought away, it only grew stronger, leaving her frustrated and restless, desperate for her mind to settle. Now, even the smallest awareness of her breath made her feel helplessly focused on something that she feared might consume her forever.

At first, it seemed like a passing thought, but as the days went by, Olivia found herself focusing on her breathing more and more. She began to feel trapped by the constant awareness, as if there was no escape from her body. Is my breathing too fast? Too slow? she wondered. What if my body isn't functioning as it should? She couldn't tell anymore. The more she tried to ignore it, the more she noticed every sensation in her chest—the rise and fall, the rhythm, and the moments when it didn't feel "just right." Each failed attempt to regain her sense of normalcy left her more frustrated, deepening the fear that she had lost control. After all, she knew that health experts recommended being attentive to bodily signals to catch early warning signs. Her sense of helplessness grew with every moment, as she became convinced she might be caught in this awareness forever, losing the freedom to relax naturally.

Before long, Olivia's focus shifted to other bodily sensations. One afternoon, she became fixated on her blinking. Am I blinking too much? she wondered. Her eyes started to feel dry and strained from paying too much attention to them. She tried to act natural, but the harder she tried, the more unnatural it all felt, leaving her exhausted and tense. Sitting through meetings became unbearable—her thoughts were consumed with the mechanics of blinking: When should it happen? How often? Are my eyelids moving at the right speed? The frustration built each time she failed to blink "correctly," and each attempt made her more certain that she was losing her ability to relax her attention. She feared that this heightened awareness would turn into a permanent state, leaving her unable to function normally.

Olivia's obsession with her bodily functions expanded further. She became acutely aware of her posture, the way she shifted her weight, and even how she gestured during presentations. This constant self-monitoring made her feel like she was at risk of embarrassing herself, unable to focus on the conversation or her clients' needs. Her concentration would waver, replaced by a desperate need to keep herself in check. Past experiences of struggling to control her focus would come to mind, making her feel vulnerable and convinced that her mind could fixate this way again, perhaps even for good. The thought of permanently losing the ability to focus naturally made her dread every social interaction, fearing that these compulsions would make her appear distracted, distant, or incapable of keeping her mind on the task at hand.

Even eating became stressful. Meals, once a time of joy and connection, now felt like a minefield of sensations she couldn't escape. Am I swallowing correctly? she wondered with every bite. She paused mid-meal, trying to determine if her throat felt normal. She feared that if she stopped paying attention, she might forget how to swallow altogether. This constant focus on the mechanics of eating exhausted her, making it feel like something she would never be able to enjoy again. With each bite, Olivia became more convinced that her natural functions were slipping away, leaving her isolated in her focus, unable to engage with the world around her.

As Olivia's focus intensified, she developed a new layer of fear. Monitoring her bodily functions became its own obsession, making her anxious that she might be stuck doing it forever. Olivia began to monitor herself monitoring, checking whether she was still thinking about breathing, blinking, or swallowing. This layer of self-monitoring made the loop even more relentless. The idea of losing control over her attention entirely felt overwhelming, leaving her trapped in a cycle that seemed impossible to break. She felt as though her mind was no longer her own, that she might live forever under a relentless gaze, constantly aware of every breath and blink.

Social interactions became increasingly difficult. Olivia would sit with friends, unable to focus on the conversation because she was too busy monitoring her body. Her sense of connection with others was replaced with feelings of vulnerability and isolation. Interactions that were once enjoyable became exhausting, deepening her frustration. This constant, unshakeable self-monitoring left her feeling disconnected and overwhelmed, making it hard to imagine a time when she might relax and experience real presence with those around her.

Even sleep offered no reprieve. At night, Olivia would lie awake, counting each breath, trying to calm herself, but it only made her more anxious. The need to monitor her body at night left her feeling restless and incapable of finding peace. Even when she managed to fall asleep, she often woke up in the middle of the night, her mind immediately fixating on her bodily functions. She found herself checking whether she was still thinking about them, adding to the emotional exhaustion. The fear that she would never again experience the deep, unbroken rest she once took for granted kept her locked in a cycle of worry and tension.

Despite all her efforts—monitoring, checking, and controlling—Olivia never felt truly reassured. The more she tried to correct her body, the more alien it felt, as if she had lost the ability to live without constant vigilance. She feared she would never stop thinking about her body. The days when her bodily functions ran smoothly without conscious thought felt distant, almost impossible to reach again. It seemed as though her mind and body were turning against her, holding her in a state of relentless self-awareness. The overwhelming belief that this hyper-focus would consume her permanently left her frustrated, restless, and trapped in a cycle of hopelessness.

OCD Related to Gender and Sexual Orientation

Gender and sexual orientation OCD are symptom dimensions that involve obsessions and compulsions related to gender identity and sexual orientation. Obsessions about sexual orientation are characterized by persistent fears that one might be, or might become gay, lesbian, bisexual, or another sexual orientation divergent from one's identified orientation (e.g., a gay person fearing they might be heterosexual). Relatedly, those with gender OCD frequently question whether they are truly the gender they identify as, or fear that their gender identity lacks genuineness (e.g., what if I am really a transsexual?).

Obsessions about one's sexual identity are not merely fleeting reflections, nor should they be confused with sexual orientation dysphoria. Those with sexual orientation dysphoria contend with feelings of conflict, anxiety, or distress about their sexual orientation, which may deviate from societal expectations or their own internalized beliefs. In contrast, individuals with sexual orientation OCD persistently doubt their true sexual orientation, leading to significant distress as a result.

Individuals with sexual orientation OCD may also experience sexual obsessions, which exacerbates their distress (e.g., "images of oneself engaged in sexual acts incongruous with one's actual sexual orientation"). This distress stems from having ego-dystonic thoughts that contradict the individual's self-concept, not from underlying homophobia. While negative attitudes, beliefs, or prejudices toward LGBTQ+ individuals remain prevalent throughout society, these biases are not inherently linked to sexual orientation or gender identity OCD.

Gender identity OCD is also not the same as gender dysphoria, a complex experience characterized by persistent discomfort or distress with one's assigned gender at birth. Unlike gender dysphoria, which aligns with the individual's core identity, obsessions in gender identity OCD are often ego-dystonic, causing significant distress by conflicting with the individual's sense of self. Ultimately, individuals with sexual orientation and gender identity OCD seek clarity about their true selves, but their obsessions hinder them from attaining it.

The predominant compulsions associated with gender and sexual orientation OCD typically revolve around mental rituals. These rituals often involve analyzing past experiences or mentally reviewing images or fantasies to affirm or deny one's sexual orientation. Situations that trigger obsessions about one's gender and sexual identity are often meticulously scrutinized in an effort to determine the validity of the obsession.

For instance, individuals with sexual orientation OCD frequently engage in heightened self-monitoring or checking. They observe their own reactions or those of others for any signs of incongruence with their gender or sexual orientation. Attempts at thought suppression may also arise when obsessions involve feared sexual mental images and impulses that contradict one's actual sexual orientation. The distress caused by such imagery is primarily because they appear to contradict one's actual sexual orientation, not because such imagery is experienced as inherently repugnant. As noted earlier, there is no evidence that those with OCD are more homophobic than anyone else, nor that such tendencies cause the onset of obsessions of this nature.

Compulsions of those with gender identity may consist of frequently checking one's appearance, body, or attire to ensure alignment with their perceived or desired gender identity. This behavior may involve frequent mirror-checking, excessive grooming, or comparisons with others of the same gender, both in real life and through social media, in an effort to assess their gender identity. Additionally, seeking reassurance through self-testing is common, with individuals engaging in stereotypical gender-specific behaviors or even sexual acts to validate their gender identity.

Seeking reassurance from loved ones can strain relationships, especially if the nature of the ego-dystonic obsession is not understood. Individuals may also seek reassurance through excessive searching for information on the internet, visiting and frequent questioning at online forums, or consuming content related to gender identity and sexual orientation. Alternatively, individuals may endure their struggles in solitude, lacking any support due to the burden of guilt and shame commonly associated with their obsessions.

Some of those with gender identity and sexual orientation OCD try to manage their obsessions and distress through avoidance. This can involve avoiding certain places, people, or situations that trigger their obsessions. For instance, someone experiencing frequent obsessions about their sexual orientation may avoid intimate relationships altogether or refrain from engaging in activities that could potentially bring their sexual orientation into question. Similarly, individuals with gender identity obsessions might avoid situations where their gender identity could be challenged, such as avoiding public restrooms or social gatherings.

Some individuals may attempt to cope with their obsession in a way that seems contrary to avoidance. For instance, a person experiencing heterosexual orientation OCD might expose themselves to gay pornography while engaging in self-stimulation to gauge their attraction to the opposite sex. Alternatively, they might seek out sexual encounters with individuals of a particular gender to assess their arousal or reactions, despite lacking genuine desire or attraction. However, like avoidance, these behaviors fail to offer any resolution; instead, they only compound the confusion.

Case Vignette 1.9.
Sexual Orientation OCD
Henry

Henry, a 24-year-old marketing consultant, had always identified as heterosexual. He had been in a long-term relationship with his girlfriend, enjoyed their time together, and felt secure in his identity. However, one day, seemingly out of nowhere, a question popped into his mind: "Maybe I'm not really heterosexual" "What if I'm attracted to the same sex?" The thought was unsettling, and Henry brushed it off as a passing idea. But the thought lingered, refusing to disappear.

Over the following days, the question resurfaced again and again. He had read that people sometimes discover hidden aspects of themselves later in life, and the thought made him wonder if his true sexuality could be one of those hidden truths. It became louder, more intrusive.

What if I'm actually gay and have been lying to myself this whole time? Henry couldn't stop thinking about it. Every time he saw another man, he found himself questioning his reaction. Did I look at him too long? Was I attracted to him? What does this mean? No matter what he told himself, the doubts persisted, gnawing at his mind.

Henry's obsessions quickly spiraled. He began to mentally review past interactions, searching for signs that he had missed. He thought back to his childhood friends, wondering if he had ever felt anything that might suggest he was gay. He recalled some experiences during adolescence when he experimented with his sexuality, and now he questioned if those were signs of a hidden attraction he'd ignored. He worried that growing up surrounded by heterosexual norms and assumptions might have shaped his self-identity more than he realized, causing him to question if his understanding of himself was based on genuine self-awareness or on societal expectations.

He analyzed his memories of being around other men, replaying conversations, glances, and body language over and over. The more he thought about it, the more unsure he became. Maybe I've been in denial all these years? Could I be lying to myself?

In his relationship, Henry started to feel a distance growing between him and his girlfriend. He found himself questioning whether his feelings for her were genuine or if he was just "playing the part." When they were together, Henry monitored his every thought and reaction: Am I really attracted to her? What if I'm just pretending? What if deep down, I'm not straight? These thoughts consumed him during intimate moments, leaving him feeling anxious and detached rather than connected to his partner. No matter how much he wanted to feel reassured, the doubts about his orientation wouldn't go away.

His compulsions became increasingly elaborate. Henry began checking his reactions to other men, both in person and online. He would purposely expose himself to pictures of attractive men, asking himself: Do I feel anything? Am I attracted to this person? The fact that these thoughts wouldn't go away made him feel that they must be telling him something important about his true self, adding to his urge to find certainty. When he couldn't detect any clear reaction, he would feel momentary relief, but it was never enough. The doubts would return, stronger than before, leading him to repeat the process again and again. He even found himself staring at strangers in public, anxiously scanning his body for any signs of attraction.

Henry also became preoccupied with how others perceived him. He feared that people might think he was gay, even if he wasn't. He worried that he might unknowingly give off signs that would make others question his orientation. At social events, he became hyper-aware of his behavior: Did I make too much *eye contact with that guy? Did my tone of voice sound different? He became so focused on how he was being perceived that he started avoiding group settings, terrified of what others might think.*

Online, Henry sought reassurance. He spent hours reading articles and forums, trying to find stories similar to his own. He looked up quizzes and tests that claimed to reveal one's true sexual orientation, but the results never satisfied him. He would take the same test over and over, hoping for a definitive answer, but every time he felt more confused than before. In moments of desperation, Henry even considered telling his girlfriend about his doubts, but the fear of hurting her—and the guilt of even having these thoughts—kept him silent.

My entire life would be a lie. I'd have to leave my current relationship and hurt everyone involved. These thoughts haunted Henry, feeding into the endless cycle of doubt. His compulsions extended beyond the mental and online realms. In an effort to "prove" his heterosexuality, Henry began testing himself with pornography. He would force himself to watch different kinds of videos, anxiously monitoring his arousal levels to see what, if anything, sparked a reaction. But this only added to his distress. When he didn't feel an immediate response, his panic deepened. What if I'm in denial? What if this proves I'm gay?

These rituals—mentally reviewing his past, testing his responses to men, and seeking reassurance online—took up more and more of Henry's time. His work began to suffer as he spent hours obsessing over his sexual orientation, unable to focus on anything else. During meetings, his mind would wander: What if I'm lying to myself and everyone around me? The more he tried to push the thoughts away, the stronger they became.

Henry's relationship with his girlfriend deteriorated as well. He pulled away emotionally, fearing that he wasn't being truthful with her or with himself. The guilt of having these doubts weighed heavily on him, and he struggled to maintain the closeness they once shared. He began to question his own identity on a deeper level. What if I've been wrong about myself all along?

Despite his best efforts to find clarity, Henry's doubts only grew more complex. Every time he thought he had found an answer, a new layer of uncertainty would appear. The cycle of questioning, testing, and reassurance never brought him the peace he desperately sought. Instead, it left him feeling more confused, more isolated, and more disconnected from the life he once knew.

Health OCD

Health OCD is characterized by excessive worry and fear about having a serious medical illness, even when there is little or no medical evidence to support this belief. Individuals with Health OCD often misinterpret normal bodily sensations or minor symptoms as signs of a severe illness, leading to persistent anxiety and distress.

Health OCD shares many similarities with Illness Anxiety Disorder (formerly known as hypochondriasis). Some suggest that in Illness Anxiety Disorder, the belief in having a specific disease is more rigid and fixed, while in Health OCD, the focus is on obsessive doubt—a recurring uncertainty about whether one might have an illness, rather than a firm conviction. Despite these subtle differences, the two conditions overlap significantly, and some researchers argue that Health OCD and Illness

Anxiety Disorder may represent different expressions of the same underlying condition. This guide adopts the view that Health OCD and Illness Anxiety Disorder are indeed very similar and can therefore be treated effectively with the same approach.

Obsessions in Health OCD go far beyond general concerns, often giving rise to compulsions that fail to alleviate anxiety and instead reinforce it. For example, individuals with Health OCD may frequently seek reassurance from healthcare professionals, undergo numerous medical tests and procedures, and constantly monitor their bodies for any signs of illness. Yet, despite receiving negative test results or reassurances from doctors, they continue to doubt their health.

Health OCD should be differentiated from contamination-related OCD, although the two can intersect or coexist. In Health OCD, health-related obsessions typically focus on specific medical conditions (e.g., brain cancer, heart disease) rather than on fear of contamination by germs, viruses, or other agents. As a result, compulsions are generally not centered on washing or cleaning but instead on attempts to confirm or disprove the presence of illness. This often includes excessive body checking, repeated reassurance seeking, undergoing medical tests and procedures, researching symptoms, and "doctor shopping."

For some individuals, medical tests and procedures offer temporary relief. For instance, someone who fears they may have contracted HIV might feel reassured after receiving a negative test result they believe is reliable. However, this relief is often short-lived, as the underlying health concerns inevitably resurface or shift to new areas. Others find no relief from medical tests at all, worrying that the tests weren't accurate or thorough enough, which perpetuates their anxiety. Some may even avoid medical tests altogether out of fear of receiving a diagnosis, leading to constant, unaddressed health worries. This avoidance may prevent them from seeking essential medical screenings they would otherwise benefit from.

Regardless of the coping strategy employed, as with other forms of OCD, these efforts rarely provide lasting relief. Instead, the cycle of obsession and compulsion continues, often intensifying over time.

Case Vignette 1.10.
Health OCD
Mia

Mia, a 30-year-old interior designer, had always been careful about her skin. She wore sunscreen, went for regular check-ups, and followed a basic skincare routine. But over the past few months, her concern about skin health had turned into an all-consuming fear. One morning, she noticed a small, irregular mole on her arm. At first, she thought nothing of it. But then, her mind took a darker turn: What if this mole is skin cancer?

Mia couldn't shake the thought. She started fixating on the mole, examining it multiple times a day. Is it changing shape? Has it gotten bigger? She would stand in front of the mirror, looking at it under different lights, convinced that the mole was a sign of something dangerous. Every time she looked, she seemed to find something new to worry about: Maybe it's darker than before. Maybe the edges look irregular. The more she checked, the more certain she became that something was wrong. If I don't catch this early enough, it could spread and become life-threatening, leaving me with limited treatment options or even an untreatable diagnosis.

Her fear didn't stop with that single mole. Soon, Mia began scanning her entire body for signs of skin cancer. She meticulously examined every mole, freckle, and blemish, searching for anything that looked suspicious. Each time she found a new spot, she would panic, thinking: What if this is cancer too? She began cataloging the spots on her skin, making mental notes of where they were and how they looked. But every time she checked, she felt more uncertain. Imagining a future cut short by a missed diagnosis haunted her constantly. Her mind filled with images of her skin changing quietly, without noticeable symptoms, just like she had read about online, feeding her fear that something dangerous could go unnoticed.

Her doubts extended beyond her visual examinations. Mia started noticing every itch, tingle, or sensation on her skin, fearing that they were symptoms of cancer. A slight itch on her leg would send her into a spiral of worry: What if this is a sign that cancer is spreading? She constantly rubbed her skin, checking for any bumps or changes in texture. Even the smallest imperfections became sources of immense anxiety.

Mia's doctor reassured her that her moles were benign during her annual check-up, but the reassurance didn't last long. Maybe the doctor missed something, she thought. What if I didn't point out the right mole? Despite the professional reassurance, Mia couldn't trust the results. She scheduled another appointment a few weeks later, hoping to feel more certain. But even after a second check, her fears persisted. The cycle of doubt had already taken root. She recalled hearing about the importance of early detection and worried that each day of delay might cost her valuable treatment options.

At home, her compulsions grew worse. She started taking photos of her moles, comparing them from one day to the next to see if anything had changed. Each time she saw even the slightest difference in color or shape, she panicked. What if the mole has gotten bigger? she thought, zooming in on the photos, hoping to spot any potential danger. But the more she analyzed her skin, the more unsure she became. Was it really different, or was her mind just playing tricks on her?

Online research became a daily routine. Mia spent hours looking up pictures of skin cancer, comparing her moles to the images she found on medical websites. She would read article after article about melanoma, desperately seeking information that would either confirm or deny her fears. But no matter how much she read, the reassurance never lasted. Perhaps I missed something important in the articles? she wondered. What if my mole looks like one of the early stages of cancer, and I didn't notice? Reading about other people who had initially ignored skin changes filled her with a sense of urgency to keep checking, as if her diligence alone could protect her from a missed diagnosis.

Her daily life began to revolve around checking her skin. At work, Mia would step into the bathroom several times a day just to look at her arms and face in the mirror, trying to spot any new moles or changes in the ones she already had. She would run her fingers over her skin, feeling for any lumps or irregularities. Her work productivity suffered, as she found it hard to focus on her projects. Even during client meetings, her mind would drift back to her skin, wondering if there was something developing that she hadn't caught in time.

Social activities also became difficult. Mia avoided going to the beach or spending time outdoors, convinced that sun exposure would make her skin cancer risk worse. She started wearing long sleeves and wide-brimmed hats, even on cloudy days, fearful that even a few minutes in the sun could cause a new mole to appear or worsen an existing one. Her friends noticed her growing anxiety about being outside, but Mia was too ashamed to explain the full extent of her fears.

Her nights were just as difficult. Before bed, Mia would spend nearly an hour checking her body for new moles, comparing them to the photos she had taken earlier. She would lay in bed, wide awake, convinced that she could feel something wrong with her skin. What if I miss something important and it's too late to treat? she thought. She even considered going to a dermatologist weekly to catch anything early, but feared being dismissed as paranoid.

Despite all the checking and doctor visits, Mia found no relief from her anxiety. Each new mole or freckle only added to her list of worries, and no amount of reassurance seemed to make a lasting difference. The fear that she was on the verge of a serious diagnosis haunted her every day. Even though she knew that constantly checking her skin wasn't helping, she couldn't stop. Her life became a never-ending cycle of checking, doubting, and searching for reassurance that never truly came.

Metaphysical and Existential OCD

Metaphysical OCD, also known as existential OCD, is a symptom dimension of OCD characterized by obsessions related to existential, philosophical, and theological themes. Individuals with metaphysical OCD may experience obsessive thoughts about the nature of reality, existence, morality, life's purpose, or the meaning of life (e.g. "What if reality does not exist?"; "What if life has no meaning"; "Am I living my life correctly?"; "What is the nature of reality?). These obsessions can lead to profound existential anxiety and distress as individuals deal with seemingly normal and commonplace questions that do not have concrete or definitive answers.

Compulsions in metaphysical and existential OCD typically consist of mental rituals and philosophical rumination through repetitive questioning or pondering existential questions without reaching resolution, often leading to heightened anxiety. Engaging in specific rituals, like prayer or magical practices, to temporarily alleviate existential anxiety is also common. Safety behaviors and reassurance seeking often involve excessive research or seeking answers from external sources, such as asking others or excessive time searching for information on the internet in an attempt to find a definitive answer to the existential questions.

Individuals with metaphysical and existential OCD often exhibit approach behavior, feeling compelled to actively engage with existential questioning rather than avoiding it. However, when symptoms become overwhelming or when specific content triggers intense fear, avoidance behaviors may emerge. This can include avoiding conversations, reading materials, or media that might evoke existential thoughts or anxiety. Similarly, individuals may shun introspection, reflection, or experiences that could prompt existential discomfort.

Metaphysical OCD often intersects with what's often termed superstitious OCD, also referred to as magical thinking OCD or magical ideation OCD. Individuals with superstitious OCD may believe that certain actions or thoughts have the power to influence events or outcomes, even when there is no logical connection between the action and the outcome (e.g. thinking a particular thought, number or object will bring on negative events or "bad luck").

On the surface, superstitious OCD may appear distinct from metaphysical OCD. However, beneath the so-called "superstitious" obsessions, individuals often carry metaphysical beliefs and models of the world (e.g., belief in karma, astrology, numerology, psychic abilities, spirits, etc.) that parallel other manifestations of metaphysical OCD, encompassing philosophical, scientific, and religious themes. For instance, individuals may obsess over the existential unreality in the face of hypothetical parallel universes, or fear that their seemingly trivial actions could trigger significant repercussions through the "butterfly effect" in quantum physics.

Furthermore, what is termed superstitious OCD has often little to do with the occurrence of the obsession itself; instead, it represents a coping mechanism aimed at managing the obsession and its associated distress through magical rituals and compulsions (e.g. arranging objects or washing one's hands a certain number of times according to a "lucky number"). Consequently, superstitious or magical thinking OCD is unlikely to represent a distinct symptom dimension of OCD but rather an idiosyncratic thread interwoven throughout various forms of the disorder.

Case Vignette 1.11.
Metaphysical OCD
Alex

Alex, a 23-year-old software developer, had always enjoyed exploring big philosophical questions. He liked pondering life's mysteries, the universe, and the nature of existence. But what once felt like intellectual curiosity began to morph into something darker—persistent doubts that clouded his mind and caused overwhelming anxiety. One night, while lying in bed, a disturbing thought hit him: Maybe reality is an illusion. Maybe nothing I experience is truly real.

At first, the idea seemed absurd, but Alex couldn't shake it. He began doubting everything around him—his experiences, his thoughts, and even his senses. He thought about how philosophers like Descartes had questioned the very nature of existence, planting the seeds of doubt even deeper. How do I know this is real? What if none of this exists? These questions would repeat in his mind, and the more he thought about them, the more disconnected he felt from the world. He started questioning everything: his relationships, his surroundings, and the very nature of reality.

As the weeks passed, the doubts deepened. Alex began to feel like he was living in a dream or a simulation. Everyday experiences became filled with uncertainty. While having coffee with a friend, he'd think: Is this actually happening, or is it all in my mind? Even simple activities, like brushing his teeth or going to the store, would trigger questions about existence. He thought of how, in nature, humans and animals perceive only fragments of reality, and he wondered if perhaps he, too, was only perceiving a small sliver of something much larger and unknowable. How do I know any of this is real? The possibility that reality itself could be an illusion haunted him, casting a shadow over everything he valued. If nothing is real, then life has no meaning, he thought, grappling with a deep-seated dread that stripped away the significance of his relationships, ambitions, and sense of self.

At work, Alex struggled to focus. His thoughts were constantly interrupted by philosophical doubts. What's the point of doing this work if nothing is real? He found it difficult to concentrate on his coding projects, often stopping mid-task to question the reality of what he was doing. His productivity suffered as his mind became preoccupied with existential questions, and his colleagues noticed his growing distraction.

Social interactions became a challenge as well. During conversations with friends, Alex felt detached, as though he were watching himself from a distance. He would zone out, lost in his thoughts about the nature of reality and whether anything around him was real. Sometimes, even familiar places suddenly felt strange to him, despite knowing he had been there many times, intensifying his uncertainty about his surroundings. He started avoiding deep conversations, fearing they would trigger more doubts about existence. Even small talk felt strange to him—he would think: Why does any of this matter if none of it is real?

At home, Alex's doubts intensified. He would lie awake at night, staring at the ceiling, questioning everything. What if I'm trapped in a simulation? What if nothing exists when I fall asleep? These thoughts would keep him up for hours, unable to relax. Sometimes, he would pinch himself or touch objects around him to try and "prove" that reality was real, but the doubts always crept back in. He would find brief moments of reassurance, but they never lasted long before the questioning returned, deepening his fear that he might be trapped in these existential doubts forever, unable to find a way out. He pictured a future where he was perpetually consumed by these thoughts, distanced from the very life he wanted to live.

In an effort to find some answers, Alex turned to the internet. He spent hours reading philosophical texts, searching for explanations, watching videos about the nature of reality, and scrolling through forums where people debated existential questions. The more he researched, the more doubts arose. Every new idea only added more uncertainty to his already anxious mind. Instead of calming him, the information he found online made him question things even more. What if there's something I haven't considered?

Rituals also became part of his daily routine. Alex developed habits like tapping objects or repeating certain phrases in his head to "anchor" himself in reality. He would check and recheck things, like the solidity of objects or the feel of his clothes, hoping to find something that felt stable, something that would ground him. But nothing ever felt certain for long, and the doubts would always return.

As time went on, Alex withdrew more and more. He stopped reading books or watching movies that touched on existential themes, fearing they would trigger his obsessions. He also avoided conversations about philosophy or reality with his friends, worried they might fuel his doubts. Even meditation or mindfulness exercises, which had once helped him relax, now felt like triggers for more existential questions.

Despite all his efforts to understand and resolve these doubts, Alex found himself increasingly lost. The more he tried to find solid ground, the more he doubted everything around him. No matter how much he researched or tried to reassure himself, the doubts about reality and existence remained, leaving him feeling disconnected, anxious, and perpetually questioning the world he once felt so sure of.

Relationship OCD

Relationship OCD is a symptom dimension of OCD characterized by frequent and persistent doubts about one's relationship with significant others. While occasional relationship doubts are common, they are very frequent and persistent among those with relationship OCD, causing both distress to the sufferer and the significant other.

Similar to "just right" OCD, relationship OCD is not caused by extreme or perfectionistic beliefs about what relationships should be like. Individuals with this form of OCD are often fully aware that love doesn't have to feel perfect, passionate, or certain at all times. However, the problem lies not in their beliefs but in their doubts and relentless questioning of what they do feel. While extreme standards or beliefs about relationships might co-occur in some individuals, they are not the root cause of Relationship OCD.

Typically, individuals obsess over potential flaws within the relationship, such as questioning their love for their partner, compatibility, or loyalty. Conversely, they may doubt their partner's love and authenticity in wanting to be with them. Some may also focus on perceived flaws in their partner, such as reliability, intelligence, attractiveness, or sociability, all of which negatively impact the relationship.

Mental rituals typically involve rumination and continuous reflection on the authenticity of one's feelings towards their partner, or whether their partner reciprocates those feelings genuinely. For instance, individuals may compare their current relationship to past experiences. Moreover, self-monitoring and checking behaviors are prevalent, with individuals scrutinizing their own and their partner's thoughts, feelings, and actions in various situations, such as questioning their level of passion during intimate moments or worrying about not constantly thinking about their partner.

To cope with persistent doubts and distress, individuals with relationship OCD may resort to avoidance behaviors. This can involve avoiding situations that trigger relationship doubts or anxieties, such as steering clear of places, activities, or people associated with past doubts. They may also shy away from making long-term commitments or plans with their partner, like moving in together or getting married, as a way to avoid facing their doubts about the relationship's future. The most heartbreaking form of avoidance is when individuals prematurely end an otherwise healthy and loving relationship solely due to their obsessional doubts.

Case Vignette 1.12
Relationship OCD
Lily

Lily, a 26-year-old marketing consultant, had been dating her boyfriend, Ben, for nearly two years. From the outside, everything seemed perfect—he was kind, thoughtful, and always supportive of her career and ambitions. However, after hearing a close friend talk about the "overwhelming certainty" she felt in her own relationship, Lily found herself questioning her own feelings. What if I don't really love him? What if this isn't real love? These questions felt unsettling, and Lily began to wonder if she lacked the same certainty her friend described. She valued authenticity in relationships and felt that, to be true to herself and Ben, she had to understand her feelings fully.

At first, she tried to reassure herself, reasoning that each relationship is unique. But the questions persisted, leaving her increasingly anxious. She knew that relationships didn't always require an intense spark or constant excitement, but she couldn't shake the feeling that something was missing or unclear about her own emotions. What if this isn't real love? Maybe I'm just pretending to love him? The more she questioned her feelings, the more anxious and uncertain she became. She started wondering if she was truly attracted to him or if they were even compatible. The thought that people can sometimes be in relationships that don't feel right without initially realizing it only fueled her worries.

As the days passed, Lily's doubts expanded. She found herself obsessively analyzing every interaction with Ben. Do I feel happy enough? Did I feel connected enough? These persistent questions gnawed at her, even though she knew love could manifest differently for everyone. She wasn't searching for butterflies or sparks but instead questioning whether her feelings were genuine or strong enough. This endless cycle of self-questioning created an overwhelming sense of guilt. She felt guilty for even questioning her relationship with someone who had done nothing wrong and who deserved someone who loved him wholeheartedly. Every moment spent with Ben was scrutinized, and Lily could never find the reassurance she was looking for.

Her mind frequently wandered back to past relationships, comparing how she felt in those moments to her current relationship. She thought about her exes, even the short-term flings, and questioned whether she had felt stronger emotions for them than she did for Ben. The more she compared, the more she doubted her current relationship. Was my love stronger before? Are these feelings enough? Is there something wrong with my relationship? The thought of potentially losing Ben filled her with dread, as she couldn't imagine finding someone as supportive and caring as he was.

Lily's worries didn't stop with her feelings. She began checking her feelings relentlessly. She would spend hours mentally reviewing her thoughts about Ben, asking herself: Do I really love him? Am I attracted to him? Is this the right relationship? She would analyze her feelings during every date or conversation, hoping to find definitive proof that she was either in love or not. But no matter how much she thought about it, the doubts remained unresolved, creating a panic about the future.

Lily's compulsive checking extended to comparing Ben to other men. When she was out with friends, she would observe other couples, wondering: Do they seem happier than we are? She would compare Ben to her friends' boyfriends, worrying that he didn't measure up. Every perceived flaw in Ben—whether real or imagined—became a source of anxiety. What if he's not smart enough for me? What if he's not as good-looking as I thought? She scrutinized every aspect of him—his personality, his appearance, even his sense of humor—always trying to determine if he was "good enough." The constant need to measure Ben against others created a sense of guilt and anxiety, making her feel like she was failing him as a partner. If she did not really love him, then maybe he was better off without her.

Her fears began to affect her daily life. At work, she found it hard to concentrate on her tasks because her mind kept drifting back to her relationship doubts. She would pause in the middle of writing an email or preparing a presentation, her thoughts hijacked by the question: Do I really love him? Her productivity declined, and she became increasingly stressed, unable to focus on anything other than her obsessional worries.

Social situations also became difficult. Lily avoided spending time with couples, fearing that being around them would trigger more doubts about her relationship. When friends asked about her plans with Ben, she would feel anxious, wondering if they could tell that something was wrong. She started pulling away from Ben too. She avoided intimate conversations and didn't want to make long-term plans, fearing that committing to a future together would only solidify her doubts.

At home, the doubts intensified. Lily spent long nights awake, going over every detail of their relationship, trying to find answers. If she was wrong about her feelings for Ben, it would mean ending the relationship and facing the pain of a breakup. We would lose everything we built together. She would replay their conversations, analyze his facial expressions, and search for clues that something was wrong. She even considered breaking up with Ben several times, thinking that it might give her clarity. But the thought of ending the relationship filled her with dread, leaving her stuck in a cycle of uncertainty.

Lily also began researching relationships online. She read countless articles, watched videos, and searched forums for answers. She looked for stories of other people who had gone through similar doubts, hoping to find reassurance. But the more she read, the more confused she became. Every relationship expert seemed to have a different opinion about what love should feel like, and none of the advice seemed to apply to her situation.

As time went on, Lily found it harder to enjoy being with Ben. Even when they went on dates or spent time together, her mind was filled with questions and doubts. Maybe I am not happy enough, she wondered. Every gesture of affection felt hollow, and every laugh felt forced, as if she were performing the role of a loving girlfriend instead of living it. Despite everything she did to reassure herself, Lily couldn't escape the constant nagging feeling that something was wrong with their relationship.

Transformation ("Morphing") OCD

Transformation OCD, also sometimes referred to as "morphing" OCD, is a lesser known and underreported form of OCD, that revolves around fears of undergoing unwanted radical physical, emotional, or psychological changes. Those with morphing OCD quite literally worry about turning into someone else other than their own actual identity.

One hallmark of morphing OCD is a fixation on physical transformations. Individuals obsess over the possibility of drastic alterations in their appearance, including becoming disfigured, aging rapidly, or developing a physical illness that changes their outward appearance. These fears can escalate to the point of imagining a complete physical transformation into another person, a fictional character, or even an inanimate object.

Beyond physical transformations, morphing OCD can also involve concerns about psychological changes. Individuals may fear adopting undesirable traits, emotions, or characteristics from others, or conversely, losing their own identity when exposed to different influences. For example, they may worry about internalizing negative emotions or preferences from others, or even adopting the beliefs and behaviors of fictional characters.

Transformation OCD shares similarities with mental contamination, where individuals fear psychological or moral contamination through contact with specific people, objects, or situations. However, morphing OCD extends beyond mere contamination fears to encompass the dread of permanent integration of undesirable characteristics into one's identity.

Morphing OCD can also intersect with metaphysical OCD where individuals entertain certain metaphysical beliefs about how the transformation into something other than themselves might occur. These beliefs may range from notions of "energy", magical shapeshifting, or genetic anomalies causing sudden physical alterations. Others may conceive of transformation occurring through more conventional psychological mechanisms, such as assuming another's identity through exposure and learning.

Compulsions in morphing OCD typically manifest as repeated checking behaviors, both overt and covert. Individuals may check their appearance or specific body parts incessantly to ensure no transformation has occurred. Similarly, those fearing psychological transformation may engage in covert checking of their inner state or act out certain traits excessively to reassure themselves (e.g., being overly attentive others to prevent turning into a rude person).

Mental questioning and analysis are also common, as individuals try to ensure they have not changed into anyone else. Rituals or routines aimed at preventing the feared changes, such as visualization techniques or avoidance of triggering stimuli, are also prevalent among individuals with morphing OCD.

Due to the unusual nature of morphing OCD, individuals are sometimes misdiagnosed with something other than OCD. However, those with morphing OCD typically recognize the irrationality of their thoughts and understand that such transformations are unlikely to occur. Despite this insight, they find themselves persistently preoccupied with these concerns.

Case Vignette 1.13.
Morphing OCD
Lucas

Lucas, a 19-year-old college student, had always been a bit unsure of himself—like many his age, he was still figuring out who he was. But recently, things began to spiral into something darker. It started one afternoon when a friend casually remarked that Lucas looked a bit like a well-known actor. At first, the comment seemed harmless, just an observation. But this particular actor was someone Lucas disliked intensely, someone with values and opinions completely opposite from his own. The idea of resembling this person began to gnaw at him. What if I'm changing? What if I'm becoming someone like him?

At first, he brushed off these thoughts, trying to convince himself it was just a passing idea. But as the days went on, the thoughts became louder and more insistent. He knew that people's identities could change over time, often without them noticing at first, which made each glance in the mirror feel like an urgent need. Soon, every time Lucas passed a mirror or reflective surface, he felt compelled to check his appearance. Maybe I don't look the same as I did before? He started scanning his face for signs of change, analyzing his features in detail. Does my face look different? Are my eyes changing? He would spend long periods staring into the mirror, convinced that subtle changes were happening, though he couldn't pinpoint exactly what was different. If I'm changing into someone else, he thought, then I might eventually lose my real self entirely.

Lucas's worries weren't limited to just his appearance. He began to feel uneasy in social interactions, questioning whether his responses were genuinely his or if he was somehow "adopting" traits from others. He'd noticed in the past how easily he picked up habits from friends and family, sometimes even their mannerisms, which left him feeling he was at risk of losing the parts of him that made him unique. The fear grew that he was unknowingly transforming into someone else, not just in appearance, but in personality, thoughts, and values as well. He worried that his very identity was slipping away, being replaced by traits he didn't choose or want.

These fears soon extended to his daily activities. If he watched a TV show or read a book, he couldn't shake the feeling that it might be subtly altering his sense of self. Experts often discuss how exposure to media can subconsciously influence a person's identity, and this idea lingered in his mind each time he engaged with any form of media. What if media or conversations are influencing my identity? He started avoiding shows, movies, and even social media, worried that exposure to strong personalities or ideas would shape him in ways he couldn't control. If I keep changing under these influences, he feared, I'll eventually lose my real self—my core identity will disappear, replaced by a version of me that I don't recognize or like.

This overwhelming fear of losing himself took over his daily life. At school, Lucas found it hard to concentrate, constantly distracted by these worries. He avoided classmates and social situations, afraid that interacting with others might further "contaminate" his identity. When he walked past photos of himself taken only a few months earlier, they felt strange and unfamiliar, fueling the anxiety that he was changing beyond recognition. If I can't trust who I am today, he thought, then what will I become tomorrow?

To cope, Lucas developed a series of rituals. He would frequently check his face and body for any signs of transformation, scrutinizing his features to ensure they hadn't altered. Every time he noticed a slight difference—perhaps a new pimple, a change in hairstyle, or even just the way light reflected off his skin—he would spiral into panic, convinced that it was proof of his feared transformation. He would mentally reaffirm his identity by repeating statements like: I am Lucas. I know who I am. These rituals gave him brief moments of relief, but the doubts always returned. No matter how often he told himself he was still the same, the worry lingered: If I'm truly changing, then I'll lose myself entirely, and I'll no longer be Lucas.

Despite understanding, on some level, the irrationality of his fears, Lucas couldn't escape the feeling that his identity was slipping away. Each day brought new doubts about who he was and who he was becoming. The fear of waking up as someone else haunted him, leaving him feeling trapped in a constant state of anxiety and self-questioning.

OCD About OCD

"OCD about OCD", also known as meta-cognitive obsessions, or meta-obsessions, refers to a phenomenon where individuals with OCD develop obsessions and compulsions specifically related to their OCD itself. This can manifest in various ways. For instance, individuals may obsessively worry about whether they truly have OCD, constantly seeking reassurance or conducting mental rituals to confirm their diagnosis. This preoccupation often stems from a fear that if they don't have OCD, then their obsessions might be true or valid, such as the fear of causing harm to others or themselves. In other cases, concerns might be more related to managing symptoms, such as excessive checking of medication, constantly researching OCD treatments, or engaging in elaborate rituals to "control" symptoms.

Other forms of "OCD about OCD" may revolve around a fear of having obsessions, or that one will never able to stop having obsessions, doomed to forever be in the clutches of the OCD. These are essentially obsessions about having obsessions that usually initially develop as a secondary concern following a period of having OCD, after which they may become the central obsessional concern as the original obsession retreats to the background. These concerns may even continue after the original obsession has disappeared altogether. In fact, the person may even develop obsessions about their obsession with having obsessions, in a never-ending layering of symptomatology that can perplex both the individual and the therapist.

For instance, someone with "just right OCD" might initially obsess over arranging objects, spending hours trying to make them feel "just right." Over time, as the distress caused by these obsessions and compulsions accumulates, they may begin to fear the act of obsessing itself. They worry that encountering other arrangements might trigger a new fixation, further exacerbating their misery. In other words, the obsession shifts to the fear of developing an obsession, rather than any genuine fixation on the arrangement of objects. For example, they might see a floral arrangement and feel anxious, not because they find the arrangement itself troubling, but because they worry it could spiral into a new obsession. Essentially, they are experiencing obsessions about nonexistent obsessions.

Finally, the phenomenon known as 'OCD about OCD' can worsen the original obsession rather than stand as an independent issue. For example, individuals might fear that their OCD will escalate to a point where they fear losing control and 'go crazy,' potentially leading them to act on their obsessions, thereby causing harm to others. However, while anyone can experience a breaking point, this does not lend validity to, or heighten the legitimacy of the obsession regarding potential harm.

Case Vignette 1.14
OCD about OCD
Abigail

Abigail, a 47-year-old elementary school teacher, had been living with OCD for many years. Her primary obsessions initially revolved around contamination and cleanliness, which led to frequent handwashing and cleaning rituals. But after months of therapy and managing her symptoms, something unexpected happened: she developed a new obsession—worrying about her OCD itself.

It started when Abigail noticed herself feeling better for a few days. Instead of feeling relieved, she was overcome with doubt: Maybe this improvement means my OCD is getting worse. Perhaps this break in my symptoms is just a sign that the OCD will come back even stronger. These thoughts spiraled, and soon she was obsessively monitoring her own OCD, analyzing whether every action she took was part of her disorder or not.

Abigail found herself constantly questioning the validity of her diagnosis. What if I don't actually have OCD and I'm just making it all up? If it's not OCD, then maybe it's something far worse. She recalled reading articles that described how some mental health issues can resemble OCD, which made her doubt whether her diagnosis was accurate. The thought terrified her, filling her with an intense sense of dread.

If her symptoms didn't fit neatly into the framework of OCD, she worried that they might be a sign of something unknown and untreatable, leaving her without a path to recovery.

She feared that if she did not have OCD, then the treatment she had received might not have been appropriate, casting doubt on any progress she had made. Her mind was filled with endless questions: Maybe I'm just using the diagnosis as an excuse? Could it be that I'm not trying hard enough to get better? She also remembered how, in the past, brief moments of relief were often followed by the resurgence of symptoms, sometimes worse than before. This memory made it even harder for her to trust her progress. Each question led to more anxiety and self-doubt. If I don't truly have OCD, then treatment might be futile, and all the progress I've made will be meaningless.

Her compulsions shifted from checking physical objects to checking her own mental state. She would spend hours reviewing her thoughts, trying to figure out whether they were truly OCD-related or something else entirely. She would mentally replay past conversations with her therapist, analyzing every word to ensure that her diagnosis was accurate.

Online research became one of her primary compulsions. Abigail would spend hours reading about OCD, checking symptoms, and comparing her experiences to others. She frequently visited online forums, asking strangers to confirm whether her experiences matched their understanding of the disorder. But no matter how much reassurance she got, the doubts persisted: Perhaps I missed something important. Maybe my OCD is different from everyone else's. The thought of living with OCD forever, without ever recovering, filled her with despair. How would I get used to living like this? She had also come across articles emphasizing that relapse is common among individuals with OCD, which made her feel as though any progress she had made was fragile and temporary.

Her fear of obsessing became a central concern. Maybe my original OCD symptoms will return. Perhaps my OCD will shift focus to something else entirely. Even when she wasn't experiencing obsessions, she feared they could appear at any moment. This led to an almost constant state of hyper-vigilance, scanning her thoughts for any potential signs of a new obsession.

In her day-to-day life, Abigail's fear of obsessing led to avoidance behaviors. She avoided situations or topics that might trigger new obsessions, even if they had nothing to do with her original OCD concerns. For example, she would avoid conversations about mental health or disorders, fearing that they might give her new ideas for obsessions. She also became hesitant to talk about her OCD with her therapist, worrying that maybe focusing too much on the disorder will make it worse.

Despite her constant checking and reassurance-seeking, Abigail's doubts about her OCD remained strong. She feared she'd never fully recover and would stay trapped in this loop forever. Even moments of calm felt suspicious to her, as if they were merely a precursor to the return of her obsessions.

Abigail's life became centered around her OCD—not just the original symptoms, but the disorder itself. The more she tried to analyze and control her OCD, the more it consumed her thoughts. The once-simple goal of managing her symptoms had transformed into an obsession with her OCD, leaving her feeling stuck in a cycle of endless rumination and self-doubt.

Despite her constant checking and reassurance-seeking, Abigail's doubts about her OCD remained strong, leaving her terrified that she might spiral into something unknown and uncontrollable. If it wasn't OCD, she feared it could be a sign that her mental health was deteriorating in ways she couldn't understand, let alone fix. Even moments of calm felt suspicious to her, as if they were merely a precursor to the return of her obsessions.

Indeed, Abigail's OCD was shifting focus—but not in the way she feared. She remained blind to where the shift had actually occurred, caught in the expectation that her obsessions would transform into something external or unrecognizable. In reality, the shift had already taken place, turning her focus inward onto the disorder itself. This relentless cycle of doubting her diagnosis and monitoring her mental state kept her locked in a pattern of obsession and compulsion, leaving her unable to fully embrace the progress she had worked so hard to achieve.

Hoarding

Hoarding OCD, once considered a subtype of OCD, is now recognized as a distinct disorder. However, it remains highly similar to OCD in its mechanisms and is included within the broader spectrum of OCD and related disorders. The defining feature of hoarding OCD is a profound difficulty discarding items, driven by obsessive fears tied to potential harm, loss, or regret. These obsessions lead to compulsions to save and collect, often fueled by a deep fear of making mistakes, being unprepared for the future, or permanently losing something of value.

One key distinction between hoarding OCD and other forms of OCD is the level of conviction attached to the obsessions. While individuals with OCD commonly experience doubts and may recognize the irrationality of their fears, those with hoarding OCD often strongly believe in the necessity of retaining their possessions. This stronger conviction can make hoarding OCD more resistant to standard treatments, as individuals may feel that discarding items would truly result in catastrophic consequences.

Compulsions in hoarding OCD manifest as repetitive saving, collecting, and even acquiring additional possessions to counter the anxiety associated with their obsessive fears. For instance, a person might keep old newspapers, broken items, or expired products because of a belief that these items may someday prove useful or hold irreplaceable value. Checking behaviors are also common, with individuals repeatedly inspecting their belongings to ensure nothing important has been lost, damaged, or mistakenly discarded. Despite efforts to organize or maintain control over their environment, the accumulation of objects typically leads to overwhelming clutter that disrupts daily living and causes significant stress.

Hoarding OCD's impact extends far beyond physical spaces. The disorder often creates emotional and social difficulties, as the cluttered living conditions strain relationships and interfere with daily routines. Family members may feel frustrated or powerless, while individuals with hoarding OCD may experience guilt, embarrassment, or shame over the state of their home. This social and emotional toll often leads to isolation, as individuals avoid inviting others into their home for fear of judgment or misunderstanding.

Moreover, the consequences of severe hoarding can include physical hazards, such as fire risks, difficulty navigating cluttered spaces, and compromised hygiene. These dangers further compound the emotional and functional impairments caused by the disorder. The individual's life becomes increasingly consumed by the need to protect and monitor their possessions, leaving little room for other meaningful activities or relationships.

Case Vignette 1.15
Hoarding
Oliver

Oliver, a 45-year-old freelance writer, never considered himself particularly attached to material things. However, over the past few years, his apartment had gradually become overwhelmed with items he couldn't seem to part with. What began as a small collection of books and magazines for his writing soon expanded to include old newspapers, worn-out clothes, unused appliances, and piles of miscellaneous items. Every surface was covered, and walking through his home had become a challenge.

For Oliver, the thought of discarding anything filled him with anxiety. He was haunted by a nagging series of doubts: "Perhaps I'll need this later, and I'll regret throwing it away." "Maybe I won't be able to replace it when I need it." "What if getting rid of this prevents me from being prepared for future emergencies?" Even items he hadn't used in years suddenly seemed essential in his mind. A receipt, a broken gadget, or a magazine article—no matter how trivial—would trigger the same fear: "What if it turns out to be important after all and someone could still use it?" If it turns out to be important, then throwing it away would be irresponsible, selfish and wasteful.

These thoughts paralyzed him. Beyond the fear of making practical mistakes, Oliver also formed deep emotional attachments to his belongings. Each object seemed to carry weight, representing memories or parts of his identity. "If I throw this away, I'll be losing a piece of myself," he would think, even about small, insignificant items like an old t-shirt or a childhood keepsake. These thoughts made it nearly impossible to let go of anything, no matter how cluttered his home became.

When Oliver did try to declutter, the anxiety became unbearable. He would sort through his belongings, only to second-guess every decision. Objects he had planned to throw away often ended up back in new piles, waiting for the "right time" to let them go. Even after placing something in the trash, Oliver would occasionally retrieve it, gripped by the thought: "I could regret this later. What if it turns out to be irreplaceable?"

The fear of discarding something useful or meaningful slowly began to take over his life. His friends stopped visiting, and Oliver avoided having anyone over, embarrassed by the state of his apartment. Family members offered to help, but he waved them off, insisting that he would get organized eventually. Deep down, though, Oliver knew the clutter was out of control. Still, the fear of future regret outweighed the discomfort of living in chaos.

Over time, the anxiety extended beyond his living space. Social invitations became rare, and Oliver declined the few that came his way, reluctant to leave his home unattended. His freelance work began to suffer as well—his time and energy were consumed by the endless cycle of acquisition, avoidance, and indecision. He found it difficult to meet deadlines, distracted by thoughts of what he should keep and what he could afford to discard.

Each attempt to declutter left Oliver more frustrated. He couldn't escape the sense that throwing something away would be an irreversible mistake. Even though he knew his behavior was irrational, the thought of parting with anything was too distressing. He felt trapped—caught between the fear of regret and the fleeting comfort of holding onto everything. As his apartment grew more cluttered, his world became smaller. He avoided parts of his home altogether, confining himself to the few areas still functional amidst the chaos.

Despite recognizing the toll the hoarding was taking on his life, Oliver remained stuck. The thought of discarding anything felt more unbearable than the clutter itself. No matter how hard he tried, he couldn't bring himself to let go of his possessions. He feared that letting go would leave him unprepared, vulnerable, or without something essential in the future.

Identifying Your Themes and Principal Symptoms

Which dimensions of OCD symptoms resonate with you? Remember, OCD isn't always confined to a single theme; often, symptoms overlap or intersect. Some individuals may experience only one or two themes, while others may have more. Recognizing and documenting your themes and symptoms is an important first step towards managing your OCD. Follow the instructions below to identify and record your symptoms effectively.

Exercise 1.1.
Identifying Your Themes and Principal Symptoms

1. **Identify Major Themes:**
   o Use section 1 of Form 1.1 to identify the symptom manifestations that significantly impact you.
   o If you don't find a match, utilize the 'Other' category and describe your OCD theme.
   o If you are troubled by more than two themes, set aside the additional ones for now. Prioritize addressing the ones that bother you the most initially.

2. **List Your Obsessions:**
   o Once you've pinpointed your themes, use section 2 of the form to list all the obsessions you experience within each theme.
   o Take your time with this process; don't rush it. Over the course of about a week, observe your inner thoughts whenever you catch yourself obsessing.
   o If you notice a new obsession or preoccupation that hadn't crossed your mind before, add it to your list.
   o Don't concern yourself with the quantity of obsessions you list. The purpose of this exercise is simply to recognize and identify what's troubling you.

3. **Identify Compulsive Strategies:**
   o Just as you identify your obsessions, use Form 1.2 to list all the compulsive strategies you employ in response to them.
   o Take your time over the course of one week to observe everything you do in reaction to your obsessions.

o Duplicate the form as needed in case the provided space is insufficient. Many individuals with OCD utilize numerous types of compulsive strategies, some of which may be quite subtle.

Form 1.1:
Identifying Your Themes and Obsessions

Section 1: Symptom Dimensions	
❑ Disturbing Thoughts	❑ Health
❑ Negligence and Mistakes	❑ Metaphysical/Existential
❑ Contamination	❑ Relationship
❑ Symmetry, Order and Arrangement	❑ Transformation
❑ Sensorimotor	❑ Gender and Sexual Orientation
❑ OCD About OCD	❑ Hoarding
❑ Other:	❑ Other:
Section 2: Obsessions	
Theme 1	Theme 2
1.	1.
2.	2.
3.	3.
4.	4.
5.	5.
6.	6.
7.	7.
8.	8.
9.	9.
10.	10.
11.	11.
12.	12.

Form 1.2.
Identifying Your Compulsive Strategies

Compulsive Strategies	
Theme 1	Theme 2
Overt Compulsions	Overt Compulsions
1.	1.
2.	2.
3.	3.
4.	4.
Covert Compulsions	Covert Compulsions
1.	1.
2.	2.
3.	3.
Reassurance Seeking	Reassurance Seeking
1.	1.
2.	2.
3.	3.
4.	4.
Safety Behaviors	Safety Behaviors
1.	1.
2.	2.
3.	3.
Avoidance	Avoidance
1.	1.
2.	2.
3.	3.
Self-Testing	Self-Testing
1.	1.
2.	2.

Forging the Trail Ahead

To conclude, we have explored the range of experiences that comprise OCD, from general patterns to the unique coping methods individuals develop. While each person's experience with OCD may differ in themes, obsessions, and compulsions, there are common threads that unite these experiences. OCD often centers around repetitive, distressing thoughts and compulsive behaviors aimed at reducing that distress.

In the next chapter, we'll delve into the history of treatments for OCD, examining traditional approaches and the evolution of therapeutic models. This will include the evidence-based approach of Inference-Based Cognitive Behavioral Therapy (I-CBT), on which this manual is based. I-CBT emerged from a growing recognition of the need to address not only the behaviors but also the reasoning processes that underlie OCD. This model, which has developed alongside cognitive-behavioral approaches, offers a distinct and structured pathway to address the core of obsessional doubt.

Gaining insight into these frameworks will provide you with a solid foundation to understand and apply the I-CBT strategies in later chapters, preparing you to recognize the thought patterns and compulsive behaviors that drive OCD. This foundational understanding will be essential as you make informed, empowered choices, adapting the strategies to your unique experience and supporting your journey toward recovery.

Chapter 2

Understanding OCD Theories and Treatment Approaches

Until the 1960s, OCD was widely regarded as highly resistant to treatment. This skepticism stemmed from the dominance of psychodynamic and psychoanalytical therapies, which failed to effectively address OCD symptoms. Additionally, biological interventions such as lobotomies and electroconvulsive therapy (ECT) yielded minimal outcomes and came at enormous costs, while medications like sedatives merely managed secondary symptoms without targeting the disorder itself. As a result, individuals with OCD were often left to cope with their struggles in isolation, enduring a profoundly debilitating condition with little hope for effective relief.

Modern understanding of OCD highlights why these traditional approaches often failed—and in some cases exacerbated symptoms. Psychodynamic and psychoanalytic treatments emphasize deep intellectual analysis, a process that ironically mirrors the compulsive over-analysis common in OCD. This process can easily result in an intensification of symptoms rather than providing relief for individuals with OCD.

Furthermore, core Freudian concepts, such as the idea of unconscious impulses driving behavior, could inadvertently reinforce OCD. For instance, telling someone with harm-related obsessions that their intrusive thoughts stem from hidden impulses might make those thoughts feel more real and distressing, compounding the problem.

> The concept of the Freudian unconscious is fertile ground for OCD.

The mid-20th century saw a turning point with the introduction of tricyclic antidepressants, such as clomipramine, which demonstrated efficacy in reducing obsessions and compulsions. However, these medications came with significant side effects, including drowsiness, dry mouth, and constipation, limiting their utility. Additionally, many patients experienced only modest improvements, and some found the effects insufficient to substantially enhance their quality of life.

The 1950s also ushered in a revolutionary shift in understanding psychological disorders through behavioral models. These models framed conditions like anxiety and phobias as behaviors acquired through learning and conditioning—behaviors that, crucially, could be unlearned. This perspective stood in sharp contrast to the fatalistic view of traditional psychoanalytic approaches, offering a more hopeful outlook on human adaptability.

By the late 1960s, these behavioral foundations evolved into Exposure and Response Prevention (ERP) therapy, a generally effective intervention for OCD. ERP demonstrated that human behavior is inherently flexible, capable of change even in deeply entrenched patterns. This marked a transformative moment in OCD treatment, bringing new hope and tangible relief to individuals once thought to be beyond psychological help.

Highlight 2.1.
Key Learning Points

Up until the 1960s, OCD was considered untreatable.

Medication often only provides a partial solution.

Exposure and response prevention was the first psychological treatment to bring hope for those with OCD.

Exposure and Response Prevention

Understanding the Phobic Model and OCD

ERP, initially designed to treat anxiety and phobias, suggests that fears and anxieties develop through learned associations and reinforcement. At the core of this process is avoidance: when someone actively avoids a feared object or situation—such as spiders or social events—their anxiety temporarily decreases. However, this reduction in distress comes at a cost. Avoidance reinforces the fear, making it more likely to recur in similar situations. Over time, the avoidance becomes habitual, and the fear deepens, exacerbating symptoms.

When we apply this phobic model to OCD, obsessions act as the anxiety triggers. Compulsions—repetitive behaviors or mental acts—are then employed to relieve the anxiety that these obsessions cause. The momentary relief that comes from performing these compulsions reinforces the overall pattern, much like avoidance in phobias. In addition, people with OCD often avoid situations or stimuli that trigger their obsessions, further embedding their fears. This creates a vicious cycle where obsessions trigger compulsions, which offer only temporary relief but strengthen OCD over time (see Diagram 2.1).

Disrupting the OCD Cycle: How ERP Works

ERP is designed to break the cycle of obsessions and compulsions by systematically exposing individuals to their fears and preventing the compulsive responses. The goal is to help individuals face the feared thoughts, situations, or images that trigger their anxiety, and at the same time, resist the urge to perform compulsions. In other words, ERP targets both aspects of OCD: the "exposure" element means confronting the anxiety-triggering situation, and "response prevention" means avoiding the compulsive action that typically follows.

For example, consider someone with a fear of accidentally harming others with a knife. They might avoid handling sharp objects altogether. In ERP, they would be encouraged to handle a knife while another person is present, without engaging in any compulsive checking or asking for reassurance. The idea is that by not performing the compulsive behavior, the person learns that the feared consequence—harming someone—does not occur. Over time, their anxiety diminishes as they build confidence in their ability to tolerate the feared situation without engaging in compulsions.

Diagram 2.1.
Phobic Model of OCD

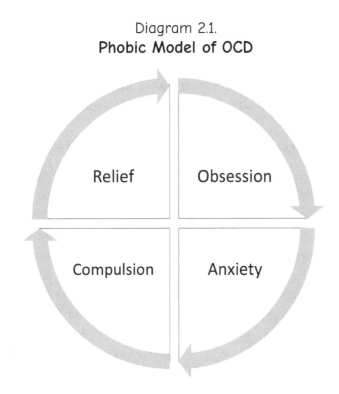

Building the "Fear Ladder": A Gradual Approach

A central concept in ERP is the use of a "fear ladder" or hierarchy of feared situations. Rather than diving headfirst into their most intense fears, individuals work through their anxiety in a structured and gradual way. They begin by identifying situations that cause varying levels of anxiety, ranking them on a scale from 0 (no distress) to 100 (extreme distress). This process allows them to face their fears step by step, starting with moderately anxiety-provoking situations and gradually moving toward more challenging tasks.

For example, someone with contamination fears might start by touching a doorknob they consider dirty, gradually moving to more anxiety-provoking tasks such as handling objects in a public restroom. This incremental process enables individuals to face their fears without resorting to compulsions, allowing their symptoms to decrease over time. Over decades of clinical application, this approach has proven effective for many, offering a structured and empowering path to overcoming OCD.

Beyond Habituation: New Insights into ERP's Mechanism

ERP's success was historically often attributed to habituation—the gradual reduction of anxiety through repeated exposure. The prevailing idea was that confronting feared stimuli repeatedly would diminish individuals' sensitivity, reducing anxiety as they "got used to" the stimuli. However, recent research has revealed that while habituation often occurs, it is not the sole factor driving ERP's effectiveness. In fact, some individuals experience little habituation yet still achieve meaningful improvements in their symptoms.

This insight has shifted the focus toward *inhibitory learning*, which explains how individuals can overcome anxiety by forming new, competing memories that weaken the influence of old, fear-based responses. Instead of focusing solely on reducing anxiety through repeated exposure (as in the habituation model), inhibitory learning emphasizes creating new, non-fearful associations that override the fear response. For example, a person with contamination OCD may repeatedly touch a doorknob they believe is "dirty" and then refrain from washing their hands. Over time, they learn that the feared consequence—becoming sick—does not occur. This new learning competes with and weakens the original fear-driven association that linked the doorknob to harm, demonstrating how inhibitory learning facilitates change without requiring anxiety to subside immediately.

Shifting Perspectives: Fear Intolerance and Uncertainty

ERP is also often described as addressing a fundamental challenge faced by many individuals with OCD: an intolerance of uncertainty and anxiety. While there is no evidence that OCD is caused by this intolerance, proponents suggest that ERP helps individuals confront and accept uncertainty as an inevitable part of life. This represents a shift in how ERP is conceptualized, placing emphasis on fostering acceptance of distressing thoughts and emotions rather than striving to eliminate fear entirely.

For example, a person might be encouraged to accept the possibility that their hands are not completely "clean" while resisting the urge to engage in repeated handwashing. This perspective reframes anxiety and uncertainty as discomforts that, while unpleasant, do not need to be fixed or resolved. Over time, this perspective is said to foster emotional flexibility and resilience, helping individuals approach intrusive thoughts and uncertainties with greater confidence and ease.

Common Ground in ERP Approaches

While different variations of ERP may emphasize distinct goals—whether fostering habituation, creating inhibitory associations, or building tolerance for uncertainty—all approaches share a fundamental principle: directly confronting one's fears. ERP encourages individuals to engage with anxiety-provoking situations while resisting compulsive behaviors, breaking the cycle of avoidance that perpetuates OCD.

At its core, ERP focuses on behavior rather than cognition as the primary mechanism for change. By leaning into anxiety as it arises—without attempting to suppress, neutralize, or escape it—individuals disrupt the cycle of avoidance and compulsion. This process can weaken the grip of intrusive thoughts and obsessions over time, regardless of whether the specific aim is reducing fear, strengthening new associations, or cultivating acceptance of uncertainty.

Advocates of ERP widely regard this shared foundation across all its approaches as essential in addressing the OCD cycle.

Effectiveness and Limitations of ERP

ERP has proven effective for many individuals with OCD, with approximately 60-70% of those who undergo treatment experiencing some level of improvement. One of its key advantages is its straightforward implementation, which can be applied through self-help methods or under the guidance of a healthcare professional. However, these numbers also reveal that 30-40% of individuals may see little to no improvement. Even for those who do benefit, residual symptoms often linger, heightening the risk of relapse over time. Complete remission, while achievable for some, is only seen in about 40-50% of individuals who complete ERP, underscoring that ERP, despite its success, is not a definitive cure for OCD.

Treatment Dropout and Resistance

Approximately one in five individuals in treatment trials either decline or discontinue ERP. While this dropout rate is similar to other treatments, it fails to account for the many individuals who avoid treatment entirely due to fear or misconceptions about ERP. Many are apprehensive about facing their deepest fears, a core component of ERP, and may feel overwhelmed by the prospect. For some, the treatment can seem too intense or daunting to even begin, let alone sustain over time.

This challenge is especially pronounced when ERP exercises conflict with deeply held personal values or moral beliefs. For example, individuals with strong religious or ethical concerns—such as those who view blasphemy as an unforgivable act—may find it profoundly distressing to engage in exposures that involve taboo thoughts. In these cases, ERP can feel not only threatening to their mental health but also to their moral integrity.

Although it is possible to adapt ERP to align with personal values, doing so is complex and requires a highly nuanced approach to maintain a balance between respecting the individual's belief system and achieving therapeutic goals.

Practical Limitations: Imaginal Exposure

In situations where real-life exposure is impractical or impossible, imaginal exposure is often employed. This technique involves having individuals vividly imagine feared scenarios, such as committing taboo acts, with the aim of reducing the emotional charge associated with intrusive thoughts. While this approach can be effective, especially if the OCD is maintained by a high level of avoidance, research on its efficacy for taboo or morally distressing thoughts remains limited. The systematic use of scripts or looped tapes for imaginal exposure has not been extensively studied in these types of OCD, and it remains unclear whether imaginal exposure alone can produce significant results without supplementary interventions.

The Risk of Compulsive Testing

One of the potential risks of ERP lies in the tendency for exposure exercises to inadvertently turn into compulsive self-tests, which can undermine the original intent of the treatment. For instance, an individual who fears microwave radiation may repeatedly test this fear by placing their head near a microwave, in an attempt to disprove the threat. Instead of alleviating their anxiety, such actions often reinforce doubts and further validate the obsession. This compulsive testing can entrench the obsessive-compulsive cycle, especially when compulsions are driven more by cognitive distortions than by behavioral avoidance.

In these cases, what is critically needed is an extensive cognitive assessment to accurately identify and address the underlying beliefs and maintaining factors contributing to the compulsions. Without this assessment, ERP's focus on behavior may overlook the cognitive distortions at the root of the issue, leading to less effective outcomes. Cognitive assessment provides the insight necessary to tailor interventions that directly target the thoughts and beliefs that fuel compulsive behaviors, ensuring a more comprehensive approach to breaking the cycle. This step is not always intuitive in a primarily behavioral approach like ERP, which can make addressing compulsions rooted in cognition more challenging without additional cognitive strategies.

ERP's Origins and Misalignment with OCD

It's important to recognize that ERP was originally developed for treating phobias, and while it has been adapted for OCD, its foundation in phobia-based techniques may not always align perfectly with the complexities of OCD. Phobias typically involve a fear of specific objects or situations, while OCD encompasses a far broader and more complex range of symptoms across a wide variety of obsessional themes. This mismatch between ERP's original intent and its application to OCD may explain why it does not always fully address the cognitive mechanisms at play in the disorder.

Conclusion: ERP's Strengths and Gaps

ERP has undoubtedly been a valuable and effective treatment for many individuals with OCD, providing significant symptom relief and helping to break the cycle of compulsions. However, its focus on behavioral exposure alone does not always address the full range of cognitive processes that drive OCD. Moving forward, it is essential to explore cognitive models of OCD that broaden the therapeutic landscape. As we shall see, one such model, inference-based cognitive behavioral therapy (ICBT), offers a transformative approach that bypasses the traditional emphasis on facing fears and anxiety induction. Before delving into ICBT, however, we will first examine the emergence and evolution of other cognitive models that have shaped modern OCD treatment, setting the stage for a deeper understanding of ICBT's distinct contributions.

Highlight 2.2.
Key Learning Points

ERP aims to break the cycle of OCD by exposing the person to their fears and preventing any responses.

ERP is an effective treatment, but not for everyone, and not everyone is able to complete the required exercises.

ERP treats OCD as if it were a phobia. Yet, OCD is not a phobia.

The Emergence and Evolution of Cognitive Models

From Behavioral Models to Cognitive Approaches

In the mid-20th century, treatments for mental health conditions, including OCD, predominantly relied on behavioral models, apart from psychodynamic and psychoanalytic approaches. Techniques such as Exposure and Response Prevention (ERP), which emerged in the 1960s, were designed to target observable actions and behaviors with minimal focus on internal thought processes. Over subsequent decades, researchers increasingly recognized the limitations of purely behavioral models, particularly in addressing the complex and nuanced cognitive aspects of mental health disorders. This growing awareness paved the way for a shift toward cognition.

By the late 1960s and 1970s, cognitive models pioneered by figures like Aaron Beck and Albert Ellis introduced a transformative perspective on mental health treatment. These models emphasized that external events or situations do not directly cause emotions or behaviors; rather, it is the individual's interpretation or appraisal of these events that ultimately shapes their response. This paradigm shift laid the foundation for modern cognitive therapy.

For instance, imagine waking up to a scratching noise at a cabin window. If you interpret the sound as the wind pushing a branch against the house, you are likely to return to sleep calmly. However, if you think the sound is a bear trying to break in, your emotional and behavioral response would be quite different. This scenario illustrates how the interpretation of an event—not the event itself—plays a crucial role in shaping feelings and behaviors. To better illustrate how thoughts, feelings, and behaviors are interconnected, the basic cognitive model can be visually represented as follows:

Diagram 2.2.
Cognitive model of thought, feeling and behavior

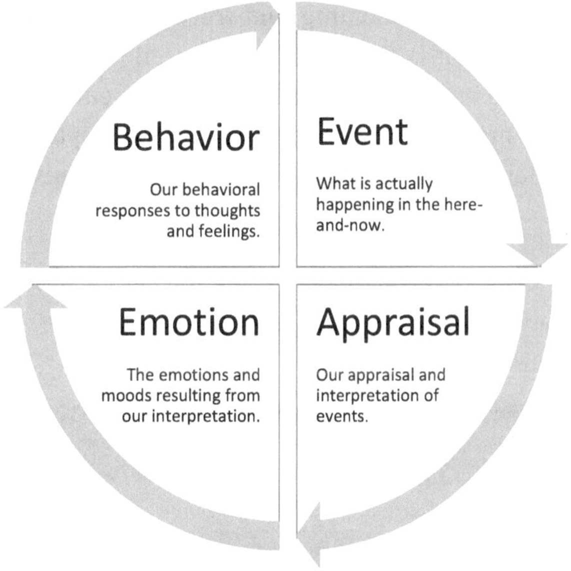

Behavior
Our behavioral responses to thoughts and feelings.

Event
What is actually happening in the here-and-now.

Emotion
The emotions and moods resulting from our interpretation.

Appraisal
Our appraisal and interpretation of events.

Cognitive Therapy's Application in Mental Health

This principle of interpretation extends directly into mental health. In psychological disorders, the way individuals appraise and interpret their experiences often triggers their emotional and behavioral responses. For example, persistent negative thoughts like "I'm a failure" or "I'm unlovable" can easily lead to feelings of sadness, hopelessness, and worthlessness, even if there is no substantial evidence supporting these beliefs. Over time, these negative interpretations can result in social withdrawal or avoidance of challenges, which only deepens feelings of incompetence and isolation.

Psychological treatment based on this cognitive model seeks to help individuals identify and challenge these negative thought patterns. The goal is to replace dysfunctional beliefs with more realistic and adaptive thoughts, thereby reducing emotional distress and modifying problematic behaviors. Therapists work collaboratively with individuals, examining their thoughts, beliefs, and interpretations of situations. This approach has proved particularly effective for conditions like depression and anxiety.

The Shift Toward Cognitive-Behavioral Therapy (CBT)

Initially, cognitive therapy clashed with traditional behavioral models, which focused solely on observable behaviors while disregarding mental processes. However, as cognitive research gained traction, the significance of thoughts and mental states became widely recognized, leading to the growing acceptance of cognitive therapy. This understanding paved the way for the development of Cognitive Behavioral Therapy (CBT), which combined the strengths of both approaches to address mental health more effectively.

CBT emphasized addressing both maladaptive thought patterns and problematic behaviors, creating an integrative framework for treating mental health disorders. This combination allowed therapists to tackle a wider range of psychological issues, making CBT one of the most widely adopted therapeutic models. Its dual focus on cognition and behavior not only expanded treatment possibilities but also provided a structured, evidence-based approach that appealed to both clinicians and researchers.

The shift from behavioral to cognitive models was a turning point in psychology, offering a broader and more nuanced approach to understanding and treating mental health conditions. By merging cognitive and behavioral techniques, CBT laid the groundwork for therapies like Exposure and Response Prevention (ERP) to be integrated into a unified treatment framework. Integrated approaches quickly became available for many disorders, as cognitive conceptualizations for specific disorders were developed. However, it took longer for OCD, with the first "cognitive" models of OCD not emerging until the late 1970s.

Highlight 2.3.
Key Learning Points

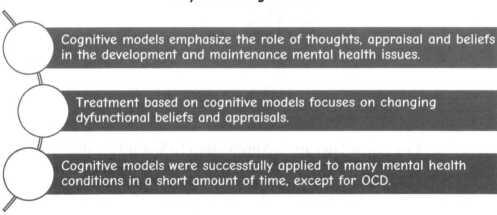

Cognitive models emphasize the role of thoughts, appraisal and beliefs in the development and maintenance mental health issues.

Treatment based on cognitive models focuses on changing dyfunctional beliefs and appraisals.

Cognitive models were successfully applied to many mental health conditions in a short amount of time, except for OCD.

Early Cognitive Models of OCD

In cognitive theory, each mental health disorder is associated with specific dysfunctional thought patterns. For example, individuals with depression often have thoughts centered around personal loss, failure, or hopelessness. In contrast, individuals with anxiety disorders typically focus on danger and threat. This principle is known as the *cognitive-specificity hypothesis*. It highlights the need to tailor therapeutic interventions to address the distinct cognitive patterns that characterize each disorder.

As the cognitive revolution gained momentum in clinical psychology, researchers were able to identify specific cognitive patterns in conditions like depression, social anxiety, and panic disorder. For instance, individuals with panic disorder tend to misinterpret physical sensations as signs of catastrophic outcomes, while those with social anxiety anticipate negative judgments from others. This allowed for the rapid development of cognitive interventions that were tailored to each disorder's unique cognitive characteristics.

However, OCD presented a far more complex challenge. Obsessions in OCD can range widely— from contamination fears to moral concerns, aggressive impulses, or a need for symmetry. This diversity raised a critical question: how could a single cognitive pattern account for such a wide array of obsessions? Experts in the field struggled to pinpoint a unifying cognitive characteristic that could explain the varied experiences of individuals with OCD, and this uncertainty echoed throughout decades of research on the disorder.

The Two-Factor Model of OCD

One of the earliest cognitive attempts to explain OCD came in the late 1970s with McFall and Wollersheim's two-factor model. This model suggested that OCD involved two key appraisal processes:

1. **Primary Appraisals**: Individuals overestimate the likelihood of negative outcomes occurring. For example, someone with contamination OCD might believe that touching a doorknob will almost certainly lead to illness.
2. **Secondary Appraisals**: Individuals underestimate their ability to cope with these perceived threats. For example, they may feel that if they contract an illness, they will be unable to recover or manage the situation.

The model further proposed that distorted beliefs, such as difficulties in dealing with uncertainty or a preoccupation with maintaining control, underpinned these appraisals. It suggested that this inability to cope with perceived threats drove individuals to assume personal responsibility for preventing harmful outcomes. This assumption of responsibility was believed to result in obsessional thoughts and compulsive behaviors as a misguided way to manage anxiety and perceived helplessness.

Limitations of the Two-Factor Model in OCD

While innovative for its time, the two-factor model of OCD had several limitations that ultimately hindered its ability to provide a complete explanation of the disorder. One significant issue was that the overestimation of threat, while central to OCD, is not unique to the disorder. Exaggerated threat perceptions are also common in many anxiety disorders, such as generalized anxiety disorder, panic disorder, and specific phobias. Thus, the model's focus on threat overestimation could not account for what specifically distinguishes OCD from these other conditions.

Additionally, the variability in the beliefs underlying primary and secondary appraisals posed another challenge. For example, some individuals with OCD may focus on beliefs about control, while others may be more concerned with perfectionism, competency, or the fear of making mistakes. This wide range of concerns made it difficult to pinpoint a consistent cognitive structure that could universally explain the development of obsessions and compulsions in a way that was specific to OCD.

The two-factor model's interpretation of obsessions and compulsions as stemming from a form of self-punishment also aligns more closely with psychodynamic theory than with cognitive theory. The idea that obsessions and compulsions are driven by a need to compensate for feelings of helplessness or guilt echoed Freudian concepts of an overly harsh superego. This psychodynamic influence complicated the model's ability to provide a clear, cognitive explanation for OCD.

Moreover, many of the concepts emphasized in the two-factor model, such as perfectionism, control, intolerance of uncertainty, and self-punishment, had already been associated with obsessive-compulsive personality disorder (OCPD) in psychoanalytic literature. However, OCD and OCPD are distinct disorders, and these concepts cannot adequately explain the complex relationship between obsessions and compulsions in OCD.

Moving Beyond the Two-Factor Model

The reliance on older psychoanalytic concepts, particularly self-punishment, left the two-factor model in a difficult position. While it incorporated cognitive elements, its psychodynamic underpinnings made it unsuitable for a modern cognitive understanding of OCD. This blend of theories highlighted the broader challenge that early cognitive models faced when applied to OCD. It reinforced the need for a more sophisticated model that could account for the unique cognitive mechanisms of OCD without relying on outdated or overly simplistic explanations.

Ultimately, these limitations paved the way for further exploration into cognitive models that could better capture the complexities of OCD. Researchers recognized that a more nuanced understanding of the disorder's cognitive underpinnings was needed to create effective therapeutic interventions. This led to the development of more refined cognitive models, such as appraisal-based models, that sought to explain how intrusive thoughts evolve into obsessions, marking a significant step forward in understanding and treating OCD.

Highlight 2.4.
Key Learning Points

The cognitive-specificity hypothesis states that each mental health condition has distinct dysfunctional beliefs and thought patterns.

Pinpointing specific cognitive patterns in OCD is complicated by the diverse range of obsessions and themes.

The two factor model is more of a psychoanalytic than cognitive model that fails to provide a specific cognitive account fo OCD.

Contemporary Appraisal-based Models

In response to dissatisfaction with earlier psychodynamic approaches, cognitive-behavioral models of OCD began to shift toward an appraisal-centered framework, also known as Appraisal-based Cognitive Behavioral Therapy (A-CBT). By the 1980s, cognitive theorists sought to apply the generic appraisal model—used successfully in other mental health conditions—to OCD.

Applying the Appraisal Model to OCD

As previously outlined, in disorders like depression or generalized anxiety, an external event (e.g., a perceived failure) triggers a cognitive appraisal (e.g., "I'm worthless" or "I'm in danger"), leading to emotional distress and maladaptive behaviors (Revisit Diagram 2.2). On the surface, it seems that this appraisal model could be easily applied to OCD by treating obsessions as a form of appraisal.

For example, in contamination-related OCD, the objective event of shaking hands with someone might lead to the appraisal, "My hands are contaminated," which then triggers anxiety and compulsive behaviors such as handwashing. Similarly, in hit-and-run OCD, a person might interpret a bump in the road with the appraisal, "I might have just killed someone," leading to compulsive checking or avoidance behaviors to ensure they haven't caused harm. In this conceptualization, appraisals like "My hands are contaminated" or "I might have just killed someone" arise directly in response to objective events, such as shaking hands or feeling a bump, and constitute the obsessions themselves.

However, for better or worse, this framework was not fully embraced, likely due to the significant theoretical and practical obstacles it presented. Any cognitive model applied to OCD had to address several major challenges:

1. Diversity of Obsessions

One of the key challenges in applying the appraisal model to OCD lies in the wide variety of obsessions, ranging from contamination fears to moral concerns, fears of harm, and symmetry compulsions. Unlike conditions such as depression or generalized anxiety, which tend to have more consistent cognitive patterns (e.g., feelings of worthlessness or catastrophic thinking), OCD's wide-ranging obsessions make it difficult to identify a unifying cognitive appraisal. Treating each obsession as a unique appraisal would result in fragmented theories, and any cohesive model of OCD would be lost in the diversity of its symptoms.

2. Overestimation of Threat: A General Feature

Another challenge is that nearly all OCD obsessions involve some form of overestimation of threat or danger. However, this is not specific to OCD, as it is common in a variety of anxiety disorders. For example, individuals with generalized anxiety disorder (GAD) may catastrophize potential future events (e.g., "What if something goes wrong?"), and people with panic disorder often misinterpret bodily sensations as signs of life-threatening conditions (e.g., "I'm having a heart attack"). Since overestimation of threat is not exclusive to OCD, it cannot serve as the unique cognitive feature needed to explain the disorder.

3. The Ego-Dystonic Nature of Obsessions

The ego-dystonic nature of OCD obsessions also complicates their classification as appraisals. Unlike typical dysfunctional thoughts seen in other disorders, such as depression or social anxiety—where thoughts tend to align with an individual's broader beliefs—obsessions in OCD feel alien and irrational. They often conflict with the person's core values and sense of self. This makes it difficult to treat obsessions through traditional cognitive models, which rely on restructuring dysfunctional thoughts that align with the individual's beliefs (e.g., "I'm unlovable" or "People will judge me"). In OCD, these obsessions are experienced as intrusive, disconnected from personal identity, and thus harder to address using standard cognitive restructuring techniques.

4. Cognitive Restructuring: Potential Risks in OCD

Cognitive restructuring is a core technique in the treatment of many mental health disorders, such as depression and anxiety. It involves challenging and reframing dysfunctional thoughts to help individuals gain insight and replace negative thinking patterns with more realistic, adaptive perspectives. In conditions like depression, cognitive restructuring can be highly effective. For instance, someone struggling with pervasive thoughts like "I'm a failure" can benefit from a structured process of evaluating evidence for and against that belief, leading to reduced emotional distress and more positive behaviors. The goal is to alter maladaptive thoughts, ultimately shifting how a person feels and behaves.

However, in the context of OCD, cognitive restructuring can present unique challenges. In particular, when this technique involves debating or disputing the content of obsessions, it risks becoming counterproductive. Conceptualizing obsessions as appraisals and attempting to directly challenge them—by weighing evidence for or against the feared scenario—can inadvertently feed into the OCD cycle.

For example, if someone is preoccupied with whether they've locked the door, engaging in a mental debate to disprove the obsession may lead to compulsive rumination. This constant cycle of disputation and mental checking reinforces the doubt, as each attempt to resolve uncertainty only strengthens the obsession. Instead of providing relief, disputing the content of obsessions can entrench the individual further into the obsessional loop.

The risk of cognitive restructuring exacerbating compulsions likely contributed to a reluctance to address obsessions directly, despite their central role in OCD. Practitioners, wary of unintentionally reinforcing the obsessional cycle, often shifted away from directly challenging the content of obsessions. Instead, the focus moved toward appraisals and beliefs detached from the obsessions themselves, effectively bypassing the need to address them in treatment.

The Intrusive Thought "Solution"

The difficulty in applying cognitive models to OCD stemmed from the disorder's complexity, including the wide variety of obsessions and their ego-dystonic nature. However, the foundational work of Dr. Jack Rachman in the 1970s and 1980s offered a new perspective. He highlighted the similarities between normal intrusive thoughts—experienced by nearly everyone—and the obsessions seen in OCD. This shift suggested that the problem in OCD was not the presence of intrusive thoughts but how these thoughts were interpreted.

The Universality of Intrusive Thoughts

A key development in this new direction was the growing recognition that intrusive thoughts are not unique to individuals with OCD but are, in fact, a universal human experience. Research by Dr. Jack Rachman and Padmal de Silva was pivotal in this regard, demonstrating that most people experience fleeting, unwanted thoughts about harm, contamination, or inappropriate behavior. In one of their studies, they found that the majority of individuals, regardless of whether they had OCD, reported occasional intrusive thoughts of this nature.

The recognition that intrusive thoughts are a normal part of human cognition shifted the focus away from the obsessions themselves to the appraisal of these thoughts. For individuals with OCD, it wasn't the intrusive thoughts that were inherently problematic, but rather how they interpreted or appraised them. For instance, where someone without OCD might have a fleeting thought about harming a loved one and quickly dismiss it, a person with OCD might view the same thought as deeply meaningful, even dangerous. They might fear that having the thought means they are capable of harm, which can then lead to obsessive ruminations and compulsive behaviors.

This shift toward focusing on the appraisals of intrusions reframed the understanding of OCD entirely. Rather than conceptualizing obsessions as independent, abnormal phenomena distinct from ordinary cognitive processes, the model emphasized that it was the significance attached to these thoughts—the faulty appraisals—that transformed otherwise harmless and fleeting experiences into sources of intense anxiety and compulsive behavior. In essence, the core issue in OCD was not the intrusive thoughts themselves, nor the obsession per se, but the distorted meanings and significance attributed to them.

Rachman and de Silva's research further demonstrated that people without OCD often experience intrusive thoughts similar in content to those of individuals with OCD. This led to the hypothesis that the key difference lies in how these thoughts are appraised: individuals without OCD may let these thoughts pass without attaching undue importance, whereas those with OCD are thought to interpret them as signals of danger, immorality, or personal responsibility, perpetuating the obsessive-compulsive cycle.

By identifying this commonality in human experience, Rachman and de Silva's work helped lay the groundwork for a cognitive approach to OCD that focused not on eradicating intrusive thoughts, but on changing how they were appraised. This provided a more cohesive framework for understanding the wide variety of obsessions seen in OCD, uniting them under a shared cognitive distortion: the misinterpretation of otherwise neutral or fleeting thoughts.

Misinterpretation and the Development of Obsessions

The notion that obsessions develop from intrusive cognitions seem to address several issues that earlier models struggled to address. First, it offered a unifying explanation for the diverse obsessions found in OCD. Whether the obsession concerns contamination, morality, or harm, the underlying mechanism is the same: a neutral or intrusive thought is misinterpreted as dangerous or deeply meaningful. This common misinterpretation provided a cohesive framework to explain the wide variety of OCD themes, from cleanliness compulsions to checking behaviors and moral concerns.

Second, the model clarified the role of overestimated threat. While overestimation of threat is common in many anxiety disorders, the model emphasized that the true issue in OCD lies in the exaggerated significance assigned to otherwise neutral thoughts. By viewing the thought itself as catastrophic, individuals with OCD become trapped in a cycle of anxiety and compulsive attempts to prevent imagined dangers. This emphasis on misinterpretation aligned closely with Rachman's earlier findings.

Third, this model helped to parsimoniously explain the ego-dystonic nature of obsessions—why OCD sufferers experience their thoughts as alien and contradictory to their core beliefs. Unlike the dysfunctional thoughts seen in disorders like depression, which often align with negative self-perceptions, OCD obsessions feel irrational and disconnected from the individual's values. By conceptualizing obsessions as originating from intrusive thoughts—often by definition ego-dystonic—the model provided an explanation for why obsessions frequently feel so foreign and unsettling.

The shift toward focusing on intrusive thoughts also prompted a change in therapeutic strategies. Instead of directly challenging the content of the obsessions—an approach that could reinforce compulsions—treatment was principally aimed at altering the appraisal process. By helping individuals reinterpret their intrusive thoughts as normal and non-threatening, the cycle of anxiety and compulsion could be interrupted. The goal became breaking the link between the intrusive thought and the compulsive behavior, rather than disputing the content of the obsession.

Diagram 2.4.
The Appraisal Model of OCD

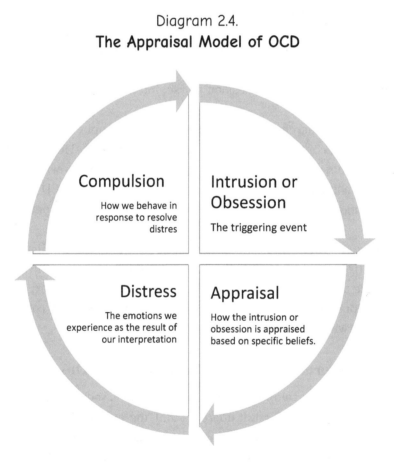

In Diagram 2.4, the misinterpretation of intrusive thoughts and the subsequent OCD cycle are illustrated, demonstrating how normal thoughts can escalate into full-blown obsessions through faulty appraisals. This model offers a clearer understanding of how intrusive thoughts and misinterpretations contribute to the development of obsessions with an appraisal framework, but as we will explore later, this approach is not without its challenges.

Highlight 2.5.
Key Learning Points

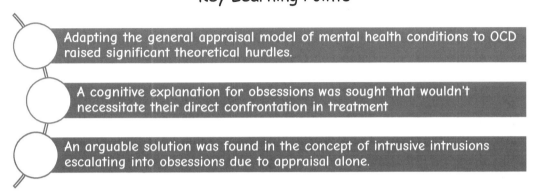

Adapting the general appraisal model of mental health conditions to OCD raised significant theoretical hurdles.

A cognitive explanation for obsessions was sought that wouldn't necessitate their direct confrontation in treatment

An arguable solution was found in the concept of intrusive intrusions escalating into obsessions due to appraisal alone.

The Search for OCD Specific Beliefs and Appraisals

Building on the limitations of earlier models and the notion that obsessions arise from the appraisal of intrusive cognitions, the focus shifted toward identifying common yet specific cognitive themes responsible for escalating intrusive thoughts into obsessions. This shift spurred deeper exploration into the appraisals and underlying beliefs contributing to OCD, a direction that gained momentum in the late 1990s. Understanding these cognitive themes became essential in refining models of OCD and distinguishing between different cognitive elements at play.

Appraisal-based models of OCD differentiate between two cognitive elements: appraisals—situation-specific interpretations of intrusive thoughts—and more enduring underlying beliefs or assumptions, which predispose individuals to certain appraisals. While appraisals reflect a person's immediate reaction to an intrusive thought, these responses are shaped by broader, more stable cognitive constructs, such as beliefs about control, perfectionism, or responsibility. This distinction laid the groundwork for a more nuanced understanding of how intrusive thoughts evolve into obsessions.

Table 2.1.
Critical concepts and definitions in the appraisal-based model of OCD.

Concept	Definition
Intrusions	"Unwanted thoughts, images, or impulses that intrude into consciousness and are called obsessions when they attain clinical severity."
Appraisal	"Expectations, interpretations, or evaluations of the meaning of particular phenomena such as unwanted intrusive thoughts."
Assumptions (beliefs)	"Relatively enduring ideas that are pan-situational and that may be specific to OCD or may be general assumptions about one's self, that are relevant to other clinical disorders."

Consensus OCCWG (1997). Cognitive assessment of obsessive-compulsive disorder. Behaviour Research and Therapy, 35(7), 667-681.

The Inflated Responsibility Model

The cognitive-behavioral model developed by Salkovskis in 1985, and refined in subsequent years, expanded on earlier conceptualizations of OCD. The concept of responsibility, already alluded to in Rachman's work, became a cornerstone in Salkovskis' model through the notion of inflated responsibility. This theory posits that individuals with OCD hold an exaggerated belief that they are personally responsible for preventing harm. This belief can become so overwhelming that it equates failing to prevent harm with directly causing it. For instance, someone with OCD might believe that leaving the door unlocked could lead to a burglary, and that if this happens, they would be as guilty as the burglar.

This heightened sense of personal responsibility becomes the lens through which intrusive thoughts are appraised. Ordinary, fleeting thoughts—such as a momentary concern about leaving the stove on—are no longer dismissed as inconsequential. Instead, they are seen as morally significant and fraught with risk. In Salkovskis' model, when these intrusive thoughts arise, the individual's inflated sense of responsibility activates appraisals such as "It would be immoral to ignore this thought" or "I must make sure that no harm occurs." These appraisals generate significant distress, leading the individual to engage in compulsive behaviors intended to neutralize the perceived threat. This model can be represented as follows:

Diagram 2.5.
The Inflated Responsibility Model of OCD

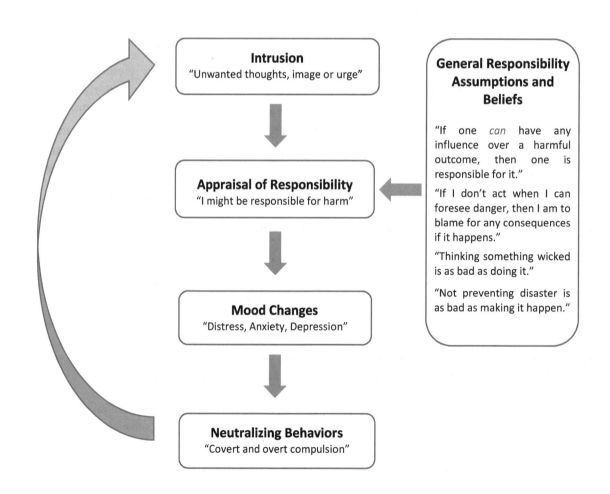

Salkovskis' model suggests that this cycle—where inflated responsibility leads to distressing appraisals, which then prompt compulsive behaviors—lies at the core of how intrusive thoughts escalate into full-blown obsessions. The compulsive behaviors, such as checking or seeking reassurance, may provide temporary relief, but they reinforce the belief that the individual has successfully prevented harm, thereby solidifying the obsessional cycle. In essence, the compulsion "proves" to the individual that their intrusive thought was valid and that their preventative action (e.g., checking the stove) was necessary. This reinforcement strengthens the belief that they hold responsibility for preventing future harm.

Additional Beliefs Domains in OCD

Salkovskis' work focused on inflated responsibility, which was later defined as "the belief that one possesses pivotal power to provoke or prevent subjectively crucial negative outcomes." This definition emphasized that the origin of negative appraisals often lies in learned assumptions, particularly assumptions about harm and responsibility. It underscored that negative appraisals are rooted in these learned assumptions, specifically regarding harm and responsibility.

However, inflated responsibility is only one perspective through which OCD has been examined. Other researchers have proposed additional beliefs that might drive the disorder. For instance, a pervasive need for control has been suggested as equally central to how individuals with OCD interpret intrusive thoughts. In this view, people with OCD may appraise such thoughts as indicators that they are losing control over their minds or lives. Thoughts like, "I'm going crazy" or "If I don't control this, something terrible will happen" can spiral into obsessive attempts to suppress or control the thought, which only intensifies anxiety.

Similarly, other theories have emphasized the role of perfectionism or intolerance of uncertainty. Many individuals with OCD find it intolerable not to have absolute certainty about whether a feared outcome will occur. This drives them to engage in compulsive checking, reassurance-seeking, or avoidance behaviors as they attempt to eliminate doubt. Even the tendency to overestimate threat was still considered important for an understanding of OCD, albeit mainly from the perspective of how intrusive cognitions are appraised.

In short, inflated responsibility was not the only factor proposed to account for the escalation of intrusive thoughts into obsessions. Nonetheless, Salkovskis' model was one of the first to outline a comprehensive cognitive-behavioral understanding of OCD and sparked significant interest in exploring specific beliefs that might explain the disorder, particularly through the lens of how intrusive thoughts are appraised. This focus on appraisals opened the door to deeper investigations into the cognitive processes that contribute to the development and persistence of obsessions, helping to refine our understanding of OCD and its treatment.

The Obsessive-Compulsive Cognitions Working Group (OCCWG)

The growing interest in understanding the cognitive mechanisms underlying OCD led to the formation of the Obsessive-Compulsive Cognitions Working Group (OCCWG) in the late 1990s. This international group of researchers aimed to systematically define and measure the appraisals and beliefs believed to drive OCD symptoms. Their collective effort resulted in the identification of six primary belief domains, including inflated responsibility, over-importance of thoughts, and intolerance of uncertainty, which were considered central to OCD's cognitive processes. The definitions of these belief domains are outlined in Table 2.2, which illustrates how they manifest in OCD.

Table 2.2.
Definitions of belief domains with examples

Belief/appraisal domain	Definition
Inflated responsibility	The belief that one has power that is pivotal to bring about or prevent subjectively crucial negative outcomes. These outcomes are perceived as essential to prevent and may have consequences in the real world and/or at a moral level.
	"To me, failing to prevent a disaster is as bad as causing it" *"If I ignore this thought, I could be responsible for serious harm."*
Over-importance of thoughts	The belief that the mere presence of a thought indicates that it is important. Beliefs may reflect thought-action fusion and magical thinking.
	"The more I think of something horrible, the greater the risk it will come true." *"Having this unwanted thought means I will act on it."*
Need to control thoughts	The overvaluation of the importance of exerting complete control over intrusive thoughts, images, and impulses and the belief that this is both possible and desirable.
	"If I don't control my unwanted thoughts, something bad is bound to happen." *"Having this intrusive thought means I'm out of control"*
Overestimation of Threat	An exaggeration of the probability or severity of harm.
	"Bad things are more likely to happen to me than to other people." *"I believe that the world is a dangerous place."*
Intolerance of uncertainty	Beliefs about the necessity for being certain, that one has poor capacity to cope with unpredictable change, and that it is difficult to functioning adequately in ambiguous situations.
	"If I'm not absolutely sure of something, I'm bound to make a mistake." *"If something unexpected happens, I will not be able to cope with it."*
Perfectionism	The belief that there is a perfect solution to every problem, that doing something perfectly is possible and necessary, and that even minor mistakes will have serious consequences.
	If I can't do something perfectly, I shouldn't do it at all. *For me, making a mistake is as bad as failing completely.*

Source: OCCWG (1997). Cognitive assessment of obsessive-compulsive disorder. Behaviour Research and Therapy, 35(7), 667-681.

The OCCWG's work was groundbreaking because it sought to create a comprehensive framework for assessing these cognitive distortions, providing clinicians and researchers with tools such as the Interpretation of Intrusions Inventory (III) and the Obsessive Beliefs Questionnaire (OBQ). These instruments were designed to measure specific appraisals and beliefs related to OCD, offering a standardized approach to evaluating the cognitive underpinnings of the disorder.

While the identification of these belief domains was initially met with enthusiasm, the research findings on their role in OCD were more complex than anticipated. The six cognitive domains were highly correlated with one another, making it difficult to isolate their individual contributions to the development and maintenance of OCD. For example, someone with elevated levels of responsibility might also score high on measures of intolerance of uncertainty, blurring the lines between these constructs. This overlap challenged the notion of cognitive specificity, raising concerns about whether these beliefs were truly distinct features of OCD.

Moreover, while the beliefs identified by the OCCWG were related to symptoms of OCD, they were not unique to it. Individuals with other mental health conditions, such as anxiety or depression, also scored high on measures of responsibility, control, and intolerance of uncertainty. This finding suggested that these beliefs might represent more general tendencies found across anxiety-related disorders, rather than being specific to OCD. Additionally, a significant proportion of individuals with OCD did not endorse these beliefs, further questioning the relevance of these cognitive constructs in fully explaining the disorder.

The lack of specificity highlighted by these findings exposed a key limitation in the OCCWG's approach: the challenge of distinguishing beliefs that are central to OCD from those that are incidental or shared across disorders. This issue was compounded by the fact that concerns with responsibility, uncertainty or control often represent common reactions to stress or anxiety, making it difficult to determine whether they are causal factors in OCD or merely secondary effects of the disorder. Furthermore, the observation that many individuals with OCD do not exhibit these beliefs suggests that alternative explanations, perhaps focusing on reasoning processes rather than belief content, may offer a more precise understanding of OCD's cognitive mechanisms.

In hindsight, the disappointing research findings in this area were perhaps not entirely surprising. The beliefs identified by the OCCWG often echoed concepts from earlier psychological models, including psychodynamic theories that emphasized a deep-seated need for control, intolerance of uncertainty, and cognitive rigidity. These traits had been long discussed in relation to anxiety and obsessive tendencies but did not introduce radically new insights specific to OCD. Relying on personality traits as a primary explanation for OCD remains problematic, given it is not a personality disorder.

One of the most significant overlaps was with the concept of inflated responsibility, where obsessions and compulsions arise from the belief in one's power to prevent negative outcomes. This idea closely mirrored mechanisms proposed in McFall and Wollersheim's two-factor model. The only difference lies in how the two-factor model conceptualizes this belief in one's own power and responsibility as a compensatory mechanism, while modern-day appraisal models attribute it to the appraisal of intrusive cognitions.

Despite these limitations, the appraisal model, with its focus on the origin of obsessions in intrusive cognitions, has persisted as a dominant framework in OCD. However, it has struggled to substantiate the idea of cognitive specificity—the notion that OCD is defined by particular, unique beliefs. This suggests that while cognitive beliefs play an important role, they may not entirely explain the disorder. Consequently, as time has passed, the allure of the appraisal model of OCD has diminished.

Highlight 2.6.
Key Learning Points

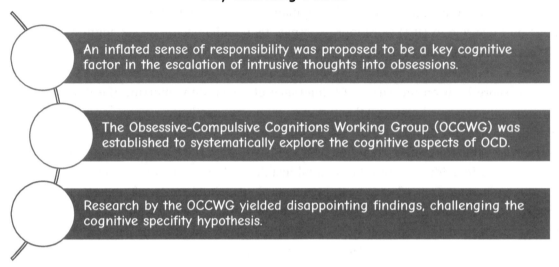

An inflated sense of responsibility was proposed to be a key cognitive factor in the escalation of intrusive thoughts into obsessions.

The Obsessive-Compulsive Cognitions Working Group (OCCWG) was established to systematically explore the cognitive aspects of OCD.

Research by the OCCWG yielded disappointing findings, challenging the cognitive specifity hypothesis.

Appraisal-Based CBT and ERP

The initial appeal of the appraisal model in treating OCD stems from its ability to address challenges faced by traditional cognitive approaches. By distinguishing intrusive thoughts from their appraisals, this model treats thoughts as neutral events without inherent meaning. This indirect approach offers a way to address OCD's cognitive mechanisms without directly confronting obsessions, thereby avoiding the perceived risk of exacerbating symptoms, similar to those in psychoanalytical approaches.

Not surprisingly, behaviorists found the appraisal model acceptable because it provided a theoretical rationale for not directly addressing obsessions, aligning with their view that cognitive elements were secondary or even inconsequential in treating OCD. Due to both models at least partially dismissing aspects of OCD cognition as irrelevant, behavioral and cognitive models for OCD shared a relatively peaceful co-existence. While behaviorists prioritized behavioral interventions, proponents of the appraisal model focused more on targeting beliefs and appraisals as crucial intervention points.

Overlapping Techniques and Limited Benefits

A-CBT primarily aims to help individuals view their intrusive thoughts as normal, insignificant occurrences. The focus is on challenging the beliefs and appraisals that give undue importance to these thoughts, rather than addressing the thoughts themselves. Techniques like *hypothesis testing* are employed to challenge dysfunctional beliefs by obtaining disconfirming evidence and supporting alternative explanations. Meanwhile, the initial intrusive thought is left untouched.

For instance, someone who feels compelled to repeatedly check the stove may hold the belief that failing to check will result in a fire. The intrusive thought, "I might have left the stove on," escalates due to this appraisal of responsibility. During hypothesis testing, the person might be asked to refrain from checking the stove to test the hypothesis that their checking prevents fires and responsibility for harm. The approach challenges the feared consequence without directly engaging with the intrusive thought.

However, hypothesis testing shares significant similarities with ERP. By requiring clients to test the validity of their fears, it mirrors ERP's exposure exercises, which involve confronting feared stimuli to habituate or learn new associations. This overlap blurs the distinction between the two approaches, suggesting that hypothesis testing may function more like ERP than as a truly distinct cognitive technique.

Such similarities highlight a shared limitation: not everyone is ready or able to confront and test their fears directly. Additionally, directly testing or confronting obsessions—even with the goal of disconfirming them—can inadvertently reinforce the obsession. This dynamic resembles self-testing in OCD, where individuals repeatedly expose themselves to obsessional situations in an attempt to disprove their fears. Instead of alleviating the obsession, this behavior often intensifies it, as repeated engagement entrenches doubt. Similarly, ERP exposure exercises can sometimes devolve into compulsive testing behaviors, diminishing their therapeutic effectiveness.

This phenomenon underscores a broader cognitive process in OCD that must be addressed to avoid unintended reinforcement of obsessions. However, it does not inherently indicate a flaw in these interventions, nor does it apply universally to all cognitive approaches. Rather, it illustrates the adaptability and complexity of OCD itself, which can undermine even well-designed treatments. To dismiss a treatment simply because OCD can exploit it would ignore this complexity; by that standard, no treatment could be considered viable.

The overlap between A-CBT and ERP also raises questions about the added value of cognitive interventions. Clinical trials have consistently shown no significant benefit in combining cognitive methods with ERP. Studies indicate that treatment outcomes for ERP alone and ERP combined with cognitive interventions are nearly identical. As a result, the appraisal model has not significantly changed OCD treatment practices, with many clinicians continuing to rely on ERP as the primary approach. Even within appraisal-based therapies, ERP often serves as a central component.

Despite regional differences, ERP remains a cornerstone of OCD treatment. In the United States, where clinical psychology traditionally leans toward behavioral approaches, ERP's structured, observable methods have made it a widely adopted standard. Cognitive interventions are often seen as complementary to ERP rather than standalone treatments, receiving less emphasis in practice. In other regions, where cognitive methods hold a more prominent role, ERP's exposure elements still frequently serve as a foundational part of treatment.

This reliance on ERP across different theoretical frameworks underscores the complex relationship between cognitive and behavioral models. While ERP has been effective in addressing OCD symptoms, this does not necessarily indicate a clear advantage over appraisal-based approaches. This landscape suggests that while ERP has become a mainstay in OCD treatment, the broader integration of cognitive and behavioral principles continues to evolve.

Theoretical Issues: Treating OCD Like a Phobia

Both behavioral and appraisal-based approaches share a fundamental principle: they treat OCD as involving exaggerated responses to stimuli. In the case of appraisal-based cognitive therapy (A-CBT), the focus is on dysfunctional appraisals of intrusive cognitions—neutral thoughts that are misinterpreted as significant or threatening. In contrast, Exposure and Response Prevention (ERP) targets the exaggerated anxiety reactions to external or internal stimuli, aiming to reduce avoidance and compulsions. While the methods differ, the underlying principle remains the same: both approaches aim to recalibrate an individual's response to what are perceived as exaggerated threats.

This shared framework stems from the historical use of cognitive and behavioral methods for treating phobias and anxiety, which were later adapted to OCD. However, OCD is not a phobia, and treating it as such introduces significant theoretical complexities, particularly in cognitive models.

In the appraisal model, intrusive thoughts are conceptualized as neutral internal events that only become distressing through the meanings attributed to them. This implies that the thoughts themselves do not need to be addressed—only the appraisal. Yet this perspective may oversimplify the issue. For example, is the thought "I might harm someone" truly neutral, or does it carry an inherent distressing quality that contributes to anxiety even before it is appraised as "I might be responsible for harm"?

In practice, the distinction between the distress triggered by the initial intrusive thought and that caused by its appraisal can be minimal. Both can elicit anxiety and compulsions, suggesting that focusing exclusively on the appraisal may overlook other crucial factors. If certain intrusive thoughts are inherently distressing due to underlying vulnerabilities or predispositions, addressing only the appraisal risks neglecting a fundamental element of OCD, potentially limiting treatment effectiveness.

Missing the Cognitive Dynamics of OCD

While intrusive thoughts are common and can reflect themes similar to those seen in OCD, there is limited evidence linking their appraisal to the development of obsessions. This suggests that obsessions may arise independently of thought appraisals, implying that the appraisal-based model does not fully capture the cognitive dynamics of OCD. By focusing primarily on appraisals, the model may leave a significant aspect of the disorder unaddressed—namely, the obsessions themselves.

Obsessions might evolve through mechanisms that are distinct from exaggerated reactions to external or internal events, as the appraisal model suggests. If this is the case, the model's focus on appraisals may only address part of the OCD puzzle. Clients sometimes express frustration that their obsessive thoughts are not adequately addressed within this framework, challenging its effectiveness as a comprehensive cognitive approach. This gap is particularly striking given the model's supposed focus on cognition.

The Need to Directly Address Obsessions

Many contemporary therapeutic models, whether appraisal-focused, behavioral, or otherwise, tend to either ignore obsessions or encourage acceptance of them. The rationale behind this is that since intrusive thoughts are a normal part of human experience, eliminating them is unrealistic. Acceptance becomes the primary strategy, based on the belief that confronting obsessive thoughts directly could worsen symptoms. In this view, if obsessions arise from normal intrusive cognitions, the logical approach seems to be accepting their presence rather than trying to eliminate them.

While disputing the content of obsessions or offering reassurance can indeed exacerbate the problem by mimicking the compulsive behaviors already present in OCD, this does not mean that obsessions should remain unexamined in treatment. Focusing exclusively on appraisals risks explaining the problem away without offering a robust or comprehensive solution. This reductive approach treats obsessions as nothing more than an extension of normal cognitive processes, potentially sidestepping the core issue and neglecting the complexity of OCD.

The limitations of the appraisal model—such as its lack of cognitive specificity and its heavy reliance on personality traits to explain OCD—highlight the need for alternative approaches. These challenges have led to the development of inference-based cognitive behavioral therapy (I-CBT), which directly addresses the reasoning processes underlying obsessions. Unlike models that focus primarily on appraisals or rely on acceptance strategies, I-CBT treats obsessions as arising from flawed inferential reasoning. By targeting these reasoning errors, ICBT offers a comprehensive and precise framework for both understanding and treating OCD.

Highlight 2.7.
Key Learning Points

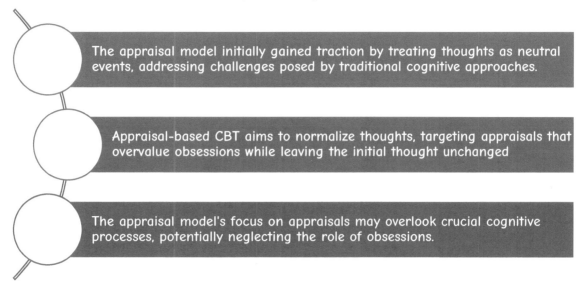

The appraisal model initially gained traction by treating thoughts as neutral events, addressing challenges posed by traditional cognitive approaches.

Appraisal-based CBT aims to normalize thoughts, targeting appraisals that overvalue obsessions while leaving the initial thought unchanged

The appraisal model's focus on appraisals may overlook crucial cognitive processes, potentially neglecting the role of obsessions.

Inference-Based Cognitive Behavioral Therapy

Initially conceptualized in the late 1990s, I-CBT represents a transformative shift in OCD treatment by focusing on the distorted reasoning processes that give rise to obsessional doubts. In I-CBT, obsessions are reframed as obsessional doubts, emphasizing the flawed reasoning and imaginative leaps that lead hypothetical possibilities to be mistaken for real threats. Rather than framing OCD solely as a fear-based or anxiety disorder, I-CBT redefines it as a condition rooted in these distorted reasoning patterns.

The Inner and Outer Wheel of OCD

To illustrate its cognitive framework, I-CBT conceptualizes OCD as operating on two interrelated levels: the *Inner Wheel* and the *Outer Wheel* (see Diagram 2.6).

- The **Inner Wheel** encompasses the obsessional narratives, flawed reasoning processes, and distorted self-concepts that sustain obsessional doubt. This is the cognitive foundation leading imagined threats to be mistaken for relevant risks.

- The **Outer Wheel** represents immediately tangible symptoms of OCD, including obsessions, feared consequences, anxiety, and compulsions that manifest as attempts to resolve the imagined threats generated by the Inner Wheel.

Diagram 2.6.
The Inner and Outer Wheel of OCD

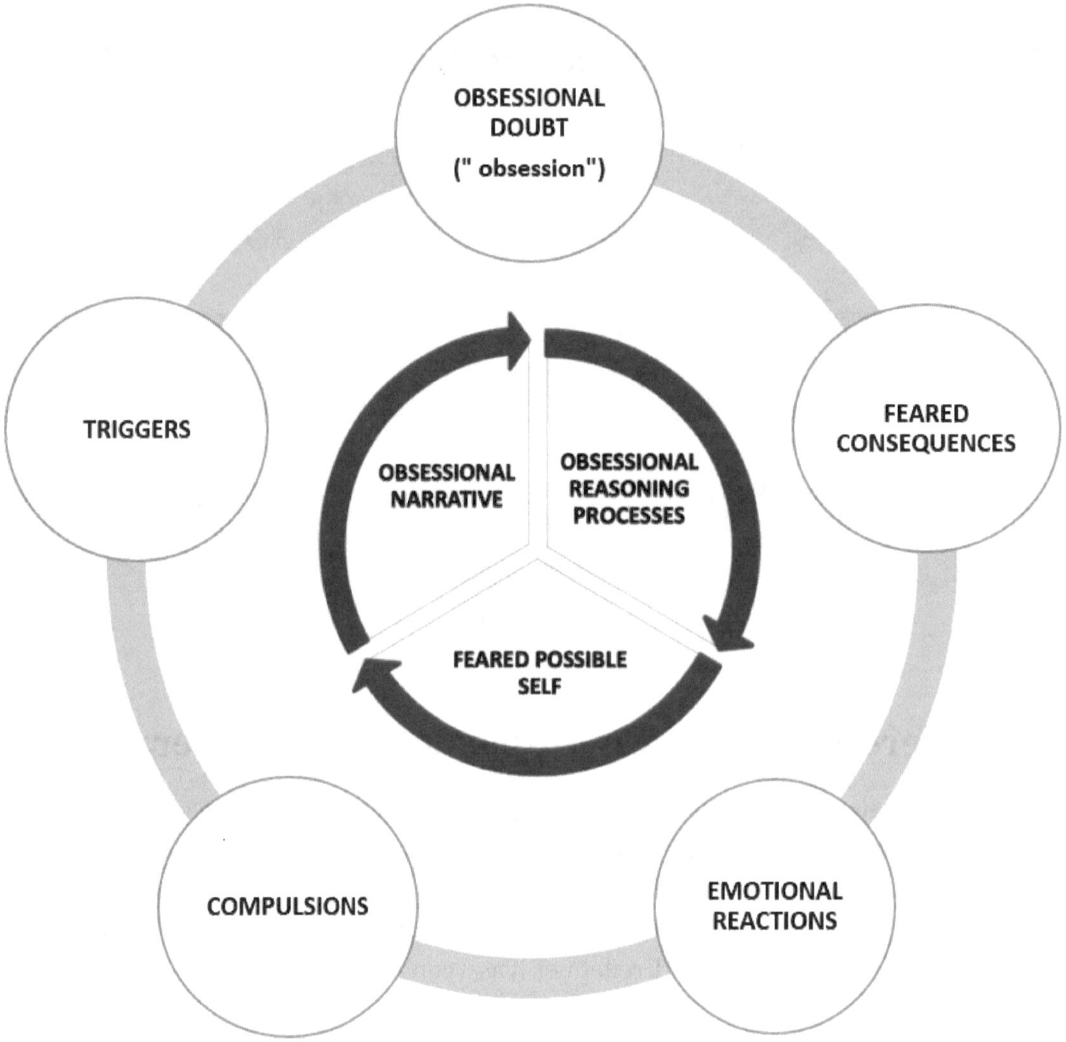

I-CBT focuses on dismantling the Inner Wheel by guiding individuals to recognize when their thinking has shifted into an imagined, obsessional narrative. By targeting this distorted reasoning structure, I-CBT helps clients understand that these narratives lead to faulty inferences about reality. This approach enables clients to address OCD at its root, without relying on direct confrontation with feared stimuli or the need to accept obsessive intrusions as part of the process.

Foundational Principles of Inference-Based CBT

I-CBT is built on five core principles that set it apart from other treatment models. It views obsessional doubt as stemming from a false narrative driven by distorted reasoning and imagination, which gives weight to hypothetical scenarios rather than reality-based judgments. These principles provide a framework for helping individuals identify and correct the reasoning errors and imaginative distortions that sustain OCD.

First Principle: Obsessions as False Inferences of Doubt

In I-CBT, obsessions are understood as false inferences—specifically, inferences of doubt. An inference is a conclusion or judgment drawn from information. In OCD, however, this reasoning process becomes distorted, generating doubts that feel real but are based on hypothetical possibilities rather than on observable reality. Rather than viewing OCD as primarily an issue of uncontrollable, fear-based thoughts, I-CBT holds that obsessions emerge from misguided reasoning that combines with imaginative processes. This reasoning shifts the individual's focus away from what is directly knowable and towards hypothetical scenarios and obsessional doubts. These inferential doubts, though compelling, are disconnected from actual evidence, leading to compulsive behaviors aimed at resolving these perceived—but unreal—problems.

Obsessions as Possibilities

A core aspect of I-CBT is recognizing that obsessional doubts are oriented around possibilities rather than certainties. People with OCD don't usually think in absolute terms like "I am contaminated." Instead, their thoughts revolve around what might be true: "What if I'm contaminated?" or "I might have left the stove on." This possibility-based thinking explains why obsessional doubts feel so compelling and persist despite rational evidence to the contrary. The doubt is about a hypothetical rather than a verified fact, rooted in what "might be" rather than "what is." This framing keeps the doubt alive and triggers compulsive responses aimed at solving a problem that exists only in possibility, not in reality.

Viewing obsessions in this way highlights the role of imagination in OCD. For example, someone with contamination fears may repeatedly wash their hands not because they see or feel dirt but because they imagine a threat. Although the content of these doubts varies across OCD themes—such as contamination, harm, moral concerns, or symmetry—the focus remains on imagined possibilities rather than tangible realities.

These imagined scenarios are difficult to dismiss because the distorted reasoning and imaginative processes make them seem as though they are supported by real evidence. This blending of imagination and reasoning creates a false sense of validity, causing the obsessional doubt to feel urgent and credible. In this way, all obsessions share a unifying framework: they revolve around what might be true, rather than what is immediately and visibly evident in the present.

The Upstream Focus of I-CBT

In I-CBT, understanding OCD requires shifting the focus upstream, beyond the idea that obsessive-compulsive symptoms primarily stem from the appraisal of unwanted intrusive thoughts, the emotional reactions they provoke, or the behaviors that follow. Instead of viewing OCD as driven by evaluations or phobic responses to intrusions, I-CBT identifies the root of symptoms as a faulty inference of doubt about reality—a primary doubt that initiates the outer wheel of the OCD.

This cycle begins with the primary doubt, which sets off a chain reaction of secondary consequences, including appraisals, feared outcomes, emotional distress, and ultimately compulsive behaviors. Yet, without this initial doubt, the OCD symptom cycle cannot activate—there are no secondary appraisals, no distress, and no compulsions. This upstream focus is a cornerstone of I-CBT. By addressing the primary doubt directly, it disrupts the OCD cycle at its starting point, making downstream effects non-essential to treat on their own.

I-CBT, however, does not stop at addressing the primary doubt. It moves even further upstream, targeting the Inner Wheel, where obsessional doubt is formed and sustained. By intervening at this deeper level, I-CBT focuses on correcting the flawed reasoning and imaginative distortions that give rise to the primary doubt.

Everyday Doubt and Obsessional Doubt

A key distinction in I-CBT is between everyday doubt and obsessional doubt. Everyday doubt is adaptive, based on sensory information, and serves a practical purpose in daily life. For example, seeing dark clouds might prompt someone to carry an umbrella. This form of doubt is situationally appropriate and typically resolves as more information becomes available.

Obsessional doubt, by contrast, lacks a foundation in reality and is disconnected from present evidence. It arises from internally constructed scenarios, often involving "what if" questions or imagined risks. This distortion leads individuals to treat hypothetical concerns as if they were immediate and urgent, even when they lack any tangible basis. For instance, someone with OCD may repeatedly check a locked door yet still feel compelled to doubt its security, despite clear sensory evidence that it is locked. Unlike everyday doubt, which is grounded in real-world cues, obsessional doubt is internally generated and fueled by imagination, creating a persistent sense of incompletion.

I-CBT's emphasis on obsessional doubt highlights that OCD is not about struggling with normal uncertainties or exaggerated dangers. Instead, it is rooted in distorted reasoning and imagination, which lead to unnecessary acts of doubting. By treating imagined possibilities as credible, individuals become locked in a cycle of compulsive checking or reassurance-seeking in an attempt to resolve what cannot be resolved.

Highlight 2.8.
Key Learning Points

ICBT views OCD as rooted in distorted reasoning and imagination, not random intrusive thoughts, their appraisals, or phobic reactions to them.

Obsessional doubts are structured inferences supported by specific justifications, making them feel plausible and urgent.

By targeting the initial obsessional doubt, ICBT aims to disrupt the OCD cycle at its source rather than managing downstream effects.

ICBT helps individuals distinguish everyday doubt, grounded in reality, from obsessional doubt, fueled by hypothetical scenarios without tangible basis.

Second Principle: Reasoning and Narrative

In I-CBT, obsessional doubts are not random intrusions or arbitrary occurrences; instead, they are conclusions formed through a structured reasoning process. Unlike other models that view obsessions as intrusive, fleeting, or unrelated thoughts, I-CBT recognizes that obsessional doubts are upheld by specific justifications that make them feel plausible and often urgent. These doubts are reinforced by various sources—abstract ideas, personal experiences, hypothetical scenarios, and sometimes societal or authoritative influences—that give them a compelling sense of credibility. Understanding that obsessional doubts are actively reasoned, rather than random, is essential in I-CBT, as it reveals the structured dynamics that give these doubts their strength and sustain their persistence.

The Reasoning Behind Obsessional Doubt

In OCD, obsessional doubt is not simply a passive feeling of uncertainty; it is an active and complex reasoning process. These doubts gain strength from specific justifications that make them seem not only plausible but essential to address. This reasoning involves layers of support, from "what if" scenarios to personal experiences, general knowledge, or abstract facts that reinforce the doubt, giving it an air of legitimacy.

In many cases, the justifications supporting the doubt are not inherently wrong—they reflect genuine concerns, abstract facts, or logical inferences that could apply to everyday life. For example, contamination fears draw on real-world knowledge that germs can spread illness. Similarly, harm-related obsessions are fueled by the reality that accidents can happen, leading the individual to feel their fears are potentially valid.

This seemingly realistic foundation is part of what gives OCD its deceptive power. OCD does not need to convince the individual that their fear or doubt is absolutely true; it only needs to make the possibility seem credible enough to warrant attention. This reasoning is not superficial or easily dismissed. Instead, it forms a cognitive structure that strengthens the obsessional doubt, making it resistant to external evidence or reassurance.

The Role of Obsessional Narratives

Obsessional doubts do not exist in isolation; they are woven into cohesive stories—obsessional narratives—that give structure and depth to the doubt. Much like how people use narratives to make sense of their experiences, these narratives shape the doubt into a logical storyline, reinforcing its credibility and grip. By linking past experiences, general knowledge, and hypothetical outcomes, they create a seamless account that makes the doubt feel both valid and urgent.

In I-CBT, the obsessional narrative is recognized as a core element of the "inner wheel" of OCD, which underpins the more visible and distressing symptoms of compulsions and obsessions in the "outer wheel." Addressing this inner narrative and the flawed reasoning that sustains it allows individuals to dismantle the foundation of OCD, rather than simply managing surface-level symptoms.

These narratives lend credibility to the doubt by transforming isolated thoughts into a persuasive storyline. For example, someone with contamination OCD might think, "The doorknob could be covered in germs; germs live on surfaces, and I read about someone getting sick from this." Here, the reasoning evolves into a structured progression, moving logically from thought to imagined consequence. This narrative framework creates a sense of urgency, making the doubt feel like an immediate threat that demands action.

The Alternative Narrative

A core component of I-CBT involves creating alternative, non-obsessional narratives that offer a balanced, reality-based perspective independent of the obsessional storyline. These alternatives are not a debate with the obsession or an attempt to disprove it; rather, they provide a perspective rooted in reality, distinct from the hypothetical layers that sustain the obsessional doubt. This approach allows individuals to see their obsessional narrative as just one possibility—a hypothetical construct—while the alternative narrative aligns more closely with real-world evidence and experience.

Importantly, I-CBT does not treat these alternative narratives as a means of reassurance or as a compulsion to soothe anxiety. Instead, it encourages individuals to practice developing alternative narratives in a non-compulsive manner, recognizing when the narrative serves reality rather than fueling OCD. This practice promotes a balanced perspective, enabling individuals to distance themselves from the obsessional story by seeing it as one interpretation of events, lacking any essential grounding in real evidence.

Through practice with alternative narratives, individuals gradually recognize that, while the obsessional narrative may feel compelling, it is not inherently more valid or urgent than other perspectives. In fact, the alternative view aligns naturally with real-world evidence, while the obsessional story remains a hypothetical construct detached from sensory and contextual information. This shift in perspective gradually reduces the dominance of obsessional doubt, allowing individuals to approach their experiences from a more balanced position.

Unlike approaches that emphasize "accepting uncertainty" generated by OCD, I-CBT teaches individuals that OCD-driven doubt lacks a real foundation and doesn't need to be accepted or endured. Instead, I-CBT helps individuals see that these hypothetical uncertainties are fabrications, enabling them to distinguish between thoughts grounded in reality and those arising purely from OCD's internal logic. As this understanding deepens, the hypothetical nature of the obsessional narrative becomes clearer, giving individuals the freedom to let it go without feeling compelled to act on it.

Highlight 2.9.
Key Learning Points

Obsessional doubt is reinforced by justifications—such as real-world knowledge or hypothetical scenarios—that lend it a strong sense of credibility.

Obsessional narratives form cohesive storylines that heighten the doubt's urgency and coherence, making it harder to dismiss.

Creating reality-based narratives helps individuals see obsessional narratives as hypothetical, reducing OCD-driven doubt and compulsions.

Third Principle: Confusion Between Imagination and Reality

At the absolute core of I-CBT is the insight that OCD is driven by a fundamental confusion between imagined possibilities and real-world probabilities—referred to as *inferential confusion*. This confusion is central to I-CBT's approach: hypothetical "what if" scenarios are mistaken for realistic probabilities, causing imagined threats to feel immediate and pressing. Rather than grounding itself in actual sensory information or present circumstances, this confusion shifts attention into an imagined realm, where hypothetical dangers are felt as tangible risks. This shift is the driving force behind the persistent obsessional doubt that fuels the OCD cycle, making inferential confusion the principal target in I-CBT.

Differentiating Between Narrative Content and Process

Inferential confusion is a central aspect of OCD's "inner wheel" and combines with the obsessional narrative to create and sustain obsessional doubts. Here, flawed reasoning processes shape a narrative that lends urgency and significance to doubts, making them feel immediate and meaningful. However, it's not the specific content of these narratives—whether focused on contamination, harm, morality, or another theme—that drives OCD. Rather, it is the reasoning processes themselves, consistent across different themes, that turn abstract possibilities into obsessional doubts. I-CBT addresses these distorted reasoning patterns, helping individuals distinguish between imagined threats and reality-based probabilities. Consequently, treatment focuses on correcting faulty reasoning rather than debating or refuting the specific narrative content, allowing individuals to break the obsessive cycle without reinforcing it by engaging with the details of their fears.

The Three Main Components of Inferential Confusion

Inferential confusion in OCD is driven by three key components: Distrust of Senses and Self, Unchecked and Boundless Imagination, and Misapplied Reality and Personal Logic. These elements intertwine to reinforce obsessional doubt, transforming abstract possibilities into what feels like probable, pressing realities. Together, they form what I-CBT calls the "OCD Trifecta," a powerful mechanism that coverts hypothetical scenario into a probable reality, making imagined fears feel as credible and immediate as real threats.

First Component: Distrust of Senses and Self

This component forms the basis for inferential confusion by undermining trust in sensory information and personal judgment. When individuals doubt what they see, hear, feel, think, or intend, a void opens up where hypothetical fears can take root. This initial distrust "breaks the dam" of reality, creating a space where ungrounded possibilities can flood in.

Second Component: Unchecked and Boundless Imagination

Once sensory and inner trust are compromised, imagination takes over, generating endless hypothetical scenarios. Detached from present sensory grounding, these fears—unanchored in the here and now—begin to feel plausible and relevant. Imagination becomes a driving force, allowing abstract possibilities to overshadow actual evidence, leading to obsessional doubts that feel urgent and real.

Third Component: Misapplied Reality and Personal Logic

Finally, OCD selectively misapplies real-world evidence or personal values to validate initial doubts, further embedding them in the mind. This component "slingshots" hypothetical concerns back to reality by cherry-picking facts or creating false equivalences that support imagined fears. By distorting reality in this way, OCD creates the illusion that these abstract scenarios are rooted in evidence, making obsessional doubts feel credible and pressing.

These components of inferential confusion fuel OCD's inner mechanisms, creating a cycle where imagined fears are experienced with the same urgency as real threats. I-CBT's approach to breaking this cycle involves helping individuals recognize these reasoning tricks and understand how the OCD Trifecta constructs an illusion of relevance and probability that has no foundation in present reality. This shift in understanding allows individuals to step back from compulsions and manage OCD with greater clarity and control.

The Role of Imaginative Sensations and Phantom Evidence

Inferential confusion does more than turn hypothetical "what ifs" into seemingly plausible scenarios; it also generates sensations and experiences that feel real. Once obsessional doubt takes hold, the mind produces imaginative sensations—such as a feeling of contamination or a sense of disconnection in relationships—that mimic genuine sensory input. These sensations, though created by focused immersion in the doubt, reinforce the perception that the imagined scenario is actually happening. For example, a person with health-related obsessions might experience chest tightness when fearing a heart condition. These sensations are the mind's response to intense focus on the doubt, not actual evidence of the feared outcome. By making the imagined feel real, these sensations intensify the obsession, reinforcing the illusion of a concrete problem needing resolution.

Reversing Causal Direction: Misinterpreting Effects as Causes

OCD's ability to create immersive, realistic sensations or thoughts around an obsessional doubt often leads to a critical trap known as reversing causal direction. In this process, the mind interprets anxiety effects—such as physical tension or intrusive thoughts—as evidence that the doubt itself is valid. For instance, if hands feel sticky after repeated thoughts about contamination, OCD may distort this sensation into "proof" of actual contamination. This reversal amplifies the obsession, making it seem that sensations caused by worry or focus are signs that the feared scenario is real. This creates a feedback loop, where each bodily response or consequence appears to confirm the doubt, trapping the mind in the illusion that hypothetical fears are unfolding in reality.

Highlight 2.10.
Key Learning Points

ICBT identifies inferential confusion as a core issue in OCD, where hypothetical "what if" scenarios are mistaken for real probabilities.

Inferential confusion is the outcome of the OCD Trifecta: Distrust of Senses and Self, Unchecked Imagination, and Misapplied Reality and Personal Logic.

Imaginative sensations and "phantom evidence" further blur the line between imagination and reality, making imagined threats feel tangible.

Reversing causal direction is a common trap in OCD that leads individuals to misnterpret these sensations as proof for the obsessional doubt

Fourth Principle: The Feared Possible Selves

The feared possible self represents an identity-based dimension within the inner wheel of OCD, shaped by the same inferential confusion that drives obsessional doubt. Just as inferential confusion leads individuals to mistake hypothetical scenarios for real probabilities, it also enables the creation of a feared self—a hypothetical and unsettling version of oneself that OCD frames as plausible. This feared self does not reflect the individual's true character but represents a distorted identity constructed through OCD's reasoning and imaginative processes. It embodies traits the person dreads becoming, such as being immoral, harmful, or inadequate, making it a profoundly distressing construct within OCD's cognitive framework.

While feared possible selves can appear in other disorders, OCD's distinct reasoning and imaginative patterns make this construct particularly potent. Inferential confusion lends the feared self emotional intensity and a false sense of immediacy, creating the illusion that it might be a "latent" or "hidden" part of the person's real identity.

The Feared Possible Self as a Construct of Self-Doubt

The feared possible self functions as an exaggerated form of self-doubt, yet it remains an illusion, disconnected from the individual's actual character. It arises not from genuine self-reflection but from OCD's imaginative distortions, resulting in a hypothetical self-concept rooted in the traits the individual fears most. While emotionally charged, this feared self lacks any grounding in reality or the person's true identity. Recognizing this self as a fictional creation of OCD helps individuals separate their true character from the distorted, hypothetical image that OCD presents.

The Role of Vulnerable Self-Themes in Directing Obsessional Focus

In addition to the feared self, OCD often targets vulnerable self-themes—areas where the individual feels a particular lack of confidence or sensitivity to self-doubt. These themes reflect perceived weaknesses in personal ideals such as morality, competence, or responsibility. For example, someone who lacks confidence in their moral judgment may develop obsessions about causing harm, while a person who doubts their ability to be thorough might fixate on fears of negligence or failure.

OCD's focus is not random; it centers on what the individual cares about most, exploiting the values and qualities they hold dear. What you care about is what you obsess about. This explains why certain obsessions feel so deeply personal and emotionally charged—they strike at the heart of the individual's identity and values.

Together, the vulnerable self-theme and the feared possible self explain the selectivity of OCD's focus, targeting areas where individuals feel the least confident. OCD amplifies these insecurities by connecting them to their most dreaded outcomes, creating doubts that feel intensely personal and emotionally charged. Recognizing how vulnerable self-themes guide OCD's attention helps clarify why certain obsessions feel so powerful while others hold little relevance.

By exploiting areas where confidence is lacking, OCD creates doubts that are compelling and difficult to dismiss. Understanding the interplay between the vulnerable self-theme and the feared possible self underscores the deeply personal nature of OCD, illustrating how it distorts the individual's sense of self by preying on perceived weaknesses.

Highlight 2.11.
Key Learning Points

- The feared possible self in OCD is a disturbing, imagined identity created by inferential confusion, appearing plausible despite being unreal.
- OCD's feared self reflects self-doubt, embodying qualities the individual fears but does not truly possess.
- OCD targets vulnerable self-themes—areas of personal significance—to amplify obsessions, making certain fears feel deeply compelling and impactful.

Fifth Principle: A Path to Complete Resolution

The fifth principle of I-CBT introduces a groundbreaking insight: obsessional doubt is not an inevitable or permanent condition but a construct of flawed reasoning that can be dismantled entirely. Resolution hinges on I-CBT's focus on the Inner Wheel of OCD, where obsessional narratives, distorted reasoning, and feared possible selves converge. By targeting these mechanisms, I-CBT empowers individuals to disrupt the cycle of doubt and compulsion at its foundation.

Unlike everyday uncertainty, obsessional doubt stems from a fundamental misunderstanding of hypothetical possibilities as probable realities. This confusion makes imagined threats feel immediate and urgent, fueling obsessions and compulsions. Through targeted questioning, restructuring narratives, and developing alternative, reality-based perspectives, I-CBT helps individuals recognize these doubts as hypothetical constructs rather than genuine threats. By correcting these reasoning errors, individuals can rebuild trust in their perception of reality and regain control over their thoughts.

Rather than focusing on merely tolerating or learning to live with these doubts, I-CBT seeks to eliminate them entirely. This shift moves the focus from accepting intrusions or uncertainties to addressing the root cause of OCD, offering individuals the possibility of complete resolution. By showing that obsessional doubts are inherently false, irrelevant, and disconnected from reality, I-CBT provides a clear and compassionate pathway to freedom from OCD's grip.

Summing Up: A Transformative Framework

I-CBT offers a comprehensive framework for understanding and resolving OCD by addressing its core mechanisms. The five principles—grounded in the recognition of obsessional doubt as a product of flawed reasoning and imagination—provide individuals with a path to dismantle the OCD cycle at its foundation. By targeting the root causes of doubt rather than merely managing its symptoms, I-CBT empowers individuals to:

1. **Reframe Obsessions as False Inferences**: Recognize obsessional doubt as a product of reasoning distortions rather than uncontrollable thoughts or fears.

2. **Identify and Restructure Obsessional Narratives**: Understand how obsessional doubts are upheld by logical-sounding but flawed stories and replace them with balanced, reality-based narratives.

3. **Distinguish Reality from Imagination**: Correct inferential confusion by learning to separate hypothetical possibilities from real-world probabilities.

4. **Disarm the Feared Possible Self**: Recognize the feared self as a fictional construct created by OCD and detach it from their true identity.

5. **Achieve Complete Resolution**: Move beyond tolerating obsessional doubt and uncertainty to fully eliminating the cognitive distortions that sustain it.

By focusing on the root causes of OCD, I-CBT aims to provide individuals with lasting freedom from obsessional doubt. This transformative approach not only disrupts the OCD cycle but also restores clarity, confidence, and trust in reality. In this way, I-CBT demonstrates that obsessional doubt can be fully resolved without the need to accept, tolerate, or coexist with lingering obsessive thoughts.

Highlight 2.12.
Key Learning Points

ICBT holds that obsessional doubt can be fully eradicated by addressing the flawed reasoning that creates it.

The principle that obsessional doubt can be eradicated relies on understanding inferential confusion at its core.

ICBT's approach removes the need to tolerate or manage doubts, freeing individuals from obsessional thinking entirely.

Comparing I-CBT with Standard Models of OCD Treatment

I-CBT presents a distinctive approach to understanding and treating OCD, setting it apart from established models such as ERP, A-CBT, and other cognitive-behavioral frameworks. While all these models aim to alleviate the distress caused by obsessions, I-CBT differs significantly in both its theoretical foundation and methodology. Unlike other approaches, I-CBT's upstream approach emphasizes addressing the core reasoning processes that generate obsessional doubt, rather than focusing solely on downstream responses to intrusive thoughts.

Comparison with Appraisal-Based CBT (A-CBT)

I-CBT distinguishes itself from A-CBT through its focus on the reasoning and imaginative processes that create obsessional doubt, rather than on the appraisal or evaluation of intrusive thoughts. A-CBT emphasizes how individuals interpret and react to unwanted cognitions, targeting the negative appraisals that transform these thoughts into obsessions. In contrast, I-CBT intervenes at the source of obsessional doubt, addressing the reasoning and imaginative distortions that drive these doubts and preventing them from arising altogether.

Moving Beyond "Living with" Intrusions

Traditional models like appraisal-based CBT consider intrusive thoughts central to the formation of obsessions in OCD. In this framework, intrusive thoughts start as neutral mental events and become significant only through appraisal. A-CBT aims to guide individuals to reinterpret these thoughts as harmless mental noise, reducing their emotional charge.

I-CBT, however, adopts a fundamentally different perspective: obsessional doubt is seen as distinct from the random intrusive thoughts that occur in the general population. While obsessional doubts can be intrusive—and since doubts are thoughts, they can appear similar to intrusive thoughts—this does not mean they develop from the appraisal of random intrusive thoughts. Instead, obsessions in I-CBT are meaningful inferences from the outset, inherently charged with emotional intensity and relevance due to the distorted reasoning that generates them.

Given that obsessions in I-CBT do not develop from the appraisal of ordinary intrusive thoughts, the therapeutic approach diverges from models that focus on "leaning into" or coexisting with distressing cognitions. Many standard CBT methods recommend resisting engagement with intrusive thoughts and accepting them as benign mental noise. While this strategy may reduce distress and frequency, it often implies that individuals must learn to live with these thoughts indefinitely, focusing on managing their presence rather than addressing their root cause.

In contrast, I-CBT views obsessional doubt as the product of flawed reasoning stemming from inferential confusion. This approach seeks not to teach coexistence with doubt but to eliminate the distorted reasoning that generates it. By understanding these doubts as hypothetical constructs—rooted in faulty inferences rather than unavoidable aspects of cognition—individuals are guided to recognize when their thinking shifts from reality-based reasoning into imagined narratives.

This perspective redefines the role of intrusive phenomena in OCD by showing that obsessional thoughts and doubts diminish as the underlying reasoning errors are addressed. With I-CBT, individuals come to recognize obsessional doubts not as fixed elements of their thinking but as invalid constructs born of distorted reasoning. This shift in focus—from tolerating unwanted thoughts to understanding and correcting the reasoning behind them—empowers individuals to reach complete resolution without any need to adapt to or accept these doubts.

Psychoanalytic Residue in A-CBT: A Lingering Influence

A-CBT, like earlier psychoanalytic models, links OCD symptoms to underlying personality traits or beliefs. Psychoanalytic theories often blur the lines between OCD and Obsessive-Compulsive Personality Disorder (OCPD), attributing OCD behaviors to unconscious conflicts or inherent traits, such as an excessive need for control, perfectionism, responsibility, and an intolerance of uncertainty. Compulsions, in this view, are seen as attempts to manage these internal conflicts, framing OCD symptoms as reflections of unresolved personality issues. Therapy rooted in these models typically focuses on addressing these core traits or beliefs to alleviate symptoms.

A-CBT retains elements of this psychoanalytic influence, particularly in its emphasis on dysfunctional beliefs and tendencies thought to guide the appraisal of intrusive cognitions, causing them to escalate into obsessions. However, I-CBT offers a fundamentally different perspective, reframing these traits and beliefs not as root causes of OCD but as natural responses to obsessional doubt arising from distorted reasoning. According to I-CBT, the drive for certainty, control, or responsibility do not reflect inherent tendencies but arises as a reaction to doubt created by inferential confusion, emphasizing OCD's cognitive rather than dispositional roots.

This distinction is crucial. In I-CBT, the drive for certainty or control is not treated as an innate characteristic but as a situational reaction to baseless doubt. When obsessional doubt takes hold, the need to "make things right" intensifies—not due to a predisposition but as a way to resolve an imagined problem. Behaviors often labeled as overly controlling or perfectionistic should be understood as temporary strategies to neutralize doubt, rather than fixed beliefs or enduring features of one's character.

> ICBT shifts the focus from beliefs and personality traits to the cognitive **processes** that spark obsessive doubt.

Interestingly, some ERP approaches also reflect a surprising overlap with psychoanalytic and appraisal-based frameworks, particularly in their focus on intolerance of uncertainty. These approaches often encourage individuals to tolerate uncertainty, implicitly reinforcing the idea that an inability to do so is a central feature of OCD.

I-CBT challenges this assumption, proposing instead that a heightened need for certainty is not an intrinsic trait but a reactive response to unwarranted doubt created by reasoning distortions. By addressing the root cause—obsessional doubt and inferential confusion—I-CBT eliminates these reactive responses. This shift helps individuals recognize these behaviors as temporary and unnecessary, disappearing naturally once the underlying reasoning errors are corrected.

Reasoning Versus Belief: A Distinctive Focus in Treating OCD

Another distinction between A-CBT and I-CBT lies in their treatment focus. A-CBT addresses obsessive beliefs, traits, or tendencies by encouraging individuals to critically evaluate and modify specific appraisals tied to their obsessive thoughts. For instance, A-CBT might guide someone to question and reassess their beliefs about responsibility, control, or certainty. By evaluating and reshaping the validity of these beliefs, A-CBT aims to lessen their influence on a person's obsessive thoughts and compulsive behaviors.

In contrast, I-CBT takes a fundamentally different approach by focusing on the reasoning processes that give rise to obsessional doubt, rather than challenging the content of beliefs themselves. Instead of asking individuals to evaluate whether a belief is true or valid, I-CBT helps them understand how their reasoning deviated from reality, leading to unnecessary and irrelevant doubt. This insight-oriented method addresses the flawed reasoning patterns that drive obsessional doubt, allowing individuals to disengage from their obsessions at the source. By concentrating on the reasoning process rather than the specific beliefs, I-CBT eliminates the need to directly confront or modify personal beliefs, making it a less confrontational and more empowering approach.

This distinction has a significant advantage: A-CBT's direct focus on beliefs can sometimes inadvertently touch on sensitive areas tied to personal values, potentially creating discomfort or resistance. For example, questioning a belief like "I must ensure I haven't caused harm" could feel, to someone with OCD, like a challenge to their moral integrity or sense of responsibility. Similarly, for individuals with religious OCD, A-CBT might involve guiding them to tolerate or accept blasphemous thoughts as harmless mental events. While this approach can help some people, it risks clashing with deeply held spiritual values, potentially creating additional conflict by focusing on the thought content.

In contrast, I-CBT's focus on the reasoning process ensures that values and beliefs remain respected and intact. For example, rather than asking someone to tolerate blasphemous thoughts, I-CBT would guide them to recognize how these thoughts arise as byproducts of distorted reasoning and obsessional doubt. By demonstrating that such thoughts have no basis in reality and can be eliminated entirely, I-CBT removes the perceived threat without requiring the individual to compromise their spiritual values. This approach reframes the problem as a reasoning error rather than a challenge to personal beliefs, allowing individuals to resolve their obsessions while maintaining their sense of integrity.

I-CBT's Holistic Approach vs. A-CBT's Reductionism

A key distinction between I-CBT and A-CBT lies in their respective "units" of focus when addressing OCD. In A-CBT, the primary focus is on distinct thoughts or appraisals, with treatment designed to neutralize specific beliefs or interpretations that give rise to distress. This modular framework systematically breaks down the OCD experience into discrete components—such as individual appraisals or intrusive thoughts—and addresses them one by one. This method offers notable strengths, providing a clear and methodical way to understand and intervene in OCD. However, it risks losing the complexity and interconnectedness of the lived OCD experience by treating symptoms in isolation rather than as part of a cohesive whole.

While modular approaches provide clarity and the reassurance of systematic rigor, they can inadvertently overlook the broader cognitive and emotional context in which obsessional doubt operates. Obsessions do not occur in isolation; they emerge within dynamic narratives shaped by personal meanings, imaginative distortions, and emotionally charged reasoning. By focusing narrowly on individual thoughts or appraisals, A-CBT risks addressing surface-level phenomena while neglecting the deeper mechanisms that sustain obsessional doubt. As a result, interventions may feel fragmented or incomplete, failing to capture the broader lived experience of OCD.

I-CBT, in contrast, adopts a more narrative and constructionist focus, emphasizing the dynamic and interdependent nature of OCD's cognitive and emotional processes. While it acknowledges the utility of structuring experience into smaller, discrete units to help individuals better understand their OCD, I-CBT does not stop there. Instead, it integrates these smaller components into a cohesive narrative framework that reflects the interconnected and evolving nature of obsessional doubt. This approach ensures that while individuals gain clarity about specific elements of their OCD, the broader obsessional dynamic that sustains their doubts remains central to treatment.

By addressing the obsessional narrative as a whole, I-CBT avoids the pitfalls of reductionism, and better reflects the dynamic and multifaceted nature of OCD as it is experienced. It aligns treatment with the way obsessional doubt is naturally structured in the mind, addressing the root causes rather than managing isolated symptoms. This approach not only provides a more comprehensive understanding of OCD but also ensures that interventions resonate with the individual's lived experience, bridging the gap between theoretical rigor and practical application.

Comparison with Exposure and Response Prevention (ERP)

A Cognitive-Behavioral Alternative to Exposure

ERP is a well-established behavioral approach that focuses on exposing individuals to their feared stimuli while preventing compulsions. By encouraging individuals to face their fears without engaging in compulsive responses, ERP aims to reduce anxiety through habituation or by promoting new associations, gradually lessening the urge to perform compulsions.

In contrast, I-CBT offers a fundamentally different framework. Instead of focusing on fear exposure, I-CBT prioritizes the correction of reasoning errors and inferential confusion that give rise to obsessional doubt. Rather than requiring individuals to confront anxiety-inducing scenarios, I-CBT eliminates the need for such exposure by addressing the cognitive distortions that generate obsessional doubts in the first place. This cognitive-first, upstream focus targets the mechanisms driving OCD, allowing individuals to dismantle doubts at their origin and preventing them from recurring.

Cognition-Behavior Integration

While I-CBT is primarily cognitive, it incorporates behavioral components toward the end of treatment. These exercises serve a distinct purpose and differ fundamentally from ERP's rationale and application. In I-CBT, behavioral exercises naturally emerge as a continuation of cognitive corrections, seamlessly integrating action with thought clarity. They encourage clients to engage with reality from a place of certainty and confidence, free from obsessional doubt.

Unlike ERP's exposure-based methods designed to provoke anxiety or "face fears" directly, I-CBT supports clients in acting confidently on what they already know to be true, grounded in accurate reasoning. For instance, a person who previously doubted whether their hands were contaminated would naturally stop excessive washing—not by forcing themselves to tolerate anxiety, but because the doubt itself has been resolved.

This organic alignment between cognition and behavior reflects I-CBT's emphasis on resolving doubts at their source, enabling lasting behavioral change without the need for distress induction.

Not Everything is Exposure

Some argue that any therapeutic approach encouraging individuals to apply insights in real-world situations constitutes a form of "exposure." From this perspective, virtually any therapeutic intervention could be classified as ERP by another name. However, this argument confuses distinct therapeutic methods, erasing critical differences in context, intention, and application.

ERP's behavioral exercises are specifically designed to promote learning through the deliberate induction of anxiety. These exercises aim to help clients confront feared stimuli, resist compulsive responses, and form new associations—such as realizing that feared outcomes are unlikely or that distress decreases over time without compulsion.

In contrast, I-CBT's behavioral exercises focus on restoring clarity and confidence in action after resolving the reasoning errors that produce obsessional doubt. For example, once someone addresses the distorted reasoning that led them to believe they might not have turned off the stove, they can move forward without compulsions—not because they've habituated to the doubt, but because it no longer exists. These exercises are grounded in accurate reasoning rather than a need to habituate to fear or tolerate distress.

If every therapeutic intervention involving real-world action were defined as exposure, then therapy itself becomes indistinguishable from life. By this logic, a chef confronting the possibility of their soufflé collapsing could be rebranded as engaging in "culinary ERP," or a student taking an exam might be seen as exposing themselves to the possibility of failure. Under such reasoning, even psychoanalysis—where a client discusses their fears in a safe environment—could be labeled exposure, as could yoga, where one faces the "distress" of a challenging pose.

This overly broad framing dilutes the specific principles and purpose of ERP, failing to recognize the distinct goals and methodologies of other therapeutic approaches. ERP hinges on enduring uncertainty and discomfort, while I-CBT resolves the reasoning that creates such uncertainty in the first place. By eliminating these distortions, I-CBT enables individuals to act confidently and without the burden of obsessional doubt.

Real Uncertainty vs. Manufactured Obsessional Doubt

ERP often operates on the assumption that individuals with OCD have difficulty tolerating real uncertainty and discomfort, leading to compulsive reassurance-seeking or avoidance. In this framework, ERP helps clients build tolerance to uncertainty by encouraging them to face situations where complete certainty is unattainable.

I-CBT, however, distinguishes between real uncertainty and obsessional doubt. Real uncertainty arises from genuine gaps in information or knowledge and can be resolved as evidence becomes available. Obsessional doubt, on the other hand, is a product of inferential confusion—manufactured by the mind and disconnected from reality. I-CBT reframes OCD as a reasoning problem, emphasizing that obsessional doubts stem not from real uncertainties but from flawed reasoning processes.

By helping individuals recognize that their doubts are grounded in faulty reasoning rather than genuine uncertainty, I-CBT shifts the focus from tolerating doubt to understanding and resolving its cognitive origins. For example, someone might initially believe, "What if I forgot to lock the door?" ERP would guide them to accept this uncertainty, while I-CBT would address the flawed reasoning that produced the doubt in the first place. Once this reasoning is corrected, the need for uncertainty tolerance disappears altogether, as the doubt itself is eliminated.

In fact, from an inference-based perspective, asking clients to embrace intolerance to uncertainty may inadvertently give validity to the obsession as a real probability, counteracting the goal I-CBT.

Phobic versus Reasoning-Based Models

ERP is rooted in a phobic model of treatment, which assumes that OCD develops similarly to phobias. In a typical phobia, such as a fear of heights or enclosed spaces, the individual experiences an exaggerated fear response to a tangible stimulus. ERP applies this framework to OCD, treating obsessions as analogous to the feared stimulus in a phobia. Exposure exercises are then used to confront these obsessions, with the goal of diminishing anxiety over time through habituation or new learning.

However, this comparison overlooks a critical difference: an obsession is not a tangible stimulus but a cognition—or more precisely, an inference of doubt. Unlike phobic fears, which are anchored to concrete and visible stimuli, obsessional doubts arise from hypothetical or imagined scenarios, disconnected from sensory input or observable reality. For example, a person with a phobia of spiders fears an actual spider that they see, whereas a person with OCD might fear the possibility of having caused harm despite no visible evidence supporting this.

This distinction underscores a fundamental divergence between the phobic model and I-CBT. While ERP addresses exaggerated fear responses to a stimulus and seeks to reduce avoidance through exposure, I-CBT focuses on the cognitive distortions and inferential confusion that give rise to obsessional doubts. Unlike ERP, which treats an obsession as a "stimulus" to be confronted, I-CBT understands it as a flawed inference rooted in distorted reasoning. The objective is not to help individuals adapt to the presence of doubt but to eliminate the reasoning errors that sustain it.

I-CBT: Diverging from Psychoanalysis, Aligning with Behavioral Models

While I-CBT is a cognitive approach, it distinctly avoids encouraging the analysis of obsessions in any psychoanalytical sense. Psychoanalytic models often delve into the symbolic or unconscious meaning behind obsessions, linking them to unresolved conflicts or deep-seated personality traits. In contrast, I-CBT discourages such explorations, focusing instead on dismantling the reasoning errors that sustain obsessional doubt. The goal is not to uncover hidden meanings but to address the flawed inferential processes that drive OCD.

At the same time, I-CBT's ultimate aim—to remove unnecessary cognition and allow individuals with OCD to naturally trust their senses and sense of self—aligns with the goals of behavioral approaches like ERP. Both strive to free individuals from the grip of OCD, fostering confident and effortless engagement with reality. However, I-CBT achieves this through correcting reasoning rather than inducing anxiety through exposure, offering a distinct cognitive pathway to the same outcome.

I-CBT also integrates a constructionist perspective, emphasizing that beliefs and personal reality are not static entities stored in the mind but actively constructed and reconstructed through present-moment interactions and intentions. This "here and now" focus aligns with modern behavioral models, which emphasize the importance of understanding how current circumstances and triggers reinforce behavior. Behavioral contingencies—the "if-then" conditions that set the occasion for the potential occurrence of certain behaviors and their consequences—are a critical component in understanding how reasoning processes and obsessional doubt are maintained. However, I-CBT extends this perspective by adding a creative dimension, highlighting how obsessional doubts are not merely maintained but actively constructed through distorted reasoning. This approach underscores the dynamic relationship between cognition and behavior, illustrating how flawed reasoning processes continually generate and sustain obsessional doubt.

By rewriting obsessional narratives and addressing cognitive distortions, I-CBT mirrors the behavioral goal of enabling natural engagement with reality—albeit through a distinctly cognitive pathway. This integration of constructionist principles highlights the connection between thought and action, helping individuals replace obsessional doubt with clarity and confidence. Importantly, I-CBT achieves these goals without relying on the distress-centric methods of traditional behavioral models, offering a compassionate and empowering alternative to overcoming OCD.

Comparison with other Cognitive-Behavioral Treatments

Several evidence-based cognitive-behavioral treatments for OCD, such as Acceptance and Commitment Therapy (ACT) and Metacognitive Therapy (MCT), offer alternative frameworks for understanding and addressing OCD symptoms. These approaches, however, were not discussed in detail earlier, as I-CBT evolved directly from traditional behavioral and cognitive models, with its conceptual foundation established in the late 1990s. Furthermore, ACT and MCT are general therapeutic approaches not specifically designed for OCD. When applied to OCD, they have adopted many elements from A-CBT and ERP, further blurring the distinctions between these methods and their applicability as specialized treatments for OCD.

Similar to ERP, ACT encourages individuals to "lean into" their anxiety and distressing thoughts, fostering acceptance rather than aiming to resolve them. A core component of ACT is mindfulness, a practice that promotes observing thoughts non-judgmentally and with distance. This approach allows individuals to relate to their thoughts as passing mental events rather than absolute truths. The goal of ACT is to build psychological flexibility, enabling individuals to pursue meaningful actions even when intrusive thoughts persist. While effective in reducing entanglement with obsessions, ACT does not explicitly target the core obsessional doubt driving OCD; instead, it focuses on reshaping the individual's relationship with their thoughts, emphasizing coexistence rather than resolution.

Similarly, MCT aligns with traditional Appraisal-Based Cognitive Behavioral Therapy (A-CBT) in its emphasis on changing one's relationship to intrusive thoughts. MCT encourages individuals to recognize obsessive thoughts as mere mental events, fostering a sense of detachment that discourages compulsive responses. This distancing helps individuals view intrusive thoughts with less immediacy, but it does not address the reasoning processes that generate obsessional doubt. As with ACT, MCT seeks to reduce the intensity of intrusive thoughts but stops short of dismantling the mechanisms that produce these doubts in the first place.

By contrast, I-CBT shifts the focus to the reasoning processes that precede and sustain obsessional doubt, addressing them directly to reveal why they lead to faulty conclusions. Instead of altering one's relationship to thoughts, I-CBT dismantles the distorted reasoning and inferential confusion that underpin OCD, thereby addressing obsessional doubt at its root. This process-oriented approach makes I-CBT distinct in its focus on the mechanisms that generate obsessional doubt, rather than simply modifying one's response to intrusive thoughts or attempting to live with them.

I-CBT naturally incorporates a form of distancing, but it does so as a means of scrutinizing the reasoning behind the obsessional doubt—not as an end goal, as seen in ACT or MCT. This distancing does not rely on meditative techniques or a deliberate effort to detach emotionally from thoughts. Instead, it empowers individuals to step back and critically evaluate the reasoning processes that lead to their doubts. By viewing doubts from a non-compulsive stance, individuals in I-CBT can clearly identify the flaws and irrelevance in their reasoning, creating an opportunity for active rejection rather than passive acceptance.

In conclusion, unlike ACT or MCT, I-CBT does not promote flexibility or openness toward obsessional intrusions or doubts. Instead, it helps individuals identify these doubts as fundamentally flawed and irrelevant, enabling them to reject—not accept—the obsessional intrusions outright. This emphasis on resolution rather than adaptation distinguishes I-CBT as a proactive, mechanism-focused approach to OCD treatment. By correcting the faulty reasoning at the heart of OCD, I-CBT ensures that individuals are not left merely coexisting with their doubts but are empowered to dismantle them entirely, achieving clarity and confidence in their thoughts and actions.

Common Goal: Reclaiming Your Life

Each treatment model—whether I-CBT or another approach—employs unique methods and strategies, yet all share the same overarching goal: helping individuals with OCD reclaim control over their lives by diminishing the grip of obsessions. Each therapy provides tools to manage or resolve the impact of OCD on daily functioning, and all have brought relief to many individuals, though no single approach works for everyone.

I-CBT, by addressing the reasoning processes that generate obsessional doubt, offers a distinctive path to recovery. Unlike approaches that emphasize habituation, acceptance, or detachment, I-CBT targets the root cause of OCD by correcting the flawed reasoning that underpins it. This empowers individuals to see their doubts as irrelevant, restoring confidence in their ability to trust their perceptions and judgments. Research indicates that ERP and other cognitive-behavioral treatments are not superior to I-CBT. In fact, I-CBT often proves more tolerable and less distressing, making it a compassionate alternative for those seeking relief from OCD.

What matters most, however, is how individuals experience each treatment. Effectiveness may hinge less on finding the "best" approach and more on identifying the approach that aligns with an individual's unique needs, values, and preferences. The need for personalization in OCD treatment is an area that remains underexplored in research but may be critical to achieving success. The lack of choice in treatment studies could partly explain why no one therapy consistently outperforms others. Personal attraction to a specific approach may influence outcomes as much as—or even more than—the model itself.

This underscores the importance of embracing diversity in evidence-based treatment methods. Rather than striving for a single ultimate therapy, the variety of options available should be seen as a strength, allowing individuals to find what works best for them. For example, if ERP hasn't worked for you, it might be time to explore I-CBT or another approach. Repeating the same method with the expectation of different results can often lead to frustration and missed opportunities for growth.

This self-help guide, grounded in I-CBT principles, offers an effective, reason-focused pathway to addressing the core of obsessional doubt. By eliminating distorted reasoning and restoring clarity, I-CBT not only helps reduce OCD's grip but provides a means to truly reclaim your life—free from the power of obsessional doubt and the constraints it imposes.

As we move forward, the next part begins by unpacking the structured processes of OCD, starting with its outer manifestations. These are the observable cycles of obsessions, emotional reactions, and compulsions. By understanding these outer dynamics, you'll gain clarity and insight into the patterns of OCD, laying the groundwork for addressing its deeper mechanisms in later chapters.

PART 2

The Outer Wheel

Chapter 3

The Obsessional Sequence

In the previous chapter, we explored the transformative framework of Inference-based Cognitive Behavioral Therapy (I-CBT), which addresses OCD by targeting its core mechanisms—flawed reasoning and obsessional doubt—rather than merely managing symptoms. Central to I-CBT is the distinction between the inner and outer wheels of OCD: the inner wheel, where distorted reasoning and imaginative processes sustain obsessional doubt, and the outer wheel, which reflects the resulting cycle of obsessions, emotional distress, and compulsions.

This chapter marks the beginning of a deeper dive into these processes, starting with the outer wheel. While the inner wheel holds the key to resolving OCD at its core, understanding the outer wheel is an essential first step. By recognizing the patterns and dynamics of the outer wheel, you can transform the overwhelming chaos of OCD into a structured and predictable sequence. This clarity not only reduces the overwhelming nature of OCD but also ensures you are better equipped to engage with I-CBT's methods in subsequent steps.

When you have OCD, your symptoms may feel like an overwhelming and chaotic blend of fear and anxiety—irrational worries merging into a relentless cycle of distress and compulsive behavior. This emotional storm often obscures the underlying processes at play, making OCD seem like an unpredictable and uncontrollable condition. For example, on the surface, OCD might feel like the following diagram:

Diagram 3.1.
What OCD Can Feel Like

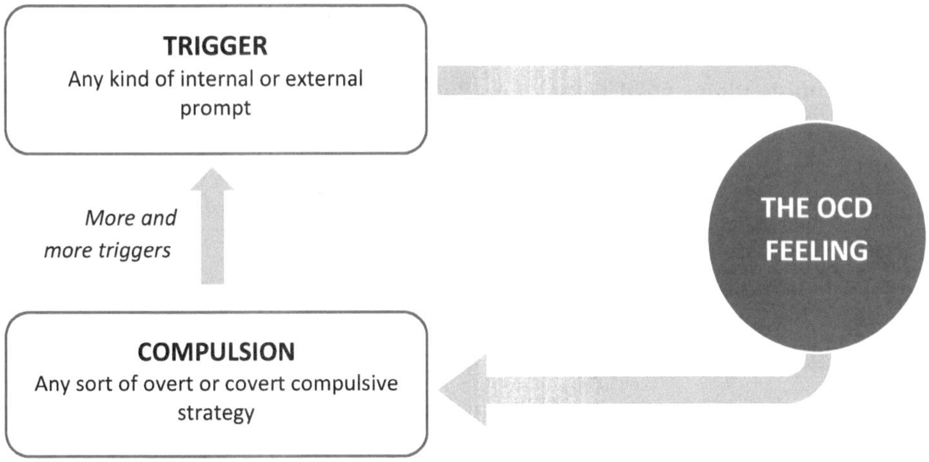

TRIGGER
Any kind of internal or external prompt

More and more triggers

COMPULSION
Any sort of overt or covert compulsive strategy

THE OCD FEELING

While OCD might feel like this tangled cycle, the reality is far more structured and predictable. Rather than a disorganized swirl of emotions and behaviors, OCD operates through a distinct and repeatable process. Each time OCD is triggered, the cycle begins with an obsession—a response to the situation that sets the entire sequence into motion. This obsession is followed by feared secondary consequences, negative emotions (the "OCD feeling"), and, finally, compulsive behaviors intended to neutralize these feelings. This predictable process is the outer wheel of OCD.

Diagram 3.2.
The Outer Wheel of the OCD

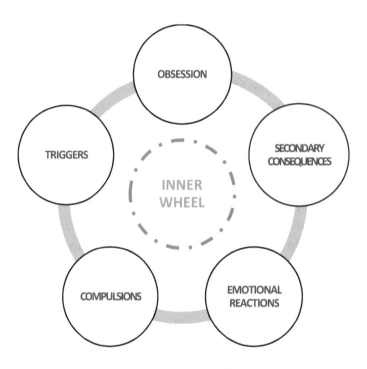

All components in the outer wheel contribute to the cycle's momentum. However, the obsession is the primary catalyst. Without the obsession, the wheel remains stagnant—secondary consequences, emotional reactions, and compulsions cannot occur. It is the obsession that assigns disproportionate significance to a situation, which would otherwise feel ordinary or inconsequential.

Triggers exist by virtue of the obsession only

Understanding and recognizing this pattern in your own symptoms is a crucial starting point. It transforms the overwhelming chaos of OCD into a manageable and predictable framework. Neglecting this vital step or overlooking the outer wheel's dynamics can impede progress by preventing a full appreciation of how OCD perpetuates itself. While the outer wheel does not represent the root cause of OCD, grasping its structure is indispensable for addressing the deeper mechanisms at play.

By enhancing your understanding of the outer wheel, you can begin to disrupt its fear-driven cycle and alleviate the anxiety it fuels. This insight allows you to break your OCD experience into distinct, comprehensible components, fostering greater clarity and control. Most importantly, this initial understanding establishes the groundwork needed to later tackle the core of OCD—the inner wheel—effectively. With this preparation in place, we will now turn to the first element in the outer wheel: the obsession.

Key Learning Points
Highlight 3.1.

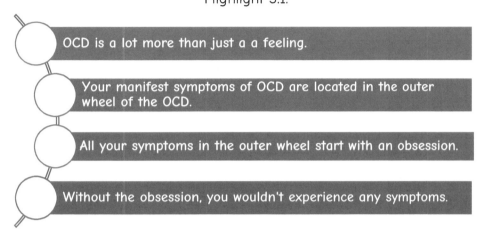

OCD is a lot more than just a a feeling.

Your manifest symptoms of OCD are located in the outer wheel of the OCD.

All your symptoms in the outer wheel start with an obsession.

Without the obsession, you wouldn't experience any symptoms.

The Form and Shape of an Obsession

Obsessions, according to textbook definitions, are often described as unwanted and persistent intrusive thoughts, images, or impulses. However, to truly understand their impact in the context of OCD, it's essential to delve deeper beyond the surface definition. Obsessions are more than just fleeting thoughts or passing images; they are the catalysts that drive the intricate web of symptoms within the outer wheel of OCD. They grip the mind with a relentless intensity, often causing distress and anxiety. Understanding the true nature of obsessions is your first step towards deconstructing and slowing down the outer wheel of the OCD.

Obsessions as Possibilities

At their core, obsessions are rooted in possibilities rather than certainties. Individuals with OCD rarely express their fears in absolute terms. For instance, someone with contamination-related OCD is unlikely to declare, "I am contaminated." Instead, they are more likely to say, "I might be contaminated," or "Perhaps I've been exposed." This emphasis on hypothetical outcomes—using terms like "might," "maybe," "could be," or "what if"—highlights the imaginative foundation of obsessions, underscoring their basis in possibility rather than reality (refer to Table 3.1).

However, some individuals with OCD express their obsessions with higher levels of conviction, appearing more certain of the reality and reasonableness of the feared possibility. Even in these cases, the obsession remains grounded in possibility rather than fact. The difference lies in the intensity of belief rather than the nature of the obsession itself.

This framing illuminates a central truth about OCD: all obsessions, regardless of their content, arise from the same underlying mechanism—the contemplation of possibilities. While the specific manifestations of obsessions may vary infinitely, from contamination fears to moral scrupulosity or harm-related concerns, they share a unifying structure. Each revolves around a hypothetical scenario, something not directly observable or verifiable, making "possibility-based thinking" the common thread across all OCD presentations.

Table 3.1.

OCD Symptom Dimensions and Related Obsessional possibilities

Symptom dimension	Obsessional Possibility "Perhaps," "Maybe," "Might be," "Could be," or "What if"	
Disturbing Thoughts	• *What if* I will hurt others? • I *might be* a pervert. • *Perhaps* I have offended God	• I *could be* a psychopath. • *Maybe* I am a racist. • *What if* I torture my children? • *Maybe* I'm a sinner.
Contamination	• There *might be* pesticides in the air. • *Maybe* that red spot is blood. • *Perhaps* my house is built on a toxic landfill. • I *might* have become infected with a parasite.	• *What if* the water is poisoned? • *Maybe* there is a deadly virus on my hands. • *What if* the doorknob is dirty? • There *could be* deadly mold behind the walls.
Negligence and Mistakes	• *Perhaps* I forgot to unlock the door. • *What if* my toaster catches fire? • *Maybe* I missed some questions on the exam. • *What if* I said something wrong during the meeting at work?	• *Maybe* I accidently hit someone with my car. • *I might* have forgotten to turn off the stove. • *Maybe* one of the water pipes is leaking.
Symmetry Order and Arrangement	• *Maybe* I did not line up the books on the shelf correctly. • I might not have placed my toothbrush correctly. • *Maybe* I did not fold my clothes just right. • *Maybe* I am not remembering everything right.	• *I might* not be dressing myself in the right order. • *Perhaps* the ornaments on the table are not properly placed. • *What if* the air in my house does not smell right? • *What if* I am using the wrong words?
Other	• *Maybe* I do not love my partner enough. • I *might be* autistic. • *What if* I turn into someone else? • *Perhaps* my heart is not beating correctly right now.	• *Maybe* I have a brain tumor. • *What if* I start obsessing again? • *What if* I do not have the right dose of medication? • *Perhaps* I am not living my life correctly.

Importantly, this focus on possibilities applies to obsessions regardless of how they manifest. Whether they appear as thoughts, images, or motor-like urges, the essence remains the same. For example, someone with harm-related obsessions may experience a vivid image of steering their car into oncoming traffic or a motor-like sensation that their arm might turn the wheel. While explicit thoughts may not accompany these experiences, the underlying preoccupation is still a possibility: "What if I lose control?" or "I might drive into traffic." In these cases, the imaginative nature of the obsession is merely expressed in a sensory or motor form, rather than through verbalized thought.

Ultimately, obsessions do not differ in kind based on their mode of expression. Whether they manifest as thoughts, images, or urges, they invariably center around hypothetical scenarios—what might be, rather than what is. Recognizing this unifying feature allows us to better understand OCD as a single, cohesive disorder rather than a collection of disparate subtypes.

Doubt and Possibility

Viewing obsessions as possibilities also highlights the pervasive doubt that defines OCD. This relentless questioning and hesitation permeate daily life, making obsessions deeply distressing and challenging to manage. Unlike fleeting uncertainties, obsessional doubt strikes at the core of an individual's sense of self, values, or assumptions about the world, forcing them to question what they usually take for granted.

For example, when a heterosexual person contemplates the possibility of being gay, they are not merely questioning their sexual identity but confronting a deeply ingrained aspect of their self-concept. Similarly, doubting whether the stove was left on goes beyond a mundane safety concern; it disrupts their trust in their own memory and sense of responsibility. These examples illustrate how obsessions compel individuals to re-evaluate fundamental aspects of their lives, leading to emotional turmoil and a destabilized sense of certainty.

This pervasive doubt is why OCD has long been described as "the doubting disease." This characteristic transcends all forms of OCD, as every obsessional cycle begins with a doubt—a question sparked by a possibility. This initial doubt sets the outer wheel in motion, calling something into question and creating a cascade of fear and compulsive responses.

Refer to diagram 3.3 for several examples of how specific obsessional doubts can call into question various aspects of an individual's life.

Diagram 3.3.
Obsessional Doubts and What They Challenge

Obsessional Doubt "I might have left the stove on."

- Calls into Question: "The stove is off."
- Calls into Question: "My home is safe."
- Calls into Question: "I am responsible."
- Calls into Question: "My memory is reliable."

Obsessional Doubt "My hands might be contaminated."

- Calls into Question: "My hands are clean."
- Calls into Question: "I am healthy."
- Calls into Question: "I am hygienic."
- Calls into Question: "I can safely touch things."

Obsessional Doubt "I might have made a mistake at work."

- Calls into Question: "My work is accurate."
- Calls into Question: "I am competent."
- Calls into Question: "My performance is satisfactory."
- Calls into Question: "I can be trusted."

Obsessional Doubt "I might suddenly harm someone."

- Calls into Question: "I am in control of my actions."
- Calls into Question: "I am safe to be around."
- Calls into Question: "I am a peaceful person."
- Calls into Question: "I respect and care for others."

Obsessional Doubt "What if I am not expressing myself correctly?"

- Calls into Question: "Others comprehend my thoughts and feelings accurately."
- Calls into Question: "I can effectively express myself verbally."
- Calls into Question: " I am being perceived as genuine and sincere."
- Calls into Question: "My expressions truly reflect my thoughts and emotions ."

Understanding the Impact of Obsessional Doubts: A Practical Exercise

We've explored how obsessional doubts call fundamental aspects of life into question—whether it's trust in memory, sense of identity, or confidence in personal integrity. These doubts don't just exist in isolation; they deeply challenge what we often take for granted, creating emotional and cognitive turmoil.

To solidify your understanding of this concept, we'll now engage in a practical exercise. This is one of the first exercises in the book, and its purpose is to help you actively explore the connection between obsessional doubts and the core aspects of life they challenge. By doing so, you'll begin to see how doubt creates its power—not through certainty but through its ability to question what feels foundational to your sense of self or worldview.

This exercise is not about achieving perfect accuracy but about fostering awareness. By practicing this skill, you'll gain insight into the mechanics of obsessional doubt, equipping yourself with the tools to eventually disrupt its influence.

Exercise 3.1.
What Do Obsessional Doubts Challenge?

1. **Retrieve Form 3.1:**
   - Have Form 3.1 ready, which contains several common obsessional doubts.
2. **Identify Underlying Questions:**
   - Underneath each obsessional doubt in Form 3.1, note what it might call into question for the person experiencing it.
   - There is no single correct answer, so don't worry about perfect accuracy.
3. **Phrase Responses Affirmatively:**
   - Aim to phrase your responses affirmatively, avoiding the use of "not" or any other form of negation.
   - For example, if someone doubts, "...my hands might be contaminated," phrase what it might call into question as "...my hands are clean" rather than using negation.
4. **Refer to Possible Answers:**
   - If you need guidance, refer to the possible answers provided in Appendix A.

Form 3.1.
What Do Obsessional Doubts Challenge

Obsessional Doubt "I might be gay."

- Calls into Question: ....
- Calls into Question: ....
- Calls into Question: ....
- Calls into Question: ....

Obsessional Doubt "What if I live in a virtual world?"

- Calls into Question: ....
- Calls into Question: ....
- Calls into Question: ....
- Calls into Question: ....

Obsessional Doubt "My heart might be beating irregular."

- Calls into Question: ....
- Calls into Question: ....
- Calls into Question: ....
- Calls into Question: ....

Obsessional Doubt "Maybe I do not love my partner enough."

- Calls into Question: ....
- Calls into Question: ....
- Calls into Question: ....
- Calls into Question: ....

Obsessional Doubt "My food might be poisoned"

- Calls into Question: ....
- Calls into Question: ....
- Calls into Question: ....
- Calls into Question: ....

Possibility, not Likelihood

Obsessional doubts hinge on possibility, not on likelihood. Whether you estimate the chance of your obsession being true at 100% or a mere 0.0001%, OCD can torment you all the same. It is impervious to arguments based on probability. Attempts to convince yourself—or be convinced by others—that your fears are unlikely may bring fleeting relief but do nothing to resolve the core issue. In fact, focusing on likelihood can make things worse. Even a slim chance can feel like validation for the obsession, reinforcing its grip.

> OCD requires only the smallest margin of likelihood to persist.

While some people with OCD may overestimate threats or exaggerate dangers, these tendencies are not the root cause of OCD symptoms. Even if you acknowledge that the likelihood of your obsession is minimal, it rarely changes how the doubt feels. Many individuals with OCD recognize how remote their fears are—yet the disorder persists, fueled not by statistical odds but by the mere possibility that the obsession might be true. If OCD were a lottery ticket with one-in-a-billion odds, it's still a "winner" every time.

OCD thrives by inflating even the faintest possibility until it feels urgent and unavoidable. This relentless focus on "what if" keeps the cycle of obsession and compulsion alive. Debating the likelihood of your fears or seeking reassurance doesn't weaken OCD's hold; it may even strengthen it by reinforcing the belief that the possibility, however remote, deserves attention and action.

To break free from OCD, the focus must shift from debating chances to dismantling the mechanisms that sustain obsessional doubt. The key lies in targeting the distorted reasoning and imaginative processes that give possibility undue weight. Only by unraveling these processes can you disrupt OCD's cycle and reclaim control.

Highlight 3.2.
Key Learning Points

- Every obsession contains the possibility of a "Perhaps," "Maybe," "Might be," "Could be," or "What if."

- Obsessional doubting characterizes all forms of OCD.

- Obsessional doubts are about possibility, not likelihood.

- OCD couldn't care less about how likely you perceive your obsessions to be.

Secondary Consequences of Obsessional Doubt

The next critical component of the outer wheel of OCD comprises the secondary consequences that arise from your obsessional doubt. These are the feared outcomes logically connected to the primary doubt. For instance, if you doubt that your hands might be contaminated with a dangerous virus, secondary consequences might include thoughts such as, "I could fall ill," "I might infect my children," or "There's a risk of death." In essence, secondary consequences are the potential outcomes you fear might occur if the obsession were true (see Table 3.2).

It's easy to become consumed by these secondary consequences to the point where the initial primary doubt fades into the background. This can make the cycle of OCD feel far more complex and overwhelming than it truly is. By shifting your focus to these feared outcomes, the initial doubt that set the cycle in motion often goes unnoticed, leading to a distorted view of what drives the outer wheel.

> Secondary consequences in OCD are like flames to a moth—easy to get drawn into, but harmful.

Table 3.2.

Examples of Secondary Consequences of Obsessional Doubts

Dimension	Obsessional Doubts	Secondary Consequences
Disturbing Thoughts	I *might be* a pervert. *What if* I suddenly hit someone?	I'm a terrible person I'll be charged for assault.
Negligence and Mistakes	*Perhaps* I forgot to unlock the door. *What if* I said something wrong during the meeting at work?	Someone could get in. People will think I'm stupid and clueless.
Contamination	*Perhaps* my house is built on a toxic landfill. I *might* be infected with a parasite.	I'll get sick over time and will die of cancer. Something disgusting will be crawling inside of me.
Symmetry, order and arrangement	*What if* I did not write that email perfectly? *Maybe* I don't remember everything as it really occurred.	People will think I'm lazy and not doing a good job. I'd be to blame for any mistakes that were made.

Individuals with OCD may experience varying levels of concern about these secondary consequences. For some, the focus on these feared outcomes becomes so intense that the primary obsessional doubt fades into the background. For instance, you might find yourself obsessing over the fear of dying without giving much thought to the initial doubt that sparked the concern, such as "I might be sick without knowing it." This shift in focus can create the impression that the obsession revolves around the consequences rather than the original doubt.

However, focusing on the consequences does not mean they replace the primary doubt as the obsession. Secondary consequences are always tied to the initial doubt, serving as logical extensions of it. The doubt acts as the foundation of the obsessional sequence, following a structured "if... then..." pattern. For example:

- **If** the stove is left on, **then** the house will burn down.

In this case, the first clause ("if the stove is left on") represents the primary doubt, while the second clause ("then the house will burn down") represents the secondary consequence. Diagram 3.4 provides more examples illustrating this logical structure.

Diagram 3.4.

The logical structure of obsessions and their consequences

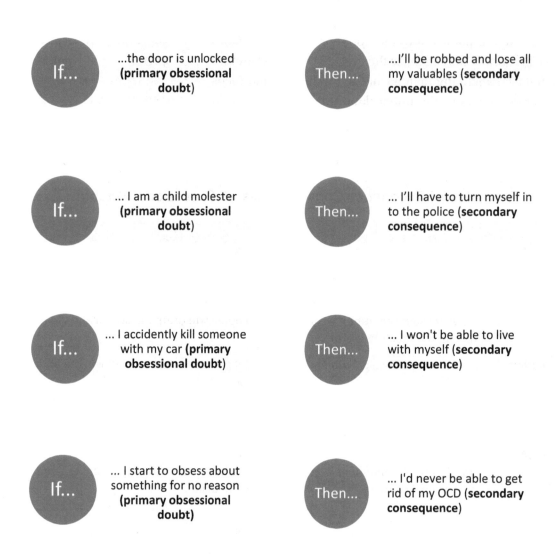

Since secondary consequences hinge entirely on the primary doubt, attempting to argue against their validity often misses the point of what drives OCD. After all, these consequences are potential outcomes if the doubt were true—they are not inherently irrational. For example, trying to reassure yourself that God will ultimately be merciful validates the doubt that you might have sinned in the first place. This inadvertently strengthens the obsessional doubt, perpetuating the OCD cycle and reinforcing its hold.

> Secondary consequences always depend entirely on the obsessional doubt being true.

The primary obsessional doubt is the engine that drives the outer wheel of OCD. Without this initial doubt, the feared secondary consequences simply cannot exist. Recognizing and addressing the primary doubt is, therefore, essential to dismantling the OCD cycle at its root.

Key Learning Points
Highlight 3.3.

Secondary consequences follow logically from the primary obsessional doubt.

Without the primary obsessional doubt, there are no secondary consequences to worry about.

OCD keeps you fixated on the secondary consequences to hide in plain sight in the present.

Emotional Reactions and Compulsive Strategies

As the OCD cycle unfolds, obsessional doubt and its secondary consequences trigger intense emotional reactions and compel strategies aimed at resolving the perceived threat. These emotions span a wide range, including distress, anxiety, discomfort, hopelessness, and depression. Feelings of shame and guilt are particularly common, though their prominence varies across different forms of OCD.

The most pervasive emotional experience in OCD, however, is an unsettling sense of uncertainty—a state of limbo created by doubting something fundamental. The more deeply entrenched the doubt, the more pronounced this uncertainty becomes. This uncertainty, coupled with other emotional reactions, fuels the compulsion to resolve the obsessional doubt.

At their essence, every compulsive action or strategy represents an attempt to "solve" the problem posed by obsessional doubt. However, as with secondary consequences, none of these emotional reactions or compulsive urges would exist without the obsessional doubt at their core. If the doubt were not obsessional, your actions would simply reflect natural responses to genuine problems rather than compulsive attempts to resolve imagined threats.

Thus, compulsions are not merely driven by anxiety or an inability to tolerate it, nor do they stem from a failure to manage uncertainty. Instead, they are a direct consequence of obsessional doubt—the central issue that sets the entire OCD cycle in motion.

Highlight 3.4
Key Learning Points

Emotional reactions and compulsions follow from the obsessional doubt and its imagined consequences.

Emotional reactions can take many different forms depending on the content of the doubt and its feared consequences.

Without the obsessional doubt, there would be no feelings of uncertainty, distress, or urge to engage in compulsions.

Triggers

Triggers encompass all the situations, events, thoughts, and feelings that precede your obsessions, ranging from mundane tasks like handling food or putting away dishes to everyday occurrences like seeing a child playing outside or getting out of your car. Depending on the nature of your OCD, these situations may or may not act as triggers for your obsessions.

For instance, if you have contamination-related OCD, shaking someone's hand might trigger an obsessional doubt ("maybe I have been contaminated"). However, it's important to understand that while triggers precede obsessional doubts, they do not cause them. Triggers are typically ordinary, neutral events—or at least, they should be. It is the obsessional doubt that transforms these situations into triggers.

> OCD is not caused by triggers, as ultimately, they are only stimuli.

Mistaking triggers as the root cause of your symptoms can lead to frustration and anger when faced with triggering situations. You might feel as though your OCD is happening because of these circumstances, as if they're to blame. In reality, triggers are merely stimuli that provide an opportunity for OCD to initiate an obsession. Whether it's shaking hands, seeing a stove, turning off lights, or encountering a red stain, the true cause lies in the underlying obsessional doubt, not the trigger itself.

Triggers are not always external stimuli or situations; they can also stem from internal states of mind. For instance, you might be reciting a prayer when the obsession arises: "What if I've offended God?" Or you might feel frustrated while waiting in line and suddenly experience the doubt: "What if I harm someone?" In these cases, the act of praying or the feeling of frustration serves as an internal trigger, while the obsessional doubt—the fear of offending God or harming someone—represents the core OCD mechanism.

It's equally important to distinguish intrusive images or urges from triggers. Intrusive images or urges are often the obsessional doubt itself, or the immediate result of it. For instance, imagine you're watching a scary movie and suddenly experience disturbing images or urges, such as a fear of harming someone. In this case, the trigger is watching the movie, while the subsequent images or urges directly embody your obsessional doubt in a vivid or motor-like format. These arise because you've become deeply absorbed in the possibility of harming someone, illustrating how OCD can translate doubt into immersive mental experiences.

Highlight 3.5.
Key Learning Points

- Triggers are never the cause for your obsessional doubt, they just precede them.

- Triggers are triggers only because you have obsessional doubts.

- Internal states of mind can act as a trigger as well, but this is never the obsessional doubt itself.

- Intrusive images or urges often represent your obsessional doubt in an imagery or motor-like format.

Unwinding The Outer Wheel

Organizing your obsessional experience within the outer wheel framework can significantly enhance your understanding of your symptoms. This method highlights that OCD symptoms do not arise randomly; they are triggered by a doubt that precedes all other elements in the outer wheel. Recognizing this initial doubt is crucial because, without this awareness, it might feel as though your symptoms occur beyond your control, fostering a sense of helplessness.

By structuring your own experience, you can heighten awareness of the individual elements and their sequential progression. This process demystifies your symptoms, which may otherwise feel like an overwhelming blend of confusion and distress. While increasing awareness won't halt your symptoms altogether, it can facilitate a clearer understanding of what you're experiencing, thereby alleviating some of the intensity.

Diagram 3.5.
Horizontal Representation of the Obsessional Sequence

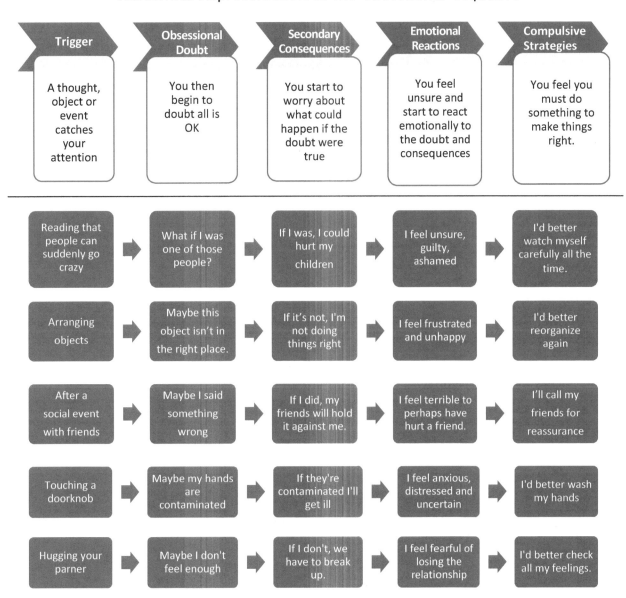

Furthermore, structuring your symptoms can help slow down the rapid pace of your OCD. The outer wheel often spins at a breakneck speed, propelling you into compulsions before you have time to reflect or intervene. OCD thrives on urgency, pressuring you to resolve doubts impulsively. However, addressing obsessional doubt through compulsions is like picking at a scab—it temporarily soothes but ultimately worsens the underlying issue, deepening the wound and making it harder to heal. By slowing down this process, you can pause long enough to recognize the patterns at play, allowing for more mindful and deliberate actions that diminish OCD's hold over your life.

Recognizing the initial doubt is the first step in unraveling your OCD symptoms. This doubt serves as the catalyst for the entire obsessional sequence, setting all subsequent reactions in motion. Pinpointing and naming this doubt transforms your experience from feeling chaotic and uncontrollable into something you can begin to understand and manage. It shifts your perspective from that of a passive victim to an active participant in the process of recovery.

Before analyzing your own obsessional sequence, it's helpful to start with those of others. Examining other people's sequences fosters a neutral perspective and creates emotional distance, which can be invaluable when reflecting on your own patterns later. Observing these predictable processes in others can also help you feel less alone in your experience, reinforcing that OCD operates through an understandable and consistent mechanism. This insight can help you feel less isolated and more confident in your ability to understand and address your symptoms.

The following exercise will guide you through this process, helping you build the skills needed to recognize and address your own OCD patterns more effectively later on.

Exercise 3.2.

Identifying the Obsessional Sequence in Others

1. **Reread and Analyze:**
   - o Revisit Chapter 1 and pick three of the case vignettes of individuals to practice with.
   - o Choose cases with themes different from those you personally experience.

2. **Use the Template (Form 3.2):**
   - o Utilize the template provided (Form 3.2) to record your findings for each case.
   - o Fill out each section of the template as thoroughly as possible based on the information given in the case descriptions.

3. **Record Multiple Answers:**
   - o Don't limit yourself to only one answer in each category if multiple triggers, obsessional doubts, etc., are evident in the individual accounts.
   - o However, there is no need to be exhaustive. Record just a few answers in each category for each case.

4. **Differentiate Primary Doubts from Secondary Concerns:**
   - o Differentiate between the primary obsessional doubts and the secondary consequences mentioned in each case description.

o Consider what prerequisites are necessary for any secondary concerns or worries to arise. These prerequisites are the obsessional doubts that precede the secondary consequences—the "Ifs..." before the "...thens."

5. **Identify Underlying Obsessional Doubts:**
   o Another way to distinguish between the obsessional doubt and the secondary consequences is to ask: "What has to be true for the worry to occur?"
   o For example, if someone worries about losing their relationship, the question to ask would be, "What would have to be true to lose that relationship?" This will typically reveal the underlying obsessional doubt, such as, "Perhaps we're not made for each other," "Maybe I don't feel enough in the relationship," or "What if my partner is not my soulmate?"

6. **Consider Various Manifestations:**
   o Obsessional doubts may manifest as images or urges in addition to thoughts.
   o Even though doubts are not always experienced as thoughts, they still represent possibilities of what could be or might be. Therefore, phrase these images and urges in terms of "what if," "could be," "maybe," or "perhaps."

7. **Review Answers in the Appendix:**
   o Answers are provided in appendix B. Since there are multiple primary doubts and possible consequences in each vignette, don't worry if your response isn't an exact match.
   o The exact nature of the obsessional sequence, including your own, will become clearer as you progress through this manual.

Highlight 3.6.
Key Learning Points

Structuring OCD symptoms into sequences transforms confusion into clarity, revealing the predictable patterns driving the disorder.

Organizing symptoms slows OCD's rapid cycle, enabling more mindful, controlled responses to obsessional doubts and compulsions.

Observing obsessional sequences in others provides emotional distance, preparing you to better analyze your own patterns.

Form 3.2

Identifying the Obsessional Sequence in Others.

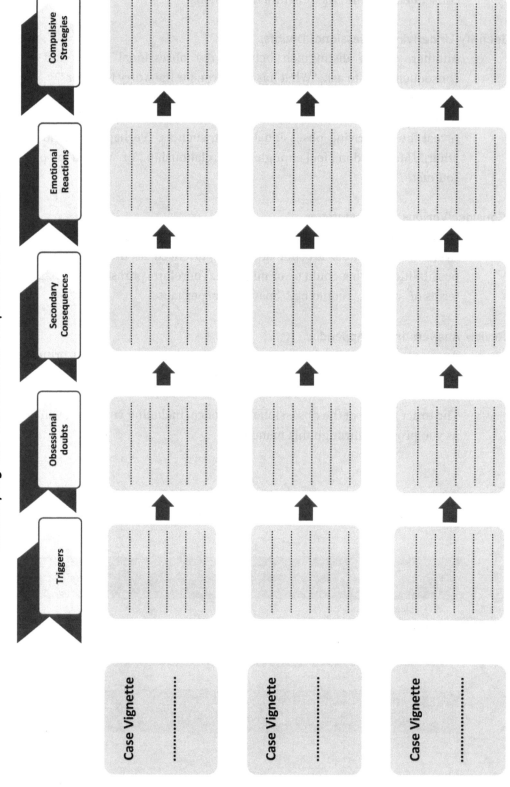

Condensing Primary Obsessional Doubts

If you've completed the previous exercise thoroughly, you may have identified several primary doubts for each case. It's uncommon to find only one obsessional doubt in any form of OCD. However, what might initially seem like numerous distinct doubts can often be simplified and condensed into one or a few overarching primary doubts.

For example, Ethan (Case Vignette 1.5) demonstrates multiple obsessional doubts that activate his outer wheel. These doubts can be succinctly condensed into two primary themes: "An appliance or fixture might not have been properly turned off" and "Maybe things are not functioning as they should" (See Diagram 3.6). This example illustrates that even when OCD presents as a complex web of doubts, these doubts often align with broader patterns or themes.

Diagram 3.6.
Condensing Multiple Primary Obsessional Doubts

Primary Obsessional Doubts	Condensed Primary Doubt(s)
Ethan Case Vignette 1.5	Maybe I forgot to turn off the stove. Perhaps the toaster is still on. Maybe the windows are left open. What if I left the light on in the bathroom? Perhaps I don't have everything I need in my wallet. What if the refrigerator isn't cooling properly? Maybe the car handbrake isn't engaged. What if the smoke detector isn't working? Perhaps my laptop could overheat and catch fire.	*I could have missed something or left something undone* *Maybe things are not functioning as they should*

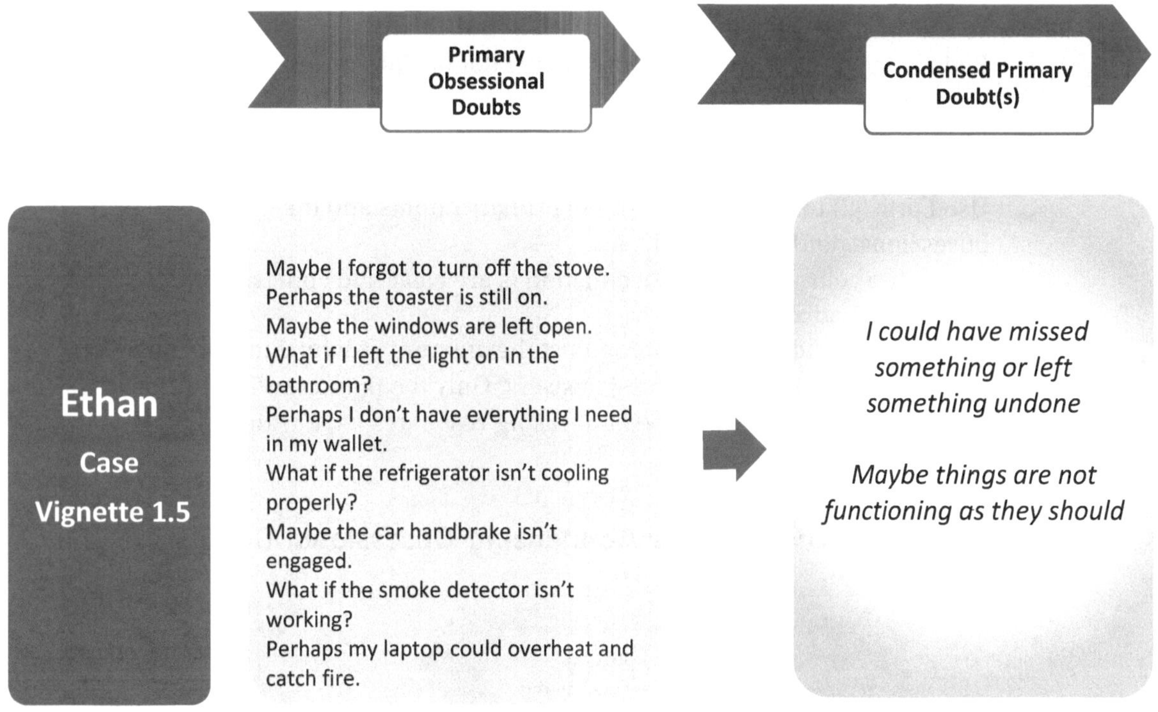

Recognizing your central doubts is a key step in managing OCD because it simplifies what often feels overwhelming. Most people with OCD have only a few central doubts, and even if there are several, one usually predominates, consuming most of their time and energy. For instance, if you compulsively wash your hands after touching doorknobs, countertops, or money, it may feel like you're responding to numerous distinct doubts tied to different triggers. However, the central doubt might simply be, "I could be contaminated." Identifying this core doubt reduces the complexity of compulsions, making them more manageable.

It's also important to recognize that not all obsessional doubts can always be reduced to a single core doubt. For individuals with more than one form of OCD, it is unlikely that all doubts can be condensed into just one. For example, if you have obsessional doubts about relationships as well as contamination, you may need at least two condensed primary doubts to capture both themes. However, condensing your doubts within each theme will still make your OCD far more manageable than leaving them scattered and unstructured.

To practice condensing your obsessional doubts, follow the steps outlined below:

Exercise 3.2.
Condensing Primary Obsessional Doubts

1. **Review the Cases:**
   - o Revisit Chapter 1 and pick two of the case vignettes of individuals to practice with.
   - o Pay attention to the details of their obsessional doubts.
2. **Identify Primary Obsessional Doubts:**
   - o For each case, identify and list the multiple primary obsessional doubts presented.
   - o Try to be thorough in identifying each primary doubt, and focus on understanding the central theme that connects them all.
   - o Write down all the primary doubts you identify in Form 3.3.
3. **Condense the Doubts:**
   - o Reduce the multiple primary obsessional doubts into one or two condensed primary obsessional doubts.
   - o Keep in mind that multiple doubts can be condensed in different ways.
4. **Complete Form 3.2:**
   - o Use Form 3.2 to record the multiple primary doubts and the condensed primary obsessional doubt(s) for each case.
   - o Make sure your condensed formulation is are clear and concise.
5. **Reference the Appendix:**
   - o Check your condensed doubts against the answers provided in Appendix C.
   - o There are no real right or wrong answers. Only the person suffering from these doubts is best able to judge what type of phrasing resonates most with them.

Form 3.3.
Exercise Template for Condensing Obsessional Doubts

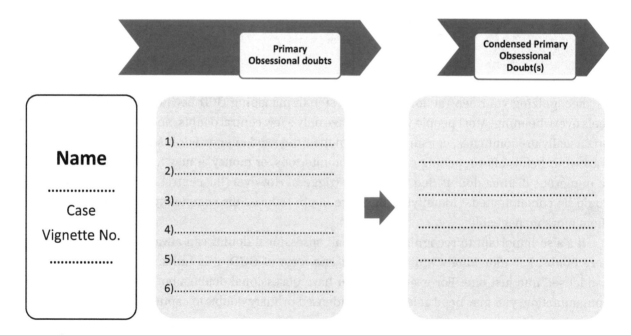

Name

....
Case
Vignette No.

....

1) ....

2) ....

3) ....

4) ....

5) ....

6) ....

....

....

....

....

Five steps Towards Identifying Your Obsessional Sequence

With the insights you've gained so far, it's now time to apply your understanding to your own experience. Identifying your obsessional sequence is a crucial step in unraveling the patterns that sustain your OCD. By tracing your symptoms back to their origins, you can begin to see how each element of the cycle connects, ultimately empowering you to disrupt it.

A clear and structured method for uncovering your obsessional sequence involves a series of focused questions designed to trace your symptoms step-by-step (refer to Diagram 3.7). This process starts with your compulsive actions—the endpoint of the sequence—and moves upstream to the initial doubt that triggers the entire cycle. Exercise 3.3 will guide you through this systematic process.

Diagram 3.7.
Five steps Towards Identifying Your Obsessional Sequence

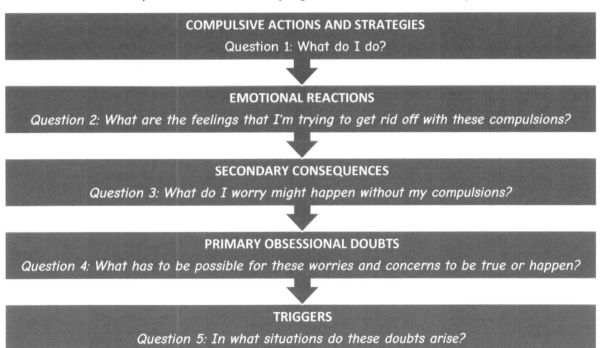

COMPULSIVE ACTIONS AND STRATEGIES
Question 1: What do I do?

EMOTIONAL REACTIONS
Question 2: What are the feelings that I'm trying to get rid off with these compulsions?

SECONDARY CONSEQUENCES
Question 3: What do I worry might happen without my compulsions?

PRIMARY OBSESSIONAL DOUBTS
Question 4: What has to be possible for these worries and concerns to be true or happen?

TRIGGERS
Question 5: In what situations do these doubts arise?

Exercise 3.3.
Identifying Your Obsessional Sequence

1. **Identify Your Compulsive Actions:**

   o **Question:** What do I do?

   o **Task:** List the compulsive behaviors that dominate your daily routine. If you've already recorded these in Form 1.2, transfer the most time-consuming actions into Form 3.4. Use separate forms for different OCD themes if needed.

2. **Determine the Emotions Behind Your Actions:**

   o **Question:** What feelings do I try to get rid of with my actions?

   o **Task:** Identify the emotions driving your compulsions—e.g., anxiety, guilt, shame, or discomfort. Record these in the "emotional reactions" section of Form 3.4 to gain insight into the motivations behind your actions.

3. **Identify Your Worries Without Compulsions:**

   o **Question:** What do I worry might happen without my compulsions?

   o **Task:** List all the potential outcomes you fear. Don't stress about distinguishing between secondary consequences and primary doubts—this will become clearer in the next step. Use Form 3.4 to record your concerns.

4. **Uncover Primary Obsessional Doubts:**

   o **Question:** What has to be true for any of my worries to happen?

   o **Task:** Reflect on the worries you listed earlier and contemplate what conditions must be met for each to materialize. This will help you uncover your primary obsessional doubts.

   o **Action:** Personalize the process by asking yourself: "What must I be absolutely certain of to alleviate all of my worries? What do I need to be sure of to resolve my OCD entirely?" The answer to this should reveal your principal obsessional doubts.

   o **Evaluate:** Use the "if...then" framework to evaluate the coherence of your answers. If discrepancies arise, one of your secondary consequences may be a primary doubt. Relocate it to your list of primary inferences.

   o **Condense:** If you have multiple primary doubts within a particular theme, combine them into a single or just a few doubts using the method described earlier. Record these condensed primary doubts in Form 3.4.

5. **Identify Situations Triggering Your Doubts:**

   o **Question:** In what situations do my primary doubts arise?

   o **Task:** Pinpoint the primary triggers for your obsessional doubts. These can be both obvious triggers (e.g., leaving home for work) and less conspicuous ones (e.g., feelings of boredom, frustration, or stress). Record your most frequently encountered triggers in Form 3.4.

Form 3.4
My Obsessional Sequence

Obsessional Theme: _____

Compulsive Actions

- .... • ....
- .... • ....
- .... • ....
- .... • ....

Emotional Reactions

- .... • ....
- .... • ....
- .... • ....
- .... • ....

Secondary Consequences

- ....
- ....
- ....
- ....

Primary Obsessional Doubts

- ....
- ....
- ....

Triggers

- .... • ....
- .... • ....
- .... • ....
- .... • ....

Additional Tips and Reminders:

1. **Time Frame Focus:**
   - Obsessional doubts typically pertain to the present (and occasionally the past) rather than the future.
   - Secondary consequences may involve all time frames. Consider what must be true in the present for a future consequence to occur, revealing the underlying obsessional doubt.

2. **Primary vs. Secondary Concerns:**
   - Obsessional doubts aren't always the thoughts that occupy you the most or cause the most anxiety. You may be predominantly preoccupied with secondary consequences while overlooking the primary doubt.

3. **Certainties vs. Possibilities:**
   - If your obsessions feel more like solid beliefs rather than possibilities or doubts, you can write them down as such, without adding a "maybe" or "what if." However, try to recognize that even this belief, no matter how convinced you feel, is still rooted in doubt. The belief is essentially a form of doubt in disguise—except that you are convinced of its reality.

4. **Sudden and Intrusive Obsessions:**
   - If you experience your obsessions as sudden and intrusive, with no apparent thought involved, slow down and carefully identify what is happening. The rapid onset of obsessional doubts makes it crucial to recognize the initial doubt.

5. **Non-Thinking Doubts:**
   - Be mindful that doubts do not always express themselves as thoughts. They can also appear as images or urges. Explicit thoughts may not always be present, but you are still contemplating possibilities that put something you value into in question.

6. **Postpone Deeper Exploration:**
   - You can always delve deeper by asking what thoughts might precede your primary obsessional doubt. For now, refrain from exploring this further; it will be addressed in greater detail later on.

Reflecting on Your Sequence

Once you've identified your obsessional sequence, take some time to review and reflect on it. Don't worry about achieving perfection on your first attempt; this is a process of discovery. Think of your sequence as a dynamic framework that evolves as your understanding deepens. You can revisit and refine it at any time, and each revision will bring greater clarity and insight into your primary obsessional doubts. Treat this reflection as an opportunity to understand the foundational role of doubt in your symptoms and to solidify your awareness of its primacy.

Exercise 3.4.
Reflection: The primacy of obsessional doubt

1. **Identify What Your Doubts Call into Question:**
   - Ask yourself: What is it that my (condensed) primary obsessional doubts call into question?

- o Use Form 3.5 to note down everything that each of your primary obsessional doubt challenge or call into question.

2. **Consider the Absence of Obsessional Doubts:**
   - o After identifying what your doubts call into question, ask yourself: What would remain of all of my symptoms in the outer wheel if I had no obsessional doubt?
   - o Don't try to get rid of your obsession or fix it; simply ask yourself the question without doing anything else.

3. **Reflect on Your Findings:**
   - o If you have identified your obsessional doubt correctly, you should be able to see that none of your symptoms should logically remain without it.
   - o Take note of these reflections and any insights gained from this exercise.

Form 3.5.
My Primary Obsessional Doubts and What They Challenge

Obsessional Doubt

- Calls into Question: ....
- Calls into Question: ....
- Calls into Question: ....
- Calls into Question: ....
- Calls into Question:..

Obsessional Doubt

- Calls into Question: ....
- Calls into Question: ....
- Calls into Question: ....
- Calls into Question: ....
- Calls into Question: ....

Obsessional Doubt

- Calls into Question: ....
- Calls into Question: ....
- Calls into Question: ....
- Calls into Question: ....
- Calls into Question: ....

Sequencing in Real Time

While identifying your obsessional sequence in a calm moment provides valuable insight, doing so during an actual episode is far more challenging. Understanding your symptoms during an episode can feel overwhelming. However, with the knowledge you've gained, you're now prepared to begin practicing real-time sequencing.

In real-time sequencing, you use the same questions for identifying your obsessional sequence, but you apply them while actively experiencing compulsive urges or behaviors. The goal is to slow down your symptoms, giving yourself the space to observe them without being consumed by their emotional intensity. This process helps create a crucial sense of separation between you and your OCD.

Remember, sequencing is just the starting point for addressing your OCD. Its purpose isn't to resolve your OCD immediately. Trying to fix or eliminate your obsession during this exercise will only hinder its primary goal: increasing awareness and establishing distance between you and your OCD. Instead, focus on asking the questions without trying to change anything—simply observe and reflect.

Exercise 3.4.

Steps for Real-Time Sequencing

1. **Hold Still:**
   - Three times a day, when you catch yourself engaging in compulsive behaviors, whether overt or covert, pause and take a moment to observe your actions closely.
   - If you can, try to postpone your compulsions during this exercise. However, if you find it difficult to delay them, it's still okay to continue to the next step.
2. **Retrace Your Steps:**
   - Identify all the elements in the sequence that prompted you to engage in compulsive actions.
   - Utilize the same five questions as previously outlined:
     1. What am I doing? [compulsive actions]
     2. What feelings am I attempting to alleviate with my actions? [emotional reactions]
     3. What worries and concerns arise if I refrain from engaging in compulsive actions? [secondary consequences]
     4. What conditions must be plausible for these worries and concerns to materialize? [the obsessional doubt]
     5. In what situation did this possibility enter my mind? [the trigger]
   - Avoid rushing or approaching it robotically; recognize that your sequence may vary with each OCD-triggering situation, resulting in different emotions, worries, and compulsions.
3. **The Primacy of Obsessional Doubt:**
   - Consider asking yourself two crucial questions: What does the doubt call into question, and how many of my symptoms would remain if I were confident that the doubt is incorrect?
   - Would any of the worries, concerns, or emotions you identified earlier still persist? Would you still feel compelled to engage in compulsive behaviors?

- o If you accurately identified the obsessional doubt, the answers to these inquiries should consistently be negative. Without the initial doubt, the outer wheel of OCD cannot be set in motion.

4. **Carry On:**
   - o Continue with whatever you were doing, even if it involves returning to your compulsive behaviors.
   - o Resist the urge to rush through the process. Trust in the gradual progress and embrace it as the most valuable gift you can give yourself at this stage. This mindful approach allows for a deeper exploration of your OCD patterns and sets the stage for lasting change.

Use the training card below as a quick reference during your practice to remind you of the steps

Training Card 3.1.

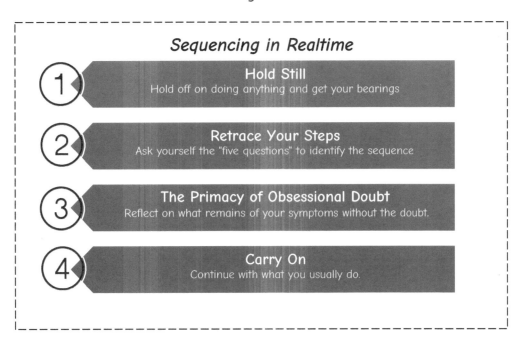

We've Only Just Begun

Practice sequencing in real-time for at least two weeks to uncover deeper insights into your OCD patterns. While the outer wheel represents the surface manifestation of your OCD, it plays a vital role in driving and sustaining the cycle. Once the outer wheel starts spinning, it gains momentum quickly, making it feel as though control is out of reach. Sequencing helps you slow down this process, creating the space needed to observe and understand your symptoms rather than being swept away by them.

Over time, sequencing provides clarity into the underlying structure of your OCD, particularly the central role of obsessional doubt. These doubts, no matter how improbable they may seem, maintain a powerful hold on your mind. Despite your logical awareness of their unlikelihood, they persist with remarkable intensity, often leading to the compulsive behaviors that sustain the cycle.

But what makes obsessional doubts different from the everyday doubts that we all experience? How can you identify an obsessional doubt the moment it surfaces? More importantly, can you uncover why it qualifies as obsessional? Answering these questions is essential to deepening your understanding of OCD. In the next chapter, we'll delve into the critical distinctions between everyday doubts and obsessional doubts, equipping you with the tools to recognize and address them more effectively.

Chapter 4

Everyday and Obsessional Doubt

Take a moment to notice how often you experience doubts in your daily life. Will I make it to work on time? Do I have enough salad left for dinner tonight? Will I meet the deadline for that project? Do I have enough money to buy that sweater? These are all doubts, and in most instances, they are entirely typical.

Everyday doubts help us navigate daily life and adapt to circumstances to ensure we reach our goals in an uncertain world. They prompt us to double-check plans, make contingency arrangements, and stay prepared for different outcomes. These doubts are practical tools for problem-solving.

Obsessional doubts, however, are different. Instead of guiding you toward solutions, they trap you in a cycle of overthinking. Rather than prompting meaningful action, they create unnecessary paralysis and fuel compulsive behaviors. Obsessional doubts don't help you achieve your goals or improve your circumstances. Instead, they hijack your attention, pulling you away from what matters most, and leave you feeling stuck.

Distinguishing between everyday and obsessional doubts is essential for overcoming OCD. However, telling them apart in the moment can be challenging, as the content of the doubt alone is not always revealing. While some obsessional doubts may seem bizarre or far-fetched (e.g., "What if a bat bites me at night?"), many are disguised as ordinary, everyday concerns (e.g., "Maybe I forgot to lock the door," "Maybe I just got contaminated," "Maybe I harmed someone").

> Obsessional doubts often disguise themselves as everyday doubts.

On the surface, these obsessional doubts appear typical, which is part of why OCD can so easily catch you off guard. When obsessional doubts mimic everyday ones, it's easy to automatically accept them as valid concerns, allowing the OCD cycle to persist. But obsessional doubts are fundamentally different—they operate in an entirely different way

Recognizing the distinction between everyday and obsessional doubts is key to further slowing the momentum of OCD's outer wheel. While this awareness won't immediately resolve the doubt—and that shouldn't be your goal at this stage—it equips you to approach the doubt with a more informed and strategic mindset. This understanding is an important step towards moving closer to recovery.

Highlight 4.1.
Key Learning Points

Unless you have an obsessional doubt, doubting is normal and functional.

OCD can trick you into thinking you are having everyday doubts.

Being able to tell the difference will slow the outer wheel of OCD and help you approach doubts with greater clarity and strategy.

Lack of Concrete Evidence in the Senses

A fundamental difference between everyday and obsessional doubt lies in the absence of concrete evidence in obsessional doubt. Obsessional doubt arises without any tangible evidence perceived by the senses in the present moment. There is never a direct link to anything you can perceive. In fact, obsessional doubts often directly contradict what your senses are telling you. For example, imagine walking past a stove and doubting whether it was left on. With obsessional doubt, there is no sensory confirmation—no warmth from the stove or smell of gas. Even after visually confirming that the stove is off, the doubt persists, defying logic and sensory information.

In contrast, everyday doubts are usually grounded in concrete evidence from the senses, such as smelling smoke and thinking there might be a fire, or questioning a sunny weather report when dark clouds are visible in the sky. These are everyday doubts because there is direct evidence in the here and now that supports the doubt. When concrete evidence is present, you are always dealing with a non-obsessional doubt, rather than an obsessional one.

For instance, doubting whether a cigarette has been properly extinguished because you see smoke rising from it is an example of an everyday doubt—your senses provide clear evidence for the concern. On the other hand, an obsessional doubt might involve worrying that a cigarette is still lit despite no smoke, smell, or other sensory evidence. This absence of tangible sensory evidence is a hallmark feature of obsessional doubt.

This distinction also separates OCD from fears seen in phobias. In most phobias, the object of fear is directly perceived. For instance, someone with arachnophobia is afraid when they see a spider, a person with hemophobia becomes anxious at the sight of blood, and someone with claustrophobia feels fear when confined in a small space. Similarly, social anxiety often arises in response to being in social situations. In all these cases, the feared object or situation is directly experienced. In OCD, however, the principal object of fear is rarely directly perceived, making obsessional doubt unique in its detachment from sensory evidence.

It's important to note that this absence of evidence doesn't mean you won't be distressed when actual evidence aligns with your doubts. For instance, if you have obsessional doubts about contaminating others, coming into direct contact with excrement will likely upset you. In such cases, the doubt shifts from obsessional to typical because sensory evidence is present, even though your reaction may still be exaggerated. The key distinction lies in whether the doubt arises without any direct evidence—if it does, it's likely an obsessional doubt.

While the absence of concrete sensory evidence isn't unique to OCD, it is especially pronounced in the disorder. Obsessional doubts arise only in situations lacking direct evidence, and this characteristic is central to understanding OCD. Moreover, this absence of evidence doesn't just apply to the outer world—it extends to the inner senses as well.

The Inner Senses

The lack of concrete evidence for obsessional doubts extends beyond our outer senses—sight, hearing, taste, touch, and smell—which inform us about the external world. It also applies to the inner senses, which convey our internal experiences, such as emotions, pain, intentions, thoughts, urges, and desires. Obsessional doubts persist without tangible evidence from either set of senses, setting them apart from everyday doubts.

Like the outer senses, the inner senses provide us with information in a very direct and immediate way, offering insight into our internal experiences. It's not about guessing or interpreting what might be inside you; it's about what you are actually experiencing at the moment. This immediate nature of the inner senses means they give us an unfiltered view of our emotional and mental state, just as the outer senses provide an unfiltered view of the physical world around us. They are the

> The inner and outer senses do not represent things as we imagine them to be. They simply present things as they are.

actual and undeniable internal experiences you have in the moment, as opposed to anything you think might be there.

Examples of concrete evidence and information coming from the inner senses include:

- Feeling happy and content while sitting in a sunny park.
- Recognizing that blue is your favorite color.
- Knowing you want to be kind and supportive to others.
- Feeling anxious about a job interview because you want to perform well.
- Seeing a beautiful painting and wanting to admire it up close.
- Wanting to congratulate a friend who has achieved something significant.
- Feeling nervous before giving a public speech.
- Feeling excited about an upcoming vacation because you love traveling.
- Seeing a delicious cake and wanting to eat it.
- Wanting to help a stranger who dropped their groceries.
- Recognizing that you dislike loud noises.
- Knowing you prefer solitude when you're feeling overwhelmed.
- Feeling proud of completing a challenging project at work.
- Seeing a familiar face and wanting to say hello.
- Wanting to share good news with your family.
- Feeling nostalgic when hearing an old song.
- Recognizing that autumn is your favorite season.
- Knowing you want to live a healthy lifestyle.
- Feeling empathy when someone shares their struggles with you.
- Seeing a messy room and wanting to clean it.

- Wanting to laugh when you hear a funny joke.
- Feeling determined to achieve your goals.
- Recognizing that you have a passion for reading books.
- Knowing you are dedicated to your hobbies and interests.
- Feeling gratitude for the support you receive from loved ones.
- Wanting to forgive someone who has apologized sincerely.
- Feeling excitement when starting a new hobby.
- Recognizing that you are an organized person.
- Knowing you value honesty and integrity in relationships.
- And so on...

The absence of evidence in the inner senses is particularly relevant for individuals experiencing obsessional doubts about their identity or self (e.g., "I might be a child molester," "I might be a deviant," "I might be a blasphemer"). In these cases, the concern revolves around what may exist within oneself rather than external realities. Just as there is never any concrete evidence in the outer senses for obsessional doubts related to external events (e.g., contamination, negligence, etc.), there is likewise no direct evidence in the inner senses for doubts regarding what you fear might be inside of you.

For example, if you doubt whether you might stab someone with a knife, this doubt does not coincide with an actual murderous urge or rage. You might fear having such an urge or feel something that resembles it in the moment, but this is not the same as direct evidence of intent or desire. Feeling frustration or anger is not concrete proof of violent intent. If it were, everyone who felt anger would need to avoid sharp objects.

Refer to diagram 4.1 for a comparison of the differences and similarities between the inner and outer senses. This comparison will help clarify how obsessional doubts persist without evidence from either set of senses.

Diagram 4.1.
Similarities and Differences Between the Inner and Outer Senses

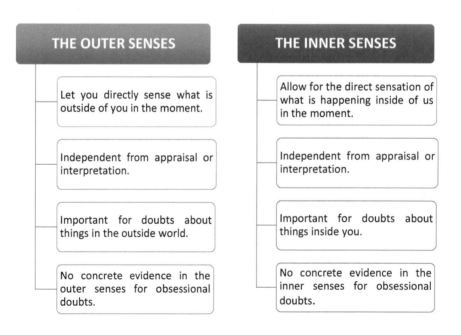

THE OUTER SENSES	THE INNER SENSES
Let you directly sense what is outside of you in the moment.	Allow for the direct sensation of what is happening inside of us in the moment.
Independent from appraisal or interpretation.	Independent from appraisal or interpretation.
Important for doubts about things in the outside world.	Important for doubts about things inside you.
No concrete evidence in the outer senses for obsessional doubts.	No concrete evidence in the inner senses for obsessional doubts.

Highlight 4.2.
Key Learning Points

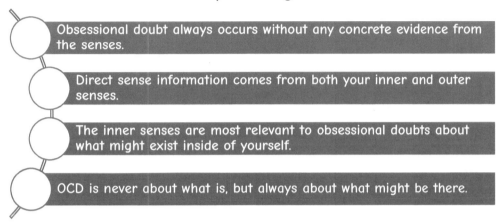

Obsessional doubt always occurs without any concrete evidence from the senses.

Direct sense information comes from both your inner and outer senses.

The inner senses are most relevant to obsessional doubts about what might exist inside of yourself.

OCD is never about what is, but always about what might be there.

Out-of-Context Occurrence

Unlike everyday doubts, obsessional doubts always arise out of context. For example, doubting it might rain when there are dark clouds in the sky is an everyday doubt because it aligns with the situation. On the other hand, worrying it might rain on a perfectly clear day is an obsessional doubt. This type of doubt is misplaced because the context does not support it, and there is no concrete evidence to back it up.

The out-of-context occurrence of obsessional doubts is closely tied to their emergence without any concrete sensory evidence. However, even everyday doubts can arise without direct evidence. For example, questioning whether your hands are sufficiently clean during a hospital visit—an environment filled with reminders to wash hands—is an everyday doubt, even without visible contamination. In such cases, the context justifies the doubt because certain environments, like hospitals, warrant extra caution. These doubts are rooted in reasonable caution or situational norms, aligning with the expectations and requirements of the environment.

Similarly, a surgeon scrubbing their hands for two or more minutes before a procedure is appropriate given the context of surgery. In these instances, doubts are based on reasonable suspicions or established safety practices, even when not directly supported by sensory information. This is never the case with obsessional doubt, which always arises in an inappropriate context.

The out-of-context occurrence of obsessional doubts is a key reason they are often experienced as intrusive and unreasonable. These doubts frequently arise in situations only tangentially related to their content, such as fearing you might harm someone while holding a knife to chop food. The inappropriate context heightens their jarring and intrusive quality. This misalignment between the doubt and the actual situation amplifies their sense of intrusion and irrationality.

However, it is important to note that the intrusive nature of obsessional doubts doesn't mean they arise without cause. These doubts don't come from nowhere; they seem disconnected because they occur outside the logical context of the senses, giving the illusion of detachment from reasoned thought. This concept will be explored in greater detail later. For now, recognizing that obsessional doubts are contextually inappropriate is an important step in distinguishing them from ordinary, everyday doubts.

Highlight 4.3.
Key Learning Points

Everyday doubts always occur in an appropriate context whereas obsessional doubts do not.

Considering the context in which a doubt occurs can help to further determine if it is obessional doubt or not.

The out-of-context occurence of obsessional doubts contributes to their intrusiveness.

The intrusiveness of obsessional doubt does not mean there are no reasons behind them.

Not About Real Uncertainty

At first glance, OCD may seem like an inability to tolerate uncertainty, with compulsions driven by a desperate need to achieve certainty. However, your symptoms don't stem from genuine difficulties with uncertainty. Instead, they arise from creating unnecessary doubt and uncertainty where none should exist.

Real uncertainty occurs when there is an actual lack of information. For instance, during the early days of the COVID-19 pandemic, there was significant uncertainty due to unreliable or incomplete information. Many people were unsure of the best precautions to take, leading to a wide range of behaviors—some of which, in hindsight, might seem exaggerated or even compulsive. However, these actions were not OCD-related because they were based on real uncertainty, where crucial information was genuinely unavailable

Obsessional doubts, by contrast, are not rooted in a lack of information or genuine uncertainty. Instead, they arise from questioning the certainty you already have. Your inner and outer senses provide all the information needed to establish certainty, but OCD leads you to question or distrust this certainty. The doubt is not caused by missing data but by the inability to trust what is already known or perceived.

> OCD does not arise from real uncertainty; it starts with doubting, which creates unnecessary uncertainty.

For example, people with checking compulsions may lock their door and see and feel themselves doing so, yet they still doubt whether it is locked. They have no problems perceiving reality correctly, and their doubt does not arise from a lack of information. They do not doubt because there is real uncertainty; rather, they doubt the certainty of what their senses tell them.

Similarly, individuals with contamination fears might wash their hands thoroughly and repeatedly; despite knowing they have already cleaned them properly. The doubt does not stem from direct perception or any in-context application of facts and knowledge when you know it is correct to wash your hands, but from persistent doubting that something might still be wrong. This relentless questioning of what they already know to be true drives their compulsive behavior.

Another example is someone with symmetry and order compulsions. They might spend hours arranging and rearranging items to achieve order, even though they can see that the items are already neatly organized. The doubt here is not about the reality of the order but about the doubt that it is not "just right," causing them to question their own perception.

In a similar way, OCD is not about striving for perfectionism. It is not the desire for perfection but the constant doubting of what is already sufficient or adequate that drives compulsive behavior. For example, someone with contamination fears doesn't wash their hands repeatedly to achieve perfect cleanliness but because they continually doubt the adequacy of their initial effort.

Therefore, what OCD seems to be about and what it truly is about are two very different things. Recognizing that your doubts are not rooted in genuine uncertainties but are instead created by the condition is crucial to addressing your symptoms. This understanding shifts the focus from misinterpreting OCD as stemming from traits like intolerance of uncertainty or perfectionism, to tackling the underlying patterns of doubt and persistent questioning that drive the disorder.

Highlight 4.4.
Key Learning Points

There is no uncertainty to tolerate if you do not doubt to start with.

Real uncertainty occurs when there is an actual lack of information, which is not the case with obsessional doubt.

Obsessional doubts are about questioning the certainty already provided by your inner and outer senses.

Having OCD does not mean that you do not perceive reality correctly. It just means that you doubt what it tells you.

Persistence and Lack of Resolution

Another important difference between everyday and obsessional doubts is that obsessional doubts worsen the more you try to resolve them. This endless cycle of attempting resolution without success is why these repetitive behaviors are termed compulsions.

Obsessional doubts cannot be resolved through compulsions because they originate without concrete evidence. Acting on an obsessional doubt that lacks a tangible basis makes it impossible to find resolution through concrete actions. The doubt inherently excludes direct evidence, creating a paradox: the more you try to resolve it, the more entrenched it becomes.

> OCD is an infinite loop command without a terminating condition.

For example, if you repeatedly check a door despite having no actual evidence that it is unlocked, no amount of checking will convince you to stop. This scenario illustrates an endless loop that continues until you consciously step away from the behavior. Similarly, someone with contamination fears may wash their hands repeatedly, even after cleaning them thoroughly according to regular standards—or even their own high standards—of hygiene and safety. However, since obsessional doubt arises from dismissing direct sensory evidence or contextual knowledge, no amount of washing can meet the criteria to stop. The loop lacks a natural endpoint.

That said, people with OCD do sometimes find ways to pause or temporarily stop their compulsions. For instance, they may set an arbitrary threshold, such as checking only three times, and stop once they've met it. External interruptions, like a phone call or another pressing task, may also disrupt the cycle momentarily. Others might stop out of sheer exhaustion or recognize the futility of their actions after repeated attempts. While these pauses can provide temporary relief, they do not resolve the obsessional doubt itself. The compulsions often return because the underlying loop of obsessional doubt remains unaddressed. These instances highlight the paradoxical nature of OCD: compulsions may occasionally cease, but the absence of any true resolution ensures the cycle persists.

Everyday doubts, on the other hand, do not lead to the same endless loop because they do not exclude concrete evidence from the onset. For example, if you see water splattering against your windshield, you have concrete evidence for the doubt that it might be raining. Gathering more information by looking around would readily resolve the doubt (i.e., are the skies clear, or is there another source for the water?). This process does not work for obsessional doubts since they do not rely on concrete evidence to begin with.

Of course, not all everyday doubts can be immediately resolved either. Some are grounded in genuine uncertainty or missing information, such as waiting for medical test results. These doubts create worry, but the worry is based on a real unknown. Similarly, a parent might feel nervous about a child climbing a tall playground structure, fearing the child might fall. While this concern could stem from an overestimation of the risk, it remains tied to a real, contextually appropriate uncertainty about the child's safety. In contrast, an obsessional doubt would question the child's safety even if they were sitting safely on the ground.

In summary, obsessional doubts and compulsions in OCD create a self-perpetuating loop due to their exclusion of concrete evidence or relevant contextual information from the outset. Recognizing this difference is yet another means to tell the difference between an everyday and obsessional doubt. If you find yourself doing things over and over, without any terminating condition, you are doing it on the basis of an obsessional doubt.

Highlight 4.5.
Key Learning Points

The more you try to fix obsessional doubts, the worse they get.

Obsessional doubts can't be resolved by acting on them because they exclude tangible evidence from the outset.

Ordinary or excessive worries do not arise from the same processes as obsessional doubts.

No Common Sense

Common sense can also be a reliable guide in determining whether a doubt is obsessional. It naturally encapsulates the key differences between everyday and obsessional doubts discussed so far. Common sense represents a basic level of practical knowledge and judgment that helps navigate daily life safely and reasonably. It relies on straightforward, intuitive assessments of situations or facts, without requiring deep analysis or overthinking.

Importantly, common sense provides an intuitive understanding of shared principles and norms that guide decision-making in typical scenarios. While common sense may vary at times between individuals or cultures, obsessional doubts often directly contradict one's own common sense. This contradiction makes common sense a valuable tool for distinguishing between everyday doubts and obsessional ones, even if your sense of "common sense" is not exactly the same as others'.

To apply common sense, take a step back from your doubt and ask yourself whether it aligns with a practical, common-sense perspective. The answer often emerges automatically and immediately, cutting through the complex web of overthinking.

This approach is particularly effective for those prone to analyzing obsessional doubts excessively. Common sense provides clear, straightforward answers. For example, if you've already locked the door and know it is secure, common sense tells you there's no need to check again. If the doubt is obsessional, common sense will reveal that you already have all the certainty and information needed. Conversely, if the doubt is everyday, common sense will prompt you to seek additional evidence or information to resolve it.

Examples of common sense include the following:

- If it's sunny, you don't need to wear a raincoat.
- Looking both ways before crossing the street ensures you don't get run over.
- If you touch a hot stove, you will get burned.
- Drinking plenty of water keeps you hydrated.
- If someone is crying, it's kind to ask if they are okay.
- If you feel no intention to harm, your fear is just a thought.
- Cover your mouth when you sneeze or cough to prevent spreading germs.
- If a plant is wilting, it likely needs water.
- If you apologized sincerely, you don't need to apologize again.
- If you turned off the light before leaving, it is off.
- If you completed and reviewed a task, it is done correctly.
- If you're feeling tired, it's a good idea to get some rest.
- You need to eat healthy foods to maintain good health.
- If you're driving and see a red light, it's a good idea to stop your car.
- Being honest builds trust with others.
- If no one is harmed and everyone is safe, you have not caused harm.
- If you followed the necessary steps to create a secure password, it is secure.
- Brush your teeth twice a day to maintain dental health.
- Helping a neighbor can foster a strong sense of community.
- Don't use electrical appliances when taking a bath.

While these examples illustrate how common sense operates, OCD often works to undermine your trust in it. OCD thrives on making you doubt what would otherwise be immediately clear through common sense. Yet, if you take the time to pause and listen, common sense will consistently provide clarity. The more you practice relying on it, the easier it becomes to recognize when OCD is trying to hijack your judgment.

For instance, if you repeatedly check whether the door is locked despite knowing it is, common sense will remind you that further checking is unnecessary and rooted in obsessional doubt. This recognition helps you see when your actions are being guided by OCD rather than genuine concern.

It's important, however, not to rush this process or try to dismiss your doubts prematurely. While common sense can help you recognize obsessional doubts, you don't yet have the full toolkit to fully disengage from them. Prematurely dismissing doubts can backfire, as OCD may amplify its efforts to undermine your confidence. For now, focus on using common sense to identify whether a doubt is obsessional or everyday. This measured approach will lay the groundwork for understanding and managing your doubts more effectively as you progress.

Highlight 4.6.
Key Learning Points

Using your common sense is the simplest and easiest way to tell if you have an obsessional doubt.

Common sense will also tell you whether or not you already have all the information you need.

Common sense will have the correct answer even though you may not yet trust it.

Focus on telling the difference btween everyday and obsessional doubt without trying to resolve it.

Telling the Difference Right Now

Based on everything you have learned so far, you should now be in a better position to differentiate between obsessional and everyday doubts. However, if you're feeling unsure or struggling to apply these distinctions, it may be because you're trying to use them on your own obsessional doubts in an attempt to resolve them. It's important to avoid this at first. It's much better to first practice with situations that are neutral to you.

This section provides various scenarios, each illustrating either an everyday or an obsessional doubt. Since no one has obsessional doubts in every area of life, at least some of these examples should feel neutral and free from emotional weight. By practicing with these neutral scenarios, you'll build a clearer understanding of the differences between everyday and obsessional doubts. This practice will make it easier to apply this knowledge to your own experiences when the time comes.

Exercise 4.1.
Differentiating Between Everyday and Obsessional Doubts

1. **Read Each Scenario:**
   - Carefully read each scenario provided in this section.
2. **Identify the Primary Doubt:**
   - Identify the primary doubt and the feared secondary consequences in each scenario.
3. **Answer the Questions:**
   - Use the following five questions to determine whether the primary doubt is everyday or obsessional:
     1. *Is there any concrete evidence in the senses for the doubt in the here-and-now?*
     2. *Does the doubt occur in an appropriate context?*
     3. *Is the doubt based on a real uncertainty?*
     4. *Does acting on the doubt help to resolve it?*
     5. *Is the doubt rooted in common sense?*
4. **Make Your Determination:**
   - Based on your answers to the question, make the determination on whether the primary doubt in each scenario is obsessional or non-obsessional.
5. **Review Example Scenario:**
   - Start with Scenario 4.1 and Sample Form 4.1 with the answers already filled in to understand the process.
6. **Record Your Answers:**
   - Use Forms 4.2 to 4.8. provided at the end of this section to record your answers for the other scenario's.
7. **Re-read Previous Sections if Needed:**
   - If you have difficulty, re-read the previous sections in this chapter on which the five questions are based.
8. **Check Your Answers:**
   - The correct answers, along with explanations, can be found in Appendix D. Review these to check your understanding.

Scenario 4.1: The Door

Michael is about to leave his home after locking the front door, but he suddenly doubts whether it is properly locked. He anxiously turns the key back and forth several times, even though the door does not open whenever he pulls the handle. His mind tells him it makes sense to be extra careful. After all, his cat once escaped through the backdoor because it didn't lock properly.

The thought of the same thing happening with the front door fills him with dread. This time, it would be even worse. The street outside is busy with traffic, and if his cat escaped, it could easily get hurt. The idea of his beloved pet getting injured or worse is unbearable. He wouldn't be able to forgive himself if something happened.

As he stands there, turning the key yet again, his heart races and his thoughts spiral. "What if the door isn't really locked?" he wonders. "What if I missed something?" Despite the door remaining firmly shut each time he tests it, the doubt persists, gnawing at him. The fear of what might happen keeps him trapped in this repetitive cycle, unable to break free and leave the house with peace of mind.

Form 4.1. Answers
Scenario 4.1: The Door

A. What is the primary doubt and the feared consequences in this scenario?

The primary doubt in this scenario is "I might not have locked the door properly" or "Perhaps the door has been left open." These thoughts are the initial triggers for his anxiety. The secondary consequences, such as the cat escaping or her inability to live with himself if something happens to the cat, are contingent upon the primary doubt being true. These secondary fears amplify the distress caused by the primary doubt, making the situation feel even more urgent and compelling, but they are not the source of the problem. Recognizing the primary doubt is crucial because it helps to pinpoint the exact source of the obsession.

1. Is there any concrete evidence in the senses for the doubt in the here-and-now?

☐ Yes ☒ No ☐ Not Sure

Elaborate on your answer and specify why:

There is no concrete evidence in the here-and-now to support the obsessional doubt that the door has been left open. His senses clearly tell him that the door is properly closed: he has turned the key, the door does not open when he pulls the handle, and he has visually confirmed that the lock is engaged. These sensory inputs provide direct evidence to confirm that the door is securely locked.

2. Does the doubt occur in an appropriate context?

☐ Yes ☒ No ☐ Not Sure

Elaborate on your answer and specify why:

Given that his senses tell him the opposite and there is nothing concrete to suggest otherwise, the doubt clearly occurs out of context. His sensory information is clear: the door is properly locked. There are no immediate signs or evidence to suggest that the door is not secure. The doubt does not align with the present situation and is therefore occurring in an inappropriate context.

3. Is the doubt based on a real uncertainty?

☐ Yes ☒ No ☐ Not Sure

Elaborate on your answer and specify why:

Real uncertainties arise when there is a genuine lack of information, which is not the case here. For example, if he had rushed out of the house without checking the door, it would be reasonable to feel uncertain about whether the door was locked. In this scenario, he doubts the information he already possesses—namely, what his senses are telling him about the door. His senses have provided clear and reliable information: the door is securely locked. This self-generated uncertainty, despite having all necessary information, is a hallmark of obsessional doubt. It contrasts sharply with real uncertainties, where genuine gaps in knowledge or information exist.

4. Does acting on the doubt help to resolve it?

☐ Yes   ☒ No   ☐ Not Sure

Elaborate on your answer and specify why:
Michael is checking repeatedly, despite concrete evidence telling him the door is locked. Acting on the doubt by checking the door again and again does not help to resolve it. The reason the doubt is not resolved with checking is because it arose without concrete evidence from his senses. Since the doubt was not based on any sensory evidence to begin with, the confirmation provided by his senses afterwards also fails to register. It's as if the sensory feedback does not matter, and the doubt persists regardless of the clear evidence that the door is locked. This persistence of doubt despite attempts to resolve it is a key indicator that it is obsessional.

5. Is the doubt rooted in common sense?

☐ Yes   ☒ No   ☐ Not Sure

Elaborate on your answer and specify why:
The doubt in this scenario is not based on common sense. Common sense naturally automatically relies on clear, direct information from our senses and rational judgment. His senses provide clear evidence that the door is locked—he has turned the key, the door doesn't open when he pulls the handle, and he can see the lock is engaged. If his doubt were based on common sense, he would trust this sensory evidence and move on, reassured that the door is secure. However, he continues to doubt and check the door repeatedly, despite this clear evidence.

B. Considering all of your answers, is the doubt obsessional?

☒ Yes   ☐ No   ☐ Not Sure

Elaborate on your answer and specify why:
The doubt in this scenario is obsessional because there is lack of direct evidence, occurs inappropriately out of context, is not based on real uncertainty, is not resolved by repeated actions, and lacks a foundation in common sense. The repetitive cycle of doubt and checking traps him in a loop of anxiety and compulsive behavior, characteristic of obsessional doubt.

Scenario 4.2: The Dog Spa

Sarah's dog is overdue for grooming. Unfortunately, the dog spa she normally goes to went out of business, so she has to find a new one. She checks online and finds another spa nearby. The reviews seem generally positive, and the website looks professional, so she books an appointment to drop off her dog the next day. Suddenly, she starts feeling uncomfortable. How does she know they will treat her dog well? What if they won't take good care of it?

Sarah fears that if the new spa doesn't take good care of her dog, it could be traumatized, leading to behavioral changes and a loss of trust. She worries that her dog might be hurt or mistreated, causing physical and emotional harm. Additionally, she's concerned that a negative experience could result in her dog developing anxiety about grooming in the future. The thought of her dog suffering because of a poor grooming experience makes her anxious and determined to ensure she chooses the right place.

As these thoughts race through her mind, she decides to go back online to find out more information about the place. She reads through more reviews, looking for any negative feedback or red flags. She checks if the spa is accredited or if the groomers are certified. She even looks up any local news stories or posts on social media about the spa. Despite finding mostly positive information, she still feels uneasy.

Sarah contemplates calling the spa to ask about their grooming process, the experience of their staff, and how they handle anxious or difficult dogs. She considers driving by the location to get a feel for the place and maybe even talking to other pet owners who are dropping off or picking up their pets. As she gathers more information, her worry starts to ease, but she still feels a lingering sense of anxiety about trying a new place.

Scenario 4.3: Asbestos Contamination

Mark recently moved into an older house and learned that asbestos was commonly used in building materials during the time his house was built. The home inspector informed him that there is asbestos in some of the building materials, but assured him that there are no health risks since it is sealed behind the floorboards and walls, which are in good condition. The inspector emphasized that there is nothing to worry about as long as the asbestos is left undisturbed. Despite this reassurance, Mark becomes increasingly anxious about the possibility of contamination. He starts thinking, "What if I do something in my everyday activities that would disturb the asbestos so that it is released?"

This thought begins to dominate his mind, including the many different ways how this might occur. He worries that walking on the floor causes vibrations that release asbestos fibers. He becomes paranoid about playing music too loudly, fearing the sound waves might dislodge asbestos particles. Mark even worries that using his vacuum cleaner could somehow cause asbestos to become airborne.

Mark starts obsessively researching asbestos and its health effects. He reads horror stories online about people getting sick from asbestos exposure. Despite finding credible information that indicates his house is safe, Mark continues to worry. He repeatedly checks areas of his home for any signs of asbestos, even though he has no training or expertise in identifying it. He also spends a lot of money on frequent asbestos test kits, which he sends to professional laboratories for analysis. These tests always turn up negative, but this does not alleviate his anxiety.

Mark begins to avoid certain rooms, fearing they might be contaminated. He wears a mask and gloves around the house, despite there being no concrete evidence of asbestos presence. He frequently calls asbestos removal companies for advice, even having multiple professionals come to inspect the house. Each time, they reassure him that there is no danger if the asbestos remains undisturbed, but Mark's anxiety does not subside.

His fear escalates to the point where he limits visitors to his home, worried they might accidentally disturb the asbestos. Mark even considers selling the house and moving, despite the significant financial and emotional costs. His daily life becomes increasingly consumed by the fear of asbestos contamination, affecting his work, relationships, and overall well-being.

Scenario 4.4: The Perfect Presentation

Alex has been invited to give a presentation at a major industry conference. He has prepared extensively, practicing his speech multiple times and fine-tuning his slides. However, as the conference date approaches, he begins to feel nervous. "What if I forget what I'm supposed to say?" or "What if the audience doesn't find my presentation engaging?" These thoughts cause him significant anxiety.

Alex worries that if he performs poorly, it could damage his professional reputation and lead to missed opportunities. To address his concerns, he decides to take additional steps to ensure he is well-prepared. He rehearses his presentation in front of friends and colleagues, asks for feedback, and makes necessary adjustments. He also researches public speaking tips and techniques to boost his confidence. All in all, Alex has spent many hours preparing, trying to cover every aspect of giving a good presentation he can think of.

As the day of the presentation approaches, Alex continues to feel nervous. He is unsure if his preparation and practice have equipped him well, and tries to focus on the positive feedback he has received from his practice sessions. Despite his thorough preparation, he still feels a lingering sense of anxiety, unsure if it will subside completely until he steps onto the stage.

Scenario 4.5: A Question of Sexual Identity

Natalie, a woman who has identified as bisexual for many years, finds herself increasingly troubled by doubts about her sexual orientation. She has always felt attracted to both men and women, and her past relationships have reflected this. Yet, doubts begin to surface: "What if I'm actually heterosexual?" or "What if I'm really gay and not bisexual at all?" These questions feel urgent, and the more Natalie tries to answer them, the more they seem to grow.

Her anxiety deepens when she recalls something she overheard at a party weeks ago: "Bisexual people eventually pick sides." The comment, though casually made, lingers in her mind, casting a shadow over her sense of identity. Natalie begins replaying her past relationships, searching for signs that might confirm or disprove her fears. She asks herself: "Did I really feel attracted to him?" or "Was I just pretending to like her?" Each memory feels like a puzzle piece, but no matter how hard she tries, the picture never seems to come together.

Natalie finds herself analyzing her present-day attractions. If she notices an attraction to a man, she questions: "Does this mean I'm straight?" If she feels drawn to a woman, she wonders: "Does this prove I'm gay?" Each attraction seems to spark a new round of questions and analysis, as though every moment of connection holds the key to unraveling her identity. But instead of gaining clarity, the doubts only seem to multiply, leaving her more confused than before.

Desperate for answers, Natalie turns to the internet. She reads articles, watches videos, and dives into forums, hoping to find someone whose experiences mirror her own. But instead of reassurance, she encounters stereotypes and conflicting narratives: "Bisexuality isn't real," or "You're just confused." Each statement feels like a blow, deepening her doubts and making her question whether she's been honest with herself all along.

Seeking reassurance, Natalie begins talking to friends and asking them: "Do you think I'm really bisexual? Have you ever doubted your identity?" While their responses are supportive, the relief is fleeting. No matter how much reassurance she gets, the doubts return, louder and more insistent, urging her to keep searching for proof.

Caught in a cycle of questioning, Natalie feels increasingly stuck. Her mind races through every relationship, attraction, and comment she's ever experienced, trying to piece together a definitive answer. The harder she searches, the more elusive it feels. She wonders if she'll ever truly know the answer, or if the doubt itself will overshadow her sense of self forever.

Scenario 4.6: Haunted by Memories

Sam values his memories and takes great care in documenting them. He keeps a detailed journal and maintains a photo album. Recently, however, he has been experiencing an overwhelming need to ensure that his memories are recorded exactly as they happened. This doubt centers around the fear that his recollections are not accurate or complete.

Every evening, Sam spends hours writing in his journal, meticulously recounting the day's events. He constantly worries: "What if I forgot an important detail?" or "What if my memory of this event isn't exactly right?"

Sam fears that if his memories are not recorded perfectly, he will lose touch with the important moments of his life. He worries that inaccurately documented memories will distort his understanding of his past and misrepresent his experiences.

These doubts and worries cause him significant distress. He repeatedly revisits his entries, erasing and rewriting parts to make sure they capture every nuance of his experiences. Despite this exhaustive verification process, he remains unsatisfied and anxious.

Sam's anxiety extends to his photo albums. He scrutinizes each picture, questioning if it truly captures the moment as he remembers it. He often rearranges the photos, trying to match them precisely with his mental image of the events. Despite his meticulous efforts, the doubt persists. "What if these photos don't represent the memory accurately?" he wonders.

Scenario 4.7: Health Scare

David, a 35-year-old man, recently noticed a persistent discomfort in his abdomen that seemed unusual to him. Concerned it could be a serious issue, such as a gastrointestinal problem, he scheduled an appointment with his physician. The doctor performed an initial examination and suggested an ultrasound to get a clearer understanding. While the physician reassured David that the symptoms could have a benign cause, they emphasized the importance of further investigation.

After undergoing the ultrasound, David was informed that no alarming signs were found, but the doctor recommended a follow-up in six months to monitor any changes. Despite this initial reassurance, David found himself worrying about the possibility of a serious health condition, and "What if it's something dangerous?" became a recurring thought.

During the waiting period, David's anxiety fluctuated. He often felt overwhelmed by speculative "what if" scenarios about his health, which seemed to dominate his focus. However, he coped by talking with friends and family, focusing on his hobbies and work, and trying to stay informed by reading reliable medical information on gastrointestinal health. He practiced relaxation techniques to manage his worry, though the intrusive doubts occasionally returned.

At the follow-up appointment, the doctor revisited the case and conducted further tests. It was eventually determined that David's discomfort was caused by a combination of mild gastritis and poor posture, which had been straining his abdominal muscles over time. The gastritis was likely triggered by stress and dietary habits, and the discomfort could be alleviated with adjustments in his diet, posture correction exercises, and stress management strategies.

Scenario 4.8: Church Service

Emily, a devoutly religious person, is attending a church service. As she participates in the service, fully engaged in worship, a disturbing doubt suddenly pops into her mind: "What if I am a blasphemer?" Almost immediately, intrusive thoughts, images, and actions that mock her religion start to flood her mind. These thoughts horrify her, as she would never intentionally say or do anything disrespectful about her faith.

Emily becomes increasingly anxious, mentally reviewing everything she said and thought during the service. She reassures herself that she hasn't done anything wrong, but the intrusive thoughts keep coming back, stronger each time. The more she tries to assure herself that she hasn't blasphemed, the more intense the doubt becomes, making it difficult for her to focus on the service.

Her heart races, and she feels a deep sense of guilt and shame. She fears judgment from her community and from a higher power, and this fear makes the service, which should be a source of comfort and solace, feel like a trial. She tries to pray for forgiveness, but the intrusive thoughts persist, leaving her trapped in a cycle of anxiety and self-recrimination.

Form 4.2.

The Dog Spa

A. *What is the primary doubt and the feared consequences in this scenario?*

Elaborate on your answer and specify why:

----

1. *Is there any concrete evidence in the senses in the here-and-now for the doubt?*

☐ Yes   ☐ No   ☐ Not Sure

Elaborate on your answer and specify why:

----

2. *Did the doubt occur in an appropriate context?*

☐ Yes   ☐ No   ☐ Not Sure

Elaborate on your answer and specify why:

----

3. *Is the doubt based on a real uncertainty?*

☐ Yes   ☐ No   ☐ Not Sure

Elaborate on your answer and specify why:

----

4. *Does acting on the doubt help to resolve it?*

☐ Yes   ☐ No   ☐ Not Sure

Elaborate on your answer and specify why:

----

5. *Is the doubt rooted in common sense?*

☐ Yes   ☐ No   ☐ Not Sure

Elaborate on your answer and specify why:

B. *Considering all of your answers, is the doubt obsessional?*

☐ Yes   ☐ No   ☐ Not Sure

Elaborate on your answer and specify why:

Form 4.3.
Asbestos Contamination

A. *What is the primary doubt and the feared consequences in this scenario?*

Elaborate on your answer and specify why:

----

1. *Is there any concrete evidence in the senses in the here-and-now for the doubt?*

☐ Yes   ☐ No   ☐ Not Sure

Elaborate on your answer and specify why:

----

2. *Did the doubt occur in an appropriate context?*

☐ Yes   ☐ No   ☐ Not Sure

Elaborate on your answer and specify why:

----

3. *Is the doubt based on a real uncertainty?*

☐ Yes   ☐ No   ☐ Not Sure

Elaborate on your answer and specify why:

----

4. *Does acting on the doubt help to resolve it?*

☐ Yes   ☐ No   ☐ Not Sure

Elaborate on your answer and specify why:

----

5. *Is the doubt rooted in common sense?*

☐ Yes   ☐ No   ☐ Not Sure

Elaborate on your answer and specify why:

B. *Considering all of your answers, is the doubt obsessional?*

☐ Yes   ☐ No   ☐ Not Sure

Elaborate on your answer and specify why:

Form 4.4.
Scenario 4.4: The Perfect Presentation

A. *What is the primary doubt and the feared consequences in this scenario?*

   Elaborate on your answer and specify why:

   ----

1. *Is there any concrete evidence in the senses in the here-and-now for the doubt?*

   ☐ Yes   ☐ No   ☐ Not Sure

   Elaborate on your answer and specify why:

   ----

2. *Did the doubt occur in an appropriate context?*

   ☐ Yes   ☐ No   ☐ Not Sure

   Elaborate on your answer and specify why:

   ----

3. *Is the doubt based on a real uncertainty?*

   ☐ Yes   ☐ No   ☐ Not Sure

   Elaborate on your answer and specify why:

   ----

4. *Does acting on the doubt help to resolve it?*

   ☐ Yes   ☐ No   ☐ Not Sure

   Elaborate on your answer and specify why:

   ----

5. *Is the doubt rooted in common sense?*

   ☐ Yes   ☐ No   ☐ Not Sure

   Elaborate on your answer and specify why:

B. *Considering all of your answers, is the doubt obsessional?*

   ☐ Yes   ☐ No   ☐ Not Sure

   Elaborate on your answer and specify why:

Form 4.5.

Scenario 4.5: A Question of Sexual Identity

A. What is the primary doubt and the feared consequences in this scenario?

Elaborate on your answer and specify why:

----

1. Is there any concrete evidence in the senses in the here-and-now for the doubt?

☐ Yes   ☐ No   ☐ Not Sure

Elaborate on your answer and specify why:

----

2. Did the doubt occur in an appropriate context?

☐ Yes   ☐ No   ☐ Not Sure

Elaborate on your answer and specify why:

----

3. Is the doubt based on a real uncertainty?

☐ Yes   ☐ No   ☐ Not Sure

Elaborate on your answer and specify why:

----

4. Does acting on the doubt help to resolve it?

☐ Yes   ☐ No   ☐ Not Sure

Elaborate on your answer and specify why:

----

5. Is the doubt rooted in common sense?

☐ Yes   ☐ No   ☐ Not Sure

Elaborate on your answer and specify why:

B. Considering all of your answers, is the doubt obsessional?

☐ Yes   ☐ No   ☐ Not Sure

Elaborate on your answer and specify why:

Form 4.6
Scenario 4.6: Haunted by Memories

A. *What is the primary doubt and the feared consequences in this scenario?*

Elaborate on your answer and specify why:

----

1. *Is there any concrete evidence in the senses in the here-and-now for the doubt?*

☐ Yes   ☐ No   ☐ Not Sure

Elaborate on your answer and specify why:

----

2. *Did the doubt occur in an appropriate context?*

☐ Yes   ☐ No   ☐ Not Sure

Elaborate on your answer and specify why:

----

3. *Is the doubt based on a real uncertainty?*

☐ Yes   ☐ No   ☐ Not Sure

Elaborate on your answer and specify why:

----

4. *Does acting on the doubt help to resolve it?*

☐ Yes   ☐ No   ☐ Not Sure

Elaborate on your answer and specify why:

----

5. *Is the doubt rooted in common sense?*

☐ Yes   ☐ No   ☐ Not Sure

Elaborate on your answer and specify why:

B. *Considering all of your answers, is the doubt obsessional?*

☐ Yes   ☐ No   ☐ Not Sure

Elaborate on your answer and specify why:

Form 4.7.

Scenario 4.7: Health Scare

A. *What is the primary doubt and the feared consequences in this scenario?*

Elaborate on your answer and specify why:

----

1. *Is there any concrete evidence in the senses in the here-and-now for the doubt?*

☐ Yes   ☐ No   ☐ Not Sure

Elaborate on your answer and specify why:

----

2. *Did the doubt occur in an appropriate context?*

☐ Yes   ☐ No   ☐ Not Sure

Elaborate on your answer and specify why:

----

3. *Is the doubt based on a real uncertainty?*

☐ Yes   ☐ No   ☐ Not Sure

Elaborate on your answer and specify why:

----

4. *Does acting on the doubt help to resolve it?*

☐ Yes   ☐ No   ☐ Not Sure

Elaborate on your answer and specify why:

----

5. *Is the doubt rooted in common sense?*

☐ Yes   ☐ No   ☐ Not Sure

Elaborate on your answer and specify why:

B. *Considering all of your answers, is the doubt obsessional?*

☐ Yes   ☐ No   ☐ Not Sure

Elaborate on your answer and specify why:

Form 4.8.
Scenario 4.8: Church Service

A. *What is the primary doubt and the feared consequences in this scenario?*
Elaborate on your answer and specify why:

----

1. *Is there any concrete evidence in the senses in the here-and-now for the doubt?*
☐ Yes   ☐ No   ☐ Not Sure
Elaborate on your answer and specify why:

----

2. *Did the doubt occur in an appropriate context?*
☐ Yes   ☐ No   ☐ Not Sure
Elaborate on your answer and specify why:

----

3. *Is the doubt based on a real uncertainty?*
☐ Yes   ☐ No   ☐ Not Sure
Elaborate on your answer and specify why:

----

4. *Does acting on the doubt help to resolve it?*
☐ Yes   ☐ No   ☐ Not Sure
Elaborate on your answer and specify why:

----

5. *Is the doubt rooted in common sense?*
☐ Yes   ☐ No   ☐ Not Sure
Elaborate on your answer and specify why:

B. *Considering all of your answers, is the doubt obsessional?*
☐ Yes   ☐ No   ☐ Not Sure
Elaborate on your answer and specify why:

Turning the Tables: Shifting Perspectives on Doubts

Now that you've practiced distinguishing between everyday and obsessional doubts, it's time to take your understanding a step further. The next exercise, "Turning the Tables," invites you to reverse scenarios—transforming an obsessional doubt into an everyday one, and vice versa.

Flipping scenarios is a powerful way to deepen your understanding of the core characteristics of everyday and obsessional doubts. By reimagining these scenarios in their opposite forms, you'll sharpen your ability to recognize the subtle differences between the two types of doubts. This exercise also provides practical insight into how doubts are influenced by factors like evidence, context, and persistence. Ultimately, this practice will reinforce your confidence in identifying and addressing obsessional doubts.

To illustrate, let's take the scenario of Michael checking his door lock and flip it into its opposite form:

Locked Door Reassurance: A Non-obsessional Scenario

Michael is about to leave his home after locking the front door. As he pulls the handle to check, he notices that the door seems slightly loose, creating a brief doubt: "Is the door properly locked?" Remembering his cat once escaped through the backdoor due to a lock issue, he decides to double-check the front door lock. He turns the key again, confirming it is securely locked. Satisfied, he takes a deep breath and reassures himself that the door is firmly shut.

The thought of his cat escaping momentarily crosses his mind, but he reminds himself that the front door is different from the backdoor incident and he has taken appropriate precautions. The street outside is busy with traffic, and while the safety of his pet is important to him, he feels confident that he has done everything necessary to ensure the door is secure.

He leaves the house with a sense of assurance, knowing that he has taken the necessary steps to prevent his cat from escaping. As he walks away, he does not dwell on the locked door but focuses on his day ahead.

At work, Michael is productive and engaged. He attends meetings, collaborates with colleagues, and completes his tasks efficiently. During a break, a colleague mentions having trouble with their own door lock, and Michael shares his morning experience. He speaks confidently about how he handled his brief doubt and moved on, providing practical advice.

Returning home in the evening, Michael notices how peaceful he feels. He recalls how easily he dismissed his earlier doubt and appreciates his ability to handle such moments without getting stuck in a cycle of worry. Opening the door, he is greeted by his cat, safe and sound inside. This reassures him further that his approach is working.

Before going to bed, Michael double-checks the front door lock one last time as part of his usual routine. The lock is secure, and he smiles, knowing he has done everything necessary. He goes to sleep feeling calm and assured, ready to face a new day without being weighed down by unnecessary doubts.

Transforming a scenario from obsessional to non-obsessional, or vice versa, becomes straightforward when you focus on the key distinctions. In the opposite scenario, Michael's doubt about whether the door is locked shifts to an everyday doubt. This change is rooted in sensory evidence—he notices the door feels slightly loose, which justifies a brief uncertainty and prompts him to double-check.

The context is also appropriate. His concern about the cat escaping makes sense but doesn't spiral out of control. Once he confirms the door is secure, the doubt resolves, and he moves on without overthinking. His actions are guided by common sense and practical judgment, with no escalation into compulsive checking.

In contrast, the obsessional version highlights irrational and persistent doubt, disconnected from any concrete evidence. Even after multiple checks, Michael's anxiety persists, and his doubt remains unresolved. This underscores how obsessional doubts often escalate, creating a cycle of compulsions and heightened anxiety, despite no real justification.

To flip a scenario effectively, focus on these critical factors:

- **Sensory Evidence:** Is the doubt based on something tangible or purely imagined?
- **Context:** Does the doubt make sense in the given situation, or is it misplaced?
- **Real Uncertainty:** Is the doubt genuine, or is it driven by OCD's manufactured uncertainty?
- **Resolution:** Does addressing the doubt resolve it, or does it lead to repetitive compulsions?
- **Common Sense:** Does the doubt align with practical, sound judgment, or defy it?

By examining these elements, you can clearly see how obsessional and everyday doubts differ and why one leads to resolution while the other perpetuates the cycle of OCD.

Exercise 4.1.

Time to Get Creative

Now it's your turn to practice identifying and rewriting scenarios. Follow the steps below to creatively transform four scenarios into their opposites.

1. **Select Four Scenarios:**
   - Choose four scenarios from the previous examples.
   - Ensure you pick two scenarios where the doubt was obsessional and two where the doubt was non-obsessional.
2. **Pick Personal or Neutral Scenarios:**
   - You can pick scenarios that are neutral to you, as well as those that resonate more personally, if there are any.
   - Keep the exercise creative and focused solely on rewriting the scenario as if it were from a stranger.
3. **Rewrite the Scenarios:**
   - Use Forms 4.9 to 4.12 to write out each of these opposite scenarios.
   - Give each rewritten scenario an appropriate title.
   - Be as creative as possible. The more creative you are, the better!
4. **Contrast with Provided Examples:**
   - Once you're done, review the examples of oppositional scenarios in appendix E.
   - Contrast them with the originals in this chapter to further reinforce your learning.

Form 4.9.
Opposite Scenario 1

Original Title: _____

New Title: _____

_____

_____

_____

_____

_____

_____

_____

_____

_____

_____

_____

_____

_____

_____

_____

_____

_____

Form 4.10.
Opposite Scenario 2

Original Title: _____

New Title: _____

_____

_____

_____

_____

_____

_____

_____

_____

_____

_____

_____

_____

_____

_____

_____

_____

_____

Form 4.11.
Opposite Scenario 3

Original Title: _____

New Title: _____

_____

_____

_____

_____

_____

_____

_____

_____

_____

_____

_____

_____

_____

_____

_____

_____

_____

_____

Form 4.12.
Opposite Scenario 4

Original Title: _____

New Title: _____

_____

_____

_____

_____

_____

_____

_____

_____

_____

_____

_____

_____

_____

_____

_____

_____

_____

Knowing the Difference When Doubting

Now that you've practiced differentiating between everyday and obsessional doubt from a distance, it's time to apply this skill to your own doubts. Not all your doubts are obsessional. It might feel that way because obsessional doubts tend to linger and demand attention, but if you take a moment to observe, you'll likely notice that many of your daily doubts are actually non-obsessional.

Doubting is often a natural and helpful part of life. Many doubts you experience throughout the day serve a useful purpose and help you accomplish your goals. For instance, when approaching a busy intersection, you might doubt whether it's safe to cross. This doubt prompts you to wait for the pedestrian signal and carefully check for oncoming traffic before proceeding.

This process is entirely normal and rooted in practical reasoning. It is driven by rational concern, based on what you perceive through your senses. Everyday doubts are typically tied to external cues and are resolved with straightforward actions, such as observing your environment. In contrast, obsessional doubts persist despite repeated attempts at resolution and often feel disconnected from any real-world context.

When practicing telling the difference between everyday and obsessional doubt, avoid the temptation to resolve your obsessional doubts. Although it may be difficult, try not to fixate on the validity of your doubts during the exercise. The purpose of this practice is not to solve your doubts but to strengthen your ability to distinguish them based on what you've learned. Any effort to seek resolution or reassurance during the exercise undermines its value. Ironically, the more modest your goal, the more beneficial this practice will be.

To practice distinguishing between your own everyday and obsessional doubts, follow the steps outlined below six to eight times a day for at least a week:

Exercise 4.2.
Steps for Knowing the Difference When Doubting

1. **Take Notice:**
   o Take note of the various kinds of doubts you experience throughout the day, especially those that don't immediately seem obsessional.
   o Once you have identified a doubt, proceed to the next step.
2. **Five Questions:**
   o Ask yourself the five familiar questions to determine if the doubt is everyday or obsessional:
      a. *Is there any concrete evidence in the senses for the doubt in the present?*
      b. *Does the doubt occur in an appropriate context?*
      c. *Is the doubt based on a real uncertainty?*
      d. *Does acting on the doubt help to resolve it?*
      e. *Is the doubt rooted in common sense?*
3. **Obsessional or Everyday?**
   o Decide whether the doubt is everyday or obsessional based on your answers to the questions.
   o If you feel unsure at the end, don't worry about it; just take your best guess. The exercise is primarily about taking the time to ask yourself the questions, nothing else.

4. **Imagine:**
   - If you decide it is an obsessional doubt, reflect for a moment on what it would be like if you did not have the doubt.
   - Don't try to resolve your doubt. Just *imagine* what it would be like.
5. **Carry On:**
   - Continue with whatever you normally do.
   - If you had an everyday doubt, address it if it is based on a real uncertainty that can be resolved in the here-and-now.
   - If it was an obsessional doubt, respond as you usually would. The purpose of the exercise is not to try to convince yourself of anything but to go through the steps as described.
   - Use the training card below as a quick reference during your practice to remind you of the steps.

Training Card 4.1.

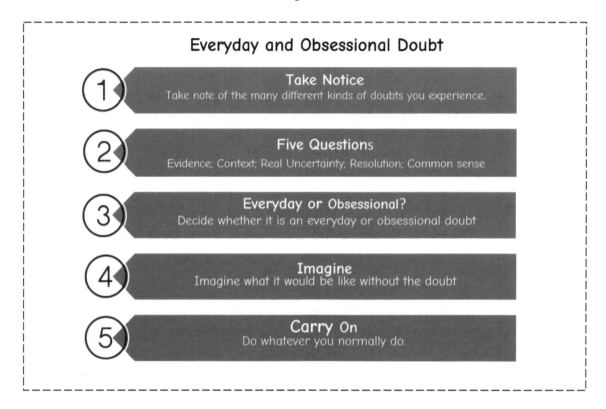

Crafting Obsessions

As you continue practicing, take note of situations and activities where you don't experience any obsessional doubts or recurring worries. Regardless of how severe your OCD may feel, there are always areas in your life untouched by obsessional doubt. These are often activities or situations you enjoy and feel confident about.

Over time, you'll likely notice an increasing number of these doubt-free moments or situations. Each time you identify one, write it down in Form 4.13. To get you started, two examples are already included—though these might not apply to everyone, they assume a non-obsessional context for most people.

Form 4.13.
List of situations and activities that I feel confident about

Ex. Going through my exercise routine	Ex. Making my favorite meal
_____	_____
_____	_____
_____	_____
_____	_____
_____	_____
_____	_____
_____	_____
_____	_____
_____	_____
_____	_____
_____	_____
_____	_____
_____	_____
_____	_____

Once you have collected several situations and activities about which you never experience any obsessional doubts, you are ready to use them for a new and creative exercise. Ask yourself, what has to happen for any of these situations to become obsessional? Just as you previously turned ordinary scenarios into obsessional ones, you can do the same with any situation on your list. All it takes is a little bit of imagination.

Rest assured, this exercise is very unlikely make these situations actually become obsessional. In areas of life where you feel confident and secure, such transformations typically do not occur. The purpose of this activity is not to create new doubts, but to deepen your understanding of how OCD operates. However, if you find that this is happening or if the exercise is causing distress, it is perfectly okay to skip it or choose a different activity instead.

Exercise 4.3.
Steps for Knowing the Difference When Doubting

1. **Select Situations for the Exercise:**
   o   Once you have collected several situations and activities where you never experience obsessional doubts, pick two from your list in Form 4.13.
2. **Imagine Obsessional Scenarios:**
   o   Ask yourself what has to happen for these situations to become obsessional.
   o   Just as you previously turned ordinary scenarios into obsessional ones, apply the characteristics that define obsessional doubts (i.e., lack of concrete evidence, out-of-context occurrence, no real certainty, no resolution, and lack of common sense).
3. **Write Out the Scenarios:**
   o   Use Forms 4.14 and 4.15 to write out the scenarios involving a person experiencing obsessional doubts and compulsions in these situations.
   o   Be creative and have some fun with it! It's okay to come up with silly scenarios, as this is often how it feels when dealing with areas of life where you are confident.
4. **Review Examples for Guidance:**
   o   To get you started, two examples are listed in appendix F. Use these as a guide to help you craft your scenarios.

By following these steps, you will gain a deeper understanding of how OCD can turn ordinary situations into obsessional ones. This exercise will help you recognize and challenge your own OCD patterns creatively and effectively. Embrace this process and have fun with it!

Form 4.14. Crafting Obsessions

First Situation or Activity: _____

Title: _____

_____

_____

_____

_____

_____

_____

_____

_____

_____

_____

_____

_____

_____

_____

_____

_____

_____

_____

_____

_____

Form 4.15. Crafting Obsessions

Second Situation or Activity: _____

Title: _____

_____

_____

_____

_____

_____

_____

_____

_____

_____

_____

_____

_____

_____

_____

_____

_____

_____

_____

_____

_____

Once you've completed Exercise 4.3, feel free to continue practicing throughout the day without needing to write everything down. You can easily adapt the exercise to your mind, using a little imagination to create and analyze obsessional doubts on the spot. After all, if imagination can fuel obsessional doubts, it can just as easily be used to practice recognizing and managing them.

This mental practice will help sharpen your awareness of when obsessional thoughts arise, deepen your understanding of their key characteristics, and improve your ability to manage symptoms. It can also boost your confidence in handling OCD while fostering a more objective perspective on your doubts, reducing their emotional intensity. Engaging in this way can provide some much-needed distance from your OCD, all while adding a touch of lightheartedness to the process.

However, fully eliminating obsessional doubts requires more than just recognizing or distinguishing them. They are not resolved by "just using common sense" or quick fixes. Obsessional doubts don't emerge out of nowhere—they are rooted in deep-seated reasoning patterns and imaginative distortions. Exploring and addressing these underlying mechanisms is the focus of the next major section in this volume: the inner wheel of OCD.

PART 3

The Inner Wheel

Chapter 5

The Obsessional Narrative

The outer wheel of OCD spins fast and furious, a relentless force driving compulsive behaviors and obsessional thoughts. You can try to stop it by resisting your compulsions, but this can be hard to sustain. You might attempt to get used to all the uncertainty and anxiety, but not everyone can. You can try to divert your attention elsewhere, but the obsession will continue to nag at you. You can even attempt to accept the obsession, but you'll be accepting something that does not deserve acceptance. None of these approaches offer real solutions.

The outer wheel is not easily stopped through direct intervention. It has tremendous velocity, making it powerful and difficult to halt. Trying to stop it is like throwing a stick at a spinning wheel, hoping it won't ricochet and hit you in the face. Often, this is exactly what happens. The more you try to fight it, the harder the OCD snaps back. Each attempt to directly stop the outer wheel can feel like a losing battle, exhausting your mental and emotional energy. Its momentum seems unstoppable, and resisting it directly often reinforces the very cycle you're trying to break. This leads to frustration and an overwhelming sense of helplessness.

Yet, despite its overwhelming presence, the outer wheel is merely a symptom of a deeper process. Real change doesn't come from attacking the surface-level problem but from addressing the underlying causes. Focusing solely on the outer wheel perpetuates the struggle. A more effective question to ask is: *Where does the outer wheel get its momentum?*

The outer wheel is not a miraculous perpetual motion machine—it doesn't drive itself. Its relentless energy comes from the inner wheel of OCD. Like any true inner wheel, the inner wheel moves slower than the outer one. However, what it lacks in speed, it makes up for in force, equal to the power of the outer wheel. This makes the inner wheel a far better target for intervention. Unlike the outer wheel, the inner wheel has less velocity, so interventions are far less likely to ricochet. A well-placed spoke in the inner wheel can bring the outer wheel to a complete halt. It may even destroy both wheels, permanently breaking the cycle of OCD.

The inner wheel is composed of three interconnected components, each playing a vital role in sustaining the obsessive-compulsive cycle:

1. **The Obsessional Narrative** – The story that provides context and plausibility to your obsessional doubt.

2. **Obsessional Reasoning Processes** – The patterns of thought that transform hypothetical fears into perceived probabilities.
3. **The Feared Possible Self** – An imagined identity one dreads becoming, adding emotional and personal significance to obsessional doubts.

These components work in unison, each reinforcing the other and sustaining the momentum that powers the outer wheel of OCD. *The obsessional narrative* provides a backdrop, painting a picture in which your doubts seem credible and emotionally charged. *Obsessional reasoning processes* are what makes you treat the obsessional doubt as a real probability rather than recognizing it as a mere hypothetical possibility. *The feared possible self* adds emotional weight and personal significance to these doubts, amplifying the urgency to engage in compulsions to avoid.

Diagram 5.1.
The Inner Wheel of OCD

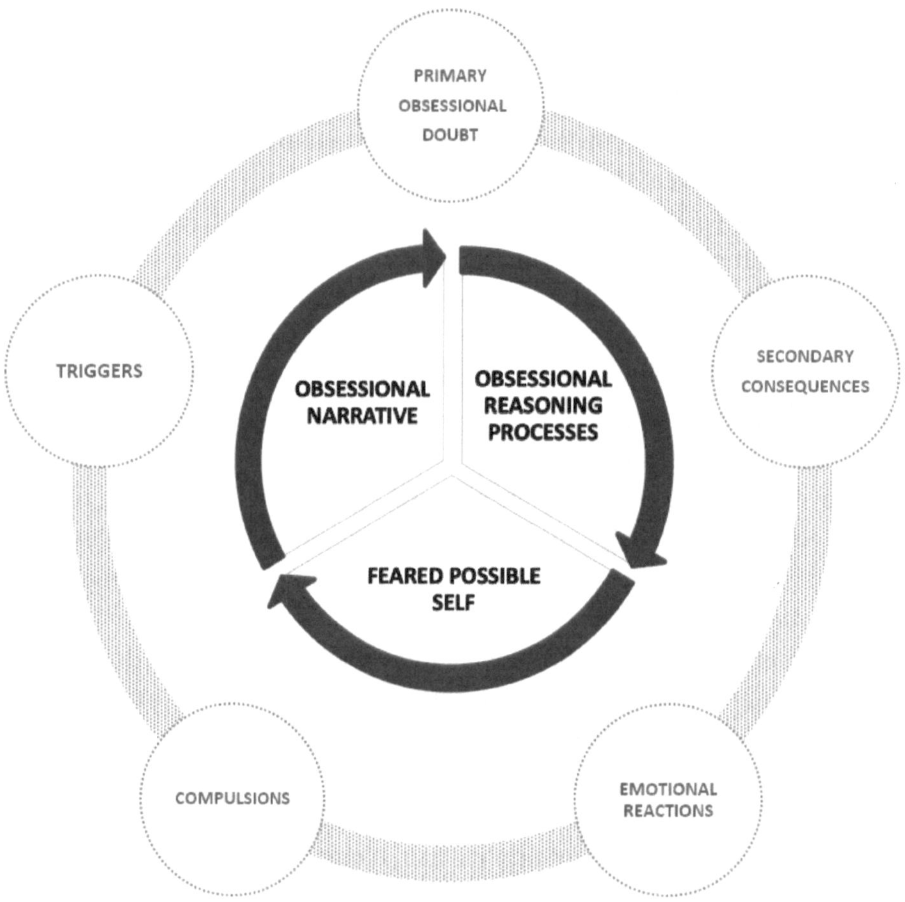

Understanding the components of the inner wheel is essential because they are the true source of the intensity, frequency, and persistence of the obsessional doubt driving the outer wheel. The outer wheel merely maintains the momentum it receives from the inner wheel. Targeting this core driver allows you to address the root causes of OCD, breaking the cycle of obsession and compulsion. This is where real, lasting change begins: disassembling the inner wheel disrupts the process that sustains obsessions and compulsions. Once the inner wheel slows or stops, the outer wheel naturally loses its force, becoming easier to manage—or even irrelevant.

This chapter begins by examining the inner wheel's intricate dynamics, starting with its first major component: the obsessional narrative. Understanding this narrative and how it fuels your doubts empowers you to dismantle the power of OCD from within.

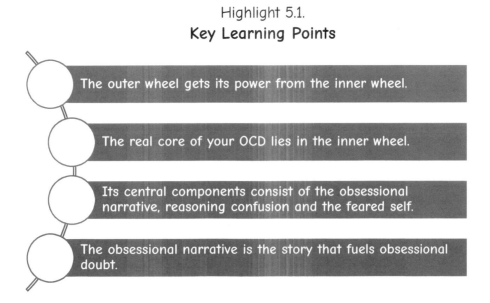

Highlight 5.1.
Key Learning Points

The outer wheel gets its power from the inner wheel.

The real core of your OCD lies in the inner wheel.

Its central components consist of the obsessional narrative, reasoning confusion and the feared self.

The obsessional narrative is the story that fuels obsessional doubt.

Intruders or Unwanted Residents?

Obsessions—the intrusive and persistent thoughts that characterize OCD—often seem to appear suddenly and without warning, disrupting daily life with their intensity. They feel as if they emerge out of nowhere, alien to you, as though they are intruders in your mind. However, a closer examination reveals that these obsessional doubts do not arise randomly. They are generated from within, by you, even if they feel disconnected from your sense of self.

Many people with OCD express sentiments like, "I know it makes no sense, but I still can't get rid of the thought," as though the obsession has no logical basis. At first glance, this may seem true. However, with introspection, most individuals with OCD can uncover reasoning behind their doubts. This reasoning might not be obvious at first, but it is not hidden or unconscious. By paying closer attention, the thought patterns that fuel these obsessions can often be identified.

A critical step in understanding obsessions is to view them not as random intrusions, but as challenges to reality—expressions of doubt about what might or could be true. This perspective shifts the focus from seeing obsessions as meaningless disruptions to recognizing them as the result of a cognitive process. While this reasoning is often distorted or biased, it follows a logical progression: specific premises lead to specific conclusions.

For example, obsessive thoughts about contamination are not random fixations on germs. They stem from an internal logic—a belief about how contamination might occur, why it might be harmful, or how it might spread. Understanding this reasoning reveals the cognitive patterns that generate and sustain these doubts.

When you start to see your obsessions as doubts or conclusions with reasoning behind them, you gain the ability to change how you interact with these thoughts. Instead of feeling helpless and at the mercy of intrusive thoughts, you can address the reasoning that gives rise to them. By viewing these doubts as unwanted residents, rather than intruders appearing out of nowhere, you can tackle the root cause of your obsessional doubts, reducing their impact—or potentially eliminating them altogether.

This transformation begins with being able identify reasons and justifications behind obsessional doubts across all forms of OCD.

Highlight 5.2.
Key Learning Points

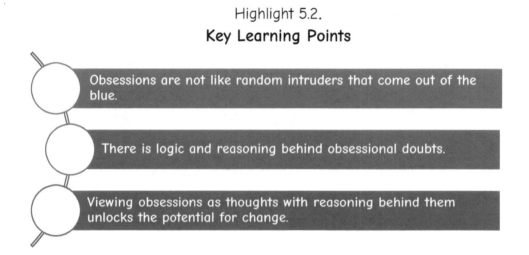

Obsessions are not like random intruders that come out of the blue.

There is logic and reasoning behind obsessional doubts.

Viewing obsessions as thoughts with reasoning behind them unlocks the potential for change.

Uncovering Reasons Behind Obsessional Doubt

OCD is not a disorder of randomness but one of misdirected logic and reasoning. People with OCD experience doubts and fears that, while seemingly irrational to others, are supported by their own internal logic. This logic can be so compelling that it feels impossible to argue against.

Take, for example, someone who has the obsessional doubt that their food might be poisoned. Instead of dismissing this fear outright, ask: *On what basis would someone think their food is poisoned?* The goal is not to find psychological explanations, such as paranoia, but to identify justifications based on logical inference. As shown in Table 5.1, there are many such reasons.

For example, someone might reason, "People sometimes tamper with food," or "Food poisoning happens in restaurants, so it could happen to me." These conclusions stem from real-world possibilities and past experiences. While the logic may not reflect the actual probability of the event, it feels compelling because it follows an internal framework rooted that makes the doubt seem plausible.

By identifying and examining these reasons, you can reframe the obsessional doubt—shifting it from an inexplicable thought to a conclusion grounded in your internal logic. These thoughts may feel disconnected from reality, but they follow a reasoning process that makes sense to the person experiencing them.

It's important to note that uncovering the logic behind your doubts doesn't mean those doubts are true. It simply highlights that they are not as random as they might initially seem. More importantly, recognizing the internal logic behind obsessional doubts gives you the ability to question their validity and weaken their hold. Dissecting the reasoning that sustains these thoughts opens the door to meaningful change. The goal isn't to dismiss obsessions as merely irrational but to understand the reasoning behind them, so you can gradually shift that reasoning over time.

Table 5.1.
Potential reasons behind an obsessional doubt

Primary Inference of Doubt *"My food might be poisonous"*

Abstract facts and ideas — Things that you know or believe to be true in general.

a. Contaminated and poisoned food is being recalled all the time.
b. Medication has tamper proof packaging yet most foods do not.
c. There are slow-acting poisons you cannot even feel or detect.
d. Everyone can access and poison unsecured food products in the supermarket.
e. Food contamination can occur at any point in the supply chain.

Personal experience — Your own personal experience, past or present

a. I once got very sick after eating out and I still don't know exactly why.
b. I have seen food being prepared next to commercial cleaning products.
c. I once bought food that smelled off and had to throw it away.
d. I found a foreign object in my food once.
e. I have a family member who got food poisoning from improperly stored food.

Values, standards and rules — The way of doing things according to an accepted principle.

a. Better safe than sorry.
b. Food has to be prepared correctly to prevent any poisoning.
c. You're not supposed to buy food in damaged packaging.
d. It's a rule to always wash fruits and vegetables before eating.
e. Avoiding food from untrusted sources is a standard precaution.

Authorities — A person, institution or organization that is perceived as important.

a. A famous doctor advised to be alert to any signs of positioning.
b. There's a national poison help hotline for a reason.
c. Health organizations regularly warn about foodborne illnesses.
d. Government agencies have stringent regulations to prevent food poisoning.
e. Food safety experts often emphasize the importance of being vigilant about potential contamination.

Hearsay and news — Information that you got from other people, substantiated or not.

a. I heard of medications being poisoned by someone.
b. My friend once told me he saw pesticides being sold right next to food.
c. I saw on the news that there is a terrorist threat aimed at poisoning food.
d. A neighbor mentioned hearing about a local food contamination incident.
e. Social media often reports on food recalls due to contamination.

Anything else — Anything that does not fit well in the previous categories

a. My intuition tells me it could happen.
b. Just by chance it is bound to happen eventually.
c. I would not have the thought if there was nothing to it.
d. My dreams sometimes feature scenarios of food being poisoned.
e. It just feels very real to me.

Before exploring the reasons behind your own doubts, it can be helpful to start by examining those of others. This exercise serves two purposes: it prepares you to identify your own reasoning later and demonstrates that even seemingly nonsensical obsessions are rooted in an underlying logic. Observing how reasoning drives others' obsessions can provide valuable insight into the processes fueling your own doubts.

Examining others' obsessions also creates emotional distance, allowing you to see how even illogical fears often have a structured basis in reasoning. While the content of their doubts might seem extreme or irrelevant, the reasoning process is often highly systematic. This perspective can help you approach your own obsessions with greater clarity and objectivity.

Exercise 5.1.
Identifying Reasons behind Obsessional doubts

1. **Select a Neutral Case:**
   o   Select a case vignette from Chapter 1 with an obsessional theme that feels neutral.
2. **Retrieve and Prepare Form 5.1:**
   o   Write the name of the individual at the top of each form.
   o   Refer to Appendix C, where the condensed primary doubt of the case is listed.
   o   Write down the condensed primary doubt of each case at the top of Form 5.1.
   o   If there is more than one primary condensed doubt, note both at the top of the form; they are usually similar enough to be analyzed together.
3. **Carefully Reread the Case Description:**
   o   Pay close attention to the justification behind the primary doubt.
   o   Identify and list any reasons you can find behind the primary doubt using Form 5.1.
   o   Expect to find only a limited number of reasons in the initial case descriptions.
4. **Generate Additional Reasons:**
   o   Come up with additional reasons for the primary obsessional doubt of up to three in each category. Add these to the form as well.
   o   Don't worry about correctly categorizing each reason. The categories are only there to help you generate ideas.
5. **Reflection:**
   o   Reflect on the reasons you have identified and added. Consider how these reasons contribute to the plausibility of the obsessional doubt and what patterns of thought they reveal. By understanding the reasoning behind obsessional doubts, you gain insight into how these thoughts are constructed and maintained.
6. **Choose Second Case**
   o   Select another case with an obsessional theme that resonates more personally or deeply. However, ensure that this case not involve exactly the same primary doubts you experience.
   o   Repeat steps one through six, documenting your reasons in Form 5.2.
7. **Optional**
   o   If you feel you need more practice, do not hesitate to list reasons behind the obsessional doubts of the other cases. Possible answers for each case are provided in Appendix G.
   o   Alternatively, just read through the reasons of each case in Appendix G. You may recognize a few that apply to your own doubts as well.

Form 5.1. First Case : _____
Potential reasons behind obsessional doubts

Condensed Primary Doubt(s)
....
....

Abstract facts and ideas — Things that you know or believe to be true in general.

    a. ....

    b. ....

    c. ....

Personal experience — Your own personal experience, past or present

    a. ....

    b. ....

    c. ....

Values, standards and rules — The way of doing things according to an accepted principle.

    a. ....

    b. ....

    c. ....

Authorities — A person, institution or organization that is perceived as important.

    a. ....

    b. ....

    c. ....

Hearsay and news — Information that you got from other people, substantiated or not.

    a. ....

    b. ....

    c. ....

Anything else — Anything that does not fit well in the previous categories

    a. ....

    b. ....

    c. ....

Form 5.2. Second Case : _____

Potential reasons behind obsessional doubts

Condensed Primary Doubt(s)
....
....
Abstract facts and ideas — Things that you know or believe to be true in general.
a. ....
b. ....
c. ....
Personal experience — Your own personal experience, past or present
a. ....
b. ....
c. ....
Values, standards and rules — The way of doing things according to an accepted principle.
a. ....
b. ....
c. ....
Authorities — A person, institution or organization that is perceived as important.
a. ....
b. ....
c. ....
Hearsay and news — Information that you got from other people, substantiated or not.
a. ....
b. ....
c. ....
Anything else — Anything that does not fit well in the previous categories
a. ....
b. ....
c. ....

Identifying Your Own Reasons

As you've seen, it's relatively easy to come up with reasons for someone else's obsessional doubts. This is because anyone can think of reasons why something might be true. Now, imagine if OCD had to actually prove its doubts were true with certainty——it would face a much harder task.

However, OCD doesn't need to prove anything. It only needs to create doubt, and reasons to do so are plentiful. Many of these reasons are even true or factual. This "low-effort" strategy ensures OCD never runs out of justifications.

But what about the reasons behind your own obsessional doubts? Is it just as easy to uncover them? This varies from person to person. Some people with OCD can quickly generate long lists of reasons why their doubts might be real, while others struggle to identify even a few. If you find yourself unable to come up with reasons, it's important to examine what might be blocking you.

Difficulties with Identifying Reasons

Avoid Freudian Analysis

One reason you might struggle to identify reasons behind your obsessional doubts is by confusing this task with uncovering the ultimate cause of your OCD. This misunderstanding can make the process feel overwhelming and unproductive. It's important to clarify that identifying reasons is not about discovering why you developed OCD or pinpointing its origins. Instead, it's about focusing on the present—on the specific thoughts and ideas that currently justify your doubts.

When we talk about the "reasons" for your doubt, we are not referring to childhood experiences, past traumas, or other deep psychological roots. Our goal is not to delve into distant causes but to address the immediate justifications that make your doubt feel plausible right now. These are the "reasons" you rely on in the moment to support the belief that your doubt might be true.

People often confuse these immediate reasons with broader explanations for OCD, thinking that uncovering past events might clarify its origins. While understanding such events can be valuable in broader therapy, they are not our focus here. What matters now is identifying the current reasoning process that keeps your doubt alive. Focusing on these immediate justifications helps you break the cycle of doubt without getting bogged down in distant causes, which rarely offer actionable insights.

It's also important to recognize the risks of becoming preoccupied with ultimate explanations for OCD. Seeking a single "root cause," whether tied to past experiences or psychological theories, can lead to endless rumination without practical results. This pursuit often mirrors the same compulsive patterns involved in trying to resolve doubts. By chasing the idea that discovering an ultimate cause will cure OCD, you risk reinforcing the very patterns you're trying to overcome.

> Reasons are justifications for your obsessional doubts, not their ultimate cause.

However, there are exceptions. If a specific past event directly relates to your current doubt—such as a traumatic experience that seems to make your doubt feel more real—it's relevant to explore as part of the reasoning behind your doubt. For example, if a past car accident justifies your current fear of driving, that event is a relevant reason to consider. But this is distinct from viewing the event as the ultimate cause of your OCD.

It's also essential to differentiate reasons from evidence or proof. The "reasons" we focus on are not definitive proof that your doubt is valid. Instead, they are the thoughts or justifications that make the doubt feel plausible in the moment. For example, if you doubt whether the stove is off, your reasons might include hearing a story about a house fire or recalling a time you nearly forgot to turn it off. These reasons make the doubt feel possible but don't confirm it as true.

Additionally, the reasoning behind obsessional doubts is not always logical. It can often be based on emotional responses rather than facts. For instance, you might feel anxious about locking the door and interpret that feeling as a reason to doubt, even without actual evidence. This shows how emotions, rather than facts, can shape the reasoning behind doubt.

Ultimately, the reasons we aim to identify are anything that justifies your doubt in the moment. By isolating these immediate justifications, you can address the processes sustaining your obsessions and free yourself from distractions tied to deeper, less actionable explanations.

Intrusiveness and Emotional Intensity

As discussed earlier, the intrusive nature of obsessional doubts often makes them feel overwhelming and uncontrollable. When combined with emotional intensity, this intrusiveness can make identifying the reasons behind your doubts particularly challenging. These doubts often appear suddenly and forcefully, disrupting your mental peace and daily activities. Their urgency demands immediate attention, leaving little room for reflection or analysis.

The emotional distress generated by these doubts adds another layer of difficulty. Anxiety and panic can shift your focus entirely to managing the immediate discomfort rather than exploring the reasoning behind the doubt itself. This reactive pattern often leads to compulsive behaviors aimed at neutralizing the doubt, which only reinforces the cycle. As a result, there's little opportunity to step back and thoughtfully examine the underlying justifications sustaining the doubt.

To address this, try to identify the reasons behind your doubts during moments of relative calm, when OCD is less active and emotional reactions are more subdued. If you find yourself reacting emotionally, refer back to Chapter 3 and practice sequencing. Sequencing helps you break down the obsessional cycle into manageable components—triggers, doubts, emotional reactions, compulsions, and consequences—so you can see the bigger picture more clearly.

By using sequencing, you create the mental space and distance needed to reflect on your doubts and uncover the reasons and justifications behind them. This deliberate approach allows you to engage with your doubts in a calmer, more thoughtful way.

Alienation, Misattribution and Externalization

Obsessional doubts in OCD often feel ego-dystonic, meaning they clash with your self-image, values, and beliefs. Because these thoughts feel so at odds with how you perceive yourself, it can be difficult to accept that they originate internally. This dissonance can make your doubts feel alien or external, as though they don't belong to you.

While you may know intellectually that your obsessions don't literally come from outside of you, it's common to externalize them as if they exist outside the realm of reasoning. You might think, "These thoughts aren't really mine," or, "Something outside of me must be causing these doubts." For example, you might attribute them to a "broken brain" or a "chemical imbalance." This externalization creates a barrier to introspection, shifting your focus away from understanding the internal processes driving your doubts and toward external explanations.

Viewing your thoughts as alien or external can also increase feelings of helplessness. You might feel like a passive victim of these doubts, making it harder to explore the reasons behind them. However, while these thoughts may feel stronger than you, they still originate from within. Acknowledging this is crucial because it means you have some control over them. You cannot begin to challenge these thoughts if you don't accept that you are the one generating them, even if you don't yet fully understand how.

To overcome this, you need to reframe your relationship with your thoughts. Recognize that obsessional doubts, no matter how alien they feel, are still part of your mental experience. This doesn't mean you have to accept them as true or that they reflect something real about you. However, acknowledging that you have reasons for considering them as valid possibilities is key to taking ownership of your thoughts and uncovering the reasoning that sustains them.

Entrenched and Automatic Cognitive Patterns

One of the challenges in identifying the reasons behind your obsessional doubts is that they often operate on autopilot. Much like other habitual behaviors, the reasoning behind your doubts becomes so automatic that it feels invisible. You may assume there are no reasons because you're not consciously thinking about them, but this isn't the case. The reasons are there—they're just so deeply ingrained that they've become hard to see.

Our brains are naturally wired to learn quickly and automate processes. Once learned, we tend to tuck away the reasoning and simply act without further thought. This is an efficient mechanism that allows us to focus on other things. However, it's a mistake to assume that, just because you're not actively thinking about the reasons behind your actions, no reasons exist.

OCD takes advantage of this natural tendency by creating entrenched cognitive patterns. These patterns become habitual, with the reasoning behind your doubts operating automatically and outside your conscious awareness. Over time, the reasoning becomes so ingrained that it feels as though the doubts are happening to you, rather than being generated by your own mind. This entrenchment makes it more difficult to unpack and identify the reasons sustaining your obsessional doubts, leaving the cycle unchecked.

Take, for example, the act of looking in your side-view mirror when changing lanes. You don't actively think through all the reasons for this behavior each time—it's automatic. But if a child were to ask, "Why do you look in the mirror?" you'd explain: "Because I want to change lanes, and there might be a car passing me right now." If pressed further, you might elaborate: "Cars are fast and heavy, so changing lanes without checking could cause an accident." While none of this goes through your mind as you perform the act, the reasoning still exists and drives your behavior.

OCD works in a similar way. Over time, the reasoning behind your doubts and compulsions becomes automatic. For example, you may not consciously think through why your hands feel contaminated or why the door might be unlocked—you simply act on the doubt. This automatization frees up mental space for other tasks but can be problematic when it comes to OCD. By leaving the reasoning unchecked, OCD thrives in the shadows, operating freely without scrutiny.

This is why uncovering the reasons behind your obsessional doubts is so important. It's fine to rely on autopilot for many everyday tasks, but not when OCD is involved. Without recognizing the underlying reasons, your efforts to stop compulsions may feel superficial and ineffective. Forcing yourself to stop a compulsion, like checking the door, won't resolve the sense that something is wrong if the underlying doubt remains unexamined. It's like asking someone to stop looking in the side-view mirror while driving without addressing the reasons why they do it.

To overcome entrenched and automatic cognitive patterns, you need to uncover the "screen of unseen logic" behind your doubts. You've taken the reasons for granted for so long that you've become blind to them. The solution doesn't lie in complex psychological explanations—it's often much simpler. Approach the reasoning as you would explain it to a child. What's the story behind your doubt? It doesn't need to be complicated. In fact, the answers are often obvious once you remove the cloak of unquestioned doubt.

Avoidance and Fear of OCD

When it comes to identifying the reasons behind your obsessional doubts, everyone reacts differently. For some, it's relatively easy—they don't feel overly anxious about exploring the reasons and find it natural to articulate them. Talking about why their doubts feel plausible might even provide relief and validation. Often, this happens because they've been told their doubts are random events that must simply be ignored to improve. Realizing that they can address these doubts without accepting them as meaningless or random can bring significant relief.

However, for others, facing their OCD feels much harder. Avoidance becomes a common coping mechanism to deal with the distress caused by obsessional doubts. You might avoid specific situations, thoughts, or objects that trigger your doubts, finding temporary relief in this avoidance. But this strategy comes with a cost: it prevents you from understanding the triggers and reasoning behind your doubts. Avoidance reinforces the idea that these thoughts are dangerous, which makes them feel even more pervasive and powerful.

Avoidance is especially problematic when it stems from a fear of OCD itself. You might worry that examining the reasons behind your doubts too closely could lead to further distress or confirm your worst fears. This fear often creates a paradox: the very thoughts and doubts you avoid are the ones that need to be understood in order to reduce their power over you.

It's important to remember that identifying the reasons behind your doubts won't make them more real. OCD doesn't deal in certainties—it thrives on doubt. Its goal isn't to confirm your fears as true but to keep you in a state of uncertainty and questioning. Looking closely at your OCD won't lead to some terrifying revelation or uncover "proof" of your doubts. Instead, it will help you recognize that these doubts are fueled by endless "what if" scenarios rather than absolute truths.

Exploring your doubts isn't a descent into a horror story where you risk uncovering a terrible secret. Instead, it's a process of examining your thoughts and recognizing their true nature—an essential step in overcoming them. By identifying the reasons behind your doubts, you open the door to seeing them for what they truly are: conclusions rooted in flawed reasoning, not accurate reflections of reality.

For some, the fear may not center on uncovering reasons in general but on engaging with specific thoughts. You might worry that thinking or writing about certain topics could somehow make them come true. If this feels overwhelming, start small. Gradually approach your doubts and their reasoning in manageable steps. If directly naming your doubts feels too difficult, writing in "code words" can be a helpful starting point. The goal is not to force yourself into distress but to gain insight into the reasons that sustain your fears.

Shame and embarrassment can also make it hard to confront your doubts. These emotions often arise from believing in the potential reality of the doubt. If this resonates with you, approach your shame as you would any other emotion linked to your OCD: acknowledge it without immediately trying to dismiss or validate it. Focus on identifying your reasons during quieter moments, and use tools like sequencing to maintain emotional distance. Remember, your goal is to understand—not to judge yourself.

If fear or avoidance feels too overwhelming, seeking professional help is essential. A therapist experienced in OCD can help you address these challenges, but they need open communication to do so. If discussing your OCD feels too difficult, let your therapist know that you're struggling to talk about it. While they're not clairvoyant, they can guide you once they understand your difficulties. Being open, even in small steps, is key to effective treatment.

Highlight 5.3.
Key Learning Points

Focus on immediate justifications for doubts, not deeper psychological causes.

Intrusive and intense doubts hinder reflection; create mental space to understand them.

Recognizing and questioning automatic cognitive patterns will help to uncover the reasoning behind your doubts.

Identifying reasons won't make your doubts more real, just more manageable.

Methods and Techniques for Identifying Your Reasons

Understanding the reasons behind your obsessional doubts is a crucial step toward managing and overcoming OCD. By examining your doubts, you can gain insight into the reasons and thought patterns that sustain them. This process involves using various techniques to explore and uncover the underlying reasons for your doubts.

The following exercises will guide you through different methods to identify the reasons you have for your own obsessional doubts. Each technique is designed to provide a different perspective, helping you build a comprehensive understanding of your doubts. Many of these techniques can be combined with each other as well.

To uncover the reasons behind your obsessional doubt, approach the process with the right perspective and attitude. Like the previous exercises, these are not intended to resolve your obsessional doubts but to uncover the reasons behind them. Act as if you are looking under the hood of your car—neutrally and calmly observing the parts that drive your OCD without immediately trying to replace or remove them. Be curious rather than trying to fix things all the time. Taking this neutral, observational approach will help prevent emotional reactions from clouding your ability to assess the reasoning behind your doubts. By staying curious and objective, you can gain a clearer understanding of the reasons fueling your obsessional doubts, enabling you to address them more effectively in the future.

Exercise 5.2.

Method 1: Daily Journal and Guided Reflection

This method builds upon the sequencing exercise and involves keeping a daily journal and setting aside time for focused reflection. By regularly documenting your thoughts and systematically questioning your doubts, you can start to uncover the underlying reasons that fuel your obsessional doubts.

1. **Daily Journal:**
   - Keep a daily journal where you record your obsessional doubts
   - Include the other elements in the obsessional sequence: the trigger, consequences, emotions, and compulsions.

2. **Reflection:**
   - Set aside time each day for focused reflection.
   - Review each journal entry to identify justifications and reasons behind each of the doubts.

3. **Questioning Doubts:**
   - If you are not immediately aware of any thoughts or ideas to justify the doubt, ask yourself questions like:
     - *"Why do I think this might be true?"*
     - *"What evidence do I have to support this doubt?"*
     - *"Why does this doubt feel real to me?"*

4. **Meaning of Triggers:**
   - Remember, triggers are never the reason for a doubt.
   - It's what the trigger means to you that connects it to the doubt.

5. **Use Reasoning Categories:**
   - Go through each of the reasoning categories to identify any reasons that resonate with you as a justification for the doubt (facts, ideas, personal experience, hearsay, news, values, standards, authorities, and anything else).

6. **Record Your Reasons:**
   - Record your justifications and reasons for the doubt using Form 5.3.
   - If you have multiple primary condensed doubts within the same theme, list them both at the top of the form, as they are typically similar enough to analyze together.
   - If you have condensed obsessional doubts across different themes, each with distinct reasons, create separate copies of the form and repeat the process for each doubt individually.

7. **Focus on Personalized Reasons:**
   - While Appendix G provides examples, try not to rely too heavily on them. The examples are generic and may not fully capture your unique experience. Instead, aim to come up with your own idiosyncratic reasons that are specific to you and your situation.
   - Write down your reasons no matter how irrational or far-fetched they may seem. Your personal reasoning is key to understanding the logic behind your doubts, even if it feels flawed or embarrassing.
   - Everyone's doubts and reasons are shaped by their own experiences, and there's no such thing as a "wrong" or "shameful" reason in this process. The goal is to bring these reasons into the open, where they can be examined and addressed.

Form 5.3
Reasons Behind my Obsessional Doubt

Condensed Primary Doubt(s)
....
....
Abstract facts and ideas — Things that you know or believe to be true in general.
a. ....
b. ....
c. ....
Personal experience — Your own personal experience, past or present
a. ....
b. ....
c. ....
Values, standards and rules — The way of doing things according to an accepted principle.
a. ....
b. ....
c. ....
Authorities — A person, institution or organization that is perceived as important.
a. ....
b. ....
c. ....
Hearsay and news — Information that you got from other people, substantiated or not.
a. ....
b. ....
c. ....
Anything else — Anything that does not fit well in the previous categories
a. ....
b. ....
c. ....

Exercise 5.3.

Method 2: OCD Unfiltered

In this exercise, you'll engage in a creative and introspective dialogue with your OCD. The aim of this method is to personify your OCD and give it a voice, allowing you to better understand its reasoning and the justifications it uses to sustain your doubts. By creating distance between yourself and your OCD, you can observe its thought patterns more clearly, without feeling the immediate pressure to solve or dismiss the doubts.

1. **Set Up the Dialogue:**
   - *Create an Empty Chair:* Place an empty chair in front of you to represent your OCD.
   - This visual aid can help make the dialogue feel more real and tangible.
   - Imagine your OCD as a separate entity that you can talk to directly.
   - If visual aids are too distracting, try having the dialogue in your mind instead.

2. **Let the OCD Speak Freely:**
   - Allow the OCD to express itself without interruption or immediate judgment.
   - Encourage it to articulate its doubts and fears openly.
   - Give it a free voice for the purpose of the exercise.
   - *Keep the Distance:* Maintain a mental distance between yourself and the OCD. Remember, you are separate from the OCD. Do not try to solve the doubt in any way during this exercise. This helps you observe the OCD without feeling personally involved, making it easier to recognize and identify the reasons behind the doubt more clearly.

3. **Ask Probing Questions:**
   - Pose questions to your OCD to understand its reasoning:
     - "What evidence supports this doubt?"
     - "What evidence contradicts it?"
     - "Why do you believe this doubt might be true?"
     - "What makes this doubt feel real to you?"

4. **Challenge the OCD's Assertions:**
   - Respond to the OCD's statements, questioning and examining its justifications:
     - "Is this evidence concrete or speculative?"
     - "Are there alternative explanations?"
     - "How does this doubt align with what I know to be true?"
   - *Keep OCD Separate:* Challenge its assertions only to gain more information, not to solve the doubt. Let the OCD speak freely without fighting it.

5. **Explore the Justifications:**
   - Delve into the reasoning behind the OCD's assertions.
   - Consider why these justifications seem convincing to the OCD.

6. **Record and Document:**
   - During the exercise, record the reasons supplied by the OCD, either by writing them down or audio-recording your conversation.
   - Use Form 5.3 to list all the reasons and justifications brought up by your OCD.
   - Document every reason, including those you feel embarrassed about. If they sustain your doubt, it's important to recognize and note them. The more reasons you uncover, the clearer the underlying structure of your doubts will become.

Exercise 5.4.
Method 3: Mind Mapping

This method involves creating a visual representation of the reasons behind your doubts. By organizing your thoughts into a mind map, you can see the bigger picture and identify connections between different doubts and reasons. This technique can be particularly effective for those who are visually oriented or find it easier to process information in a non-linear format.

1. **Create a Mind Map:**
   o Start by creating a mind map to visually organize the reasons behind one of your primary doubts.
   o Place your main doubt in the center of the map.
2. **Branch Out:**
   o From the main doubt, draw branches outward for each reason, evidence, or related thought.
   o Use lines, arrows, or connections to show relationships between the reasons surrounding your doubt.
3. **Differentiate Types of Reasons:**
   o Use different colors or symbols to differentiate between types of reasons (e.g., facts, personal experience, hearsay, news, values, standards, authorities,).
   o This helps in visually categorizing and distinguishing the various sources of your doubts.
4. **Use a Suitable Medium:**
   o Choose a medium that works best for you (e.g., app, paper, crayon, pencils, paint).
   o The goal is to create a visual that you can easily refer to and expand upon as needed.
5. **Reflect and Record:**
   o Reflect on the completed mind map.
   o Keep it in the same format, or record the reasons into Form 5.3, depending on your preference.

Exercise 5.5.
Method 4: The Gauntlet

This method involves directly challenging your OCD when you experience an obsessional doubt and feel the urge to engage in compulsions. You confront the doubt with evidence against it as it arises. By challenging and resisting your OCD in the moment, you compel it to respond, often loudly.

It's important to note that debating with your OCD is typically a compulsive activity you should not engage in, as it can strengthen your obsession. However, purposefully engaging in this exercise can quickly uncover the reasons behind your obsessional doubt. This approach is especially useful if you tend to actively avoid your OCD and have difficulty identifying the underlying reasons.

1. **Identify a Moment of Obsessional Doubt:**
   o Recognize when you experience an obsessional doubt.
2. **Resist, Challenge and Listen:**
   o Hold off on engaging with your compulsions, reminding yourself that if there are truly no reasons behind the doubt, then there's no need to act on it.
   o Try to refute the doubt by coming with evidence against the doubt.

- o Listen to the arguments of the OCD in response.
- o Continue to resist and debate the OCD to gain further insights into its reasoning.
3. **Document Your Findings:**
   - o Record all the reasons and justifications in a notebook or journal.
   - o Transfer the reasons to Form 5.3 to organize your findings systematically.

From Reason to Reasoning: The Obsessional Narrative

You should now have identified a number of reasons and justifications behind your obsessional doubt. It shows that these doubts originate within you, and there are reasons you have for having them. However, obsessional doubts are not justified by a static list of reasons that exist in isolation from each other. Instead, they are part of a dynamic and interconnected narrative that weaves together various thoughts and justifications. This is the *obsessional narrative* – the first major element in the inner wheel that gives your obsessional doubts their credibility.

Diagram 5.2.
From Reasons to Narrative

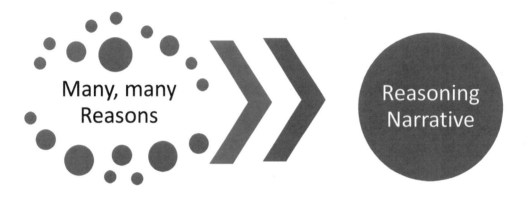

Disjointed reasons justifying
the obsessional doubt

The "narrative unit" linking up the
reasons leading up to the
obsessional doubt

A narrative is simply a story with a beginning, middle, and end. We all live within our own stories, consisting of our past, present, and future. These narratives help us make sense of the world, guiding our decisions and providing context and meaning. We understand where we come from and where we are headed, always existing in the middle of our stories. It is through narratives how we make sense of the world and our position within it. They provide context and meaning, showing the flow of events that make up our daily lives. While we might simplify our stories, or abbreviate them in communication, we cannot live without them.

For example, if I asked how you arrived at your vacation destination, you might say, "by plane," "by train," or "by boat." However, if this was really all that you remembered, you would be concerned. Your entire journey to the vacation spot, described in detail, makes up a complete story. Similarly, if I asked someone to describe their experience of cooking dinner, and they only remembered, "I made pasta," without recalling buying ingredients, preparing the food, or setting the table, it would be worrying. We need the story for the memory to make sense. We need these stories to fill in the gaps and make the experience coherent.

The stories we tell ourselves also give credibility to our beliefs and doubts. Without a reasoning narrative behind them, they wouldn't be very convincing or credible. For instance, if I simply say, "There's someone living in your attic," you probably won't believe me. But if I add, "I heard footsteps and faint whispers coming from the attic last night," you might start to feel convinced. If I continue with, "I read in the news that a man in the neighborhood has been reported missing, and some people think he might be hiding in attics to avoid being found," your belief in the story grows stronger. Notice that in all these scenarios, no one actually saw the person. Yet, the dynamic nature of the narrative—its plots and subplots—makes it persuasive.

Obsessional narratives work similarly. They encompass all the reasons that justify your obsessional doubt, forming the "why" behind your doubts. These narratives are not just a random collection of reasons but a coherent, albeit distorted, story that makes the obsessional doubt seem plausible, real, and urgent. The strength of the obsessional narrative lies in how it blends together different elements— abstract facts, personal experiences, and hypothetical scenarios—into a compelling storyline that pushes you toward compulsive actions.

For example, someone with contamination fears might create a vivid story about contracting a deadly disease from touching a doorknob. Such a narrative might blend together abstract facts, such as the knowledge that germs can survive on surfaces for extended periods, with specific information from news reports about outbreaks of contagious illnesses. Past experiences, like remembering a time they got sick after touching something in a public place, further fuel the narrative. Additionally, hypothetical scenarios, such as imagining what could happen if they didn't wash their hands immediately, add to the sense of urgency.

This intricate story is what makes the doubt feel not only reasonable but also compelling, pushing the person to take immediate action to mitigate the perceived threat. The power of the narrative lies in its ability to combine various elements into a convincing whole. The person's mind weaves together factual information, personal history, and imaginative possibilities, creating a narrative that feels both realistic and pressing. It is this compelling story that drives the obsessional doubt, strong enough to set the entire outer wheel in motion.

The Bridging Role of Narrative

Obsessional narratives drive the obsessional doubt and act as the bridge connecting external triggers or stimuli to the doubt. They make doubts feel real and urgent, even in the absence of immediate, tangible evidence. By filling the gaps between what is perceived and what is feared, they create a sense of continuity and plausibility.

Diagram 5.3 presents a very short and simplified reasoning narrative to demonstrate how narratives bridge the sensory gap from the initial trigger ("living in an old house") to the primary obsessional doubt ("my drinking water might contain lead"). By connecting the initial trigger to the obsessional doubt, the narrative makes the doubt seem credible and plausible even without direct concrete evidence for the threat.

Diagram 5.3.
Narrative Bridging Sensory Gaps

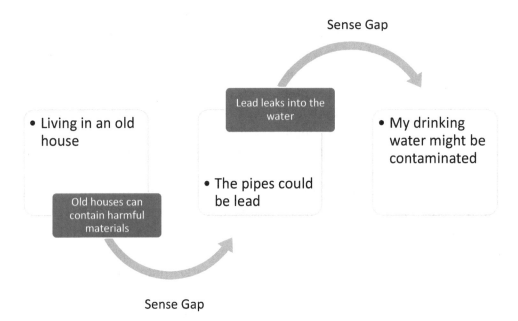

Bridging can apply to any unconnected statements, no matter how seemingly far apart. It starts with one statement and creates a series of believable events that connect it to the final statement. This way, the two statements form a seamless story with detail and flow, making the connection seem convincing.

For example, let's take the following pair of statements:

- "The light bulb was flickering."
- "Jane forgot to water the plants."

On the surface, none of these statements appear to have anything to do with each other. Yet, a bridging story is able to seamlessly connect one with the other. For example:

> Bridging story: "The light bulb was flickering because there was a problem with the electrical wiring. Jane was so preoccupied with fixing the flickering light that she forgot to water the plants."

Obviously, what creates the link between these seemingly unrelated sentences is the story, which literally fills up, or bridges the gap, between them. The richer and more detailed the bridge, the stronger the link seems.

The obsessional narrative works in the same way, except that it links up direct sensory perception with an obsessional doubt. Perception and doubt may contradict each other, but the OCD story links them together.

For example, consider these statements:

- "I see the stove is off."
- "It could still be on."

OCD bridging story: "I see the stove is off, but the control knob might be malfunctioning. Sometimes knobs can appear to be off but still let gas through. Just because it looks off doesn't mean it actually is. So, the stove could still be on.""

In reality, obsessional narratives are much longer and more complex, but they function similarly. For example, let's consider the obsessional doubt "My food might be poisonous" with the previously identified reasons to justify the doubt (see Table 5.1).

A more complete obsessional narrative that integrates and weaves together all these reasons into a compelling storyline could look something like this:

Obsessional Narrative
"Why My Food Might Be Poisonous"

Every time I sit down to eat, a familiar dread creeps into my mind: What if my food is poisonous? It's usually in the evening, after a long day at work. I'm sitting at my kitchen table, the warm glow of the overhead light casting soft shadows around the room. The aroma of freshly cooked food fills the air. There is nothing visibly wrong with the food, but the doubt still creeps in. Could something have happened to the food I prepared?

I know that food poisoning is a real threat. People have fallen ill, and some have even died due to contaminated food. Unlike medications, which come in tamper-proof packaging, most foods don't have this level of protection, making them vulnerable to tampering. Then there are the slow-acting poisons that you can't see or feel immediately, making the threat even more insidious.

I remember the time I got violently sick after eating out. To this day, I don't know what caused it, but that memory lingers, making me question every bite I take. I once saw on television that food was prepared next to commercial cleaning products, and maybe that's what happened to me. I can clearly envision those chemicals spilling carelessly onto the food—an image that has stuck in my mind. Then there was that one person who threatened me once—could they have somehow followed through in a sinister way?

"You can't be too careful with food," I tell myself. It must be prepared perfectly to prevent poisoning. I remember warnings about avoiding food with damaged packaging because it might indicate tampering. Every time I see a dented can or torn box, my anxiety spikes. I know food must be handled properly to avoid contamination, and I scrutinize every step of the process, constantly on edge.

I've always been diligent about food hygiene, making sure to wash everything thoroughly before cooking. But what if I missed something without realizing it? What if I wasn't as careful as I thought, and harmful bacteria remain on the food?

Food can be contaminated in countless ways. The water I'm using to cook might be poisoned or contain pollutants. Or what if the utensils I'm using are contaminated, even though they appear clean? Food is so exposed, with hundreds of people passing by it, having full access to tamper with it if they wanted to. It's like trusting your life to hundreds of strangers. Who would do that? It's a miracle that nothing has happened before now.

I can't ignore the experts who emphasize vigilance. A well-known doctor advised always being alert for signs of poisoning, and the existence of a national poison help hotline only reinforces my fear. Contaminated and poisoned food gets recalled all the time, a constant reminder that the threat is real and ongoing. Health organizations and government agencies regularly issue warnings about foodborne illnesses, highlighting the seriousness of the risk.

I hear stories that only add fuel to the fire. I've heard of medications being poisoned, and a friend told me once that pesticides were being sold right next to food. The news is filled with reports of terrorist threats targeting food supplies. Even my neighbor mentioned a local food contamination incident. Social media is constantly buzzing with food recalls due to contamination. These stories make my fears feel justified and tangible.

My intuition screams that it could happen, and by sheer chance, it's bound to occur eventually. I wouldn't have these thoughts if they weren't grounded in reality, right? "Better safe than sorry," I think, as I inspect every meal meticulously. I once saw a TV show where food was poisoned, and it keeps replaying in my mind. Sometimes, my dreams feature scenarios of food being poisoned, blurring the line between fiction and my waking fears. I've even read fictional books where poisoning played a central role, and those stories have embedded themselves into my thoughts, making the fear seem all the more real.

Every meal becomes a battleground. I scrutinize each bite, looking for signs of tampering, whether or not the food smells and tastes normal. Sometimes, I can almost see or taste the poison in the food, which only makes me more certain that something is wrong. My heart races if anything seems even slightly off. The thought of what might be in my food overshadows everything else. And even if I don't feel sick afterward, I still can't be sure the food wasn't poisoned—it might just be a slow-acting poison. The poison could be building up in my cells slowly, completely undetectable. In fact, many food poisonings go unnoticed, so if I feel fine after eating, that could actually mean I was poisoned.

What if my food is poisoned? This doubt spins in my mind, leading to terrifying consequences: I might fall gravely ill, or worse, die. I can vividly imagine hospital visits, severe health complications, or even death. The fear stretches further—what if I'm responsible for an outbreak that causes harm to others? The anxiety becomes overwhelming, triggering intense fear and dread.

To manage this fear, I wash my hands obsessively before handling any food. I inspect every item meticulously, avoiding eating out whenever I can. I constantly seek reassurance from others, asking if they think the food looks safe. I check labels and expiration dates repeatedly, making sure nothing seems off. Sometimes, I even throw away perfectly good food, just in case. The anxiety, compulsions, and constant vigilance overshadow every meal, transforming what should be a simple source of nourishment into a continuous source of dread and suspicion.

As you can see, a story is far more powerful in making an obsessional doubt feel real than isolated reasons alone. It's not just the reasons themselves that create a sense of urgency and distress—it's how they are woven into a cohesive, emotionally charged narrative. When reasons are considered in isolation, they may seem less compelling. But when strung together as part of a larger story, they give the obsessional doubt a sense of plausibility and immediacy. The narrative structure breathes life into the doubt, making it feel both rational and urgent.

This obsessional narrative fuels not only the primary obsessional doubt itself but also the spiraling process that leads to anxiety and compulsive behaviors in the outer wheel. Once the initial doubt is accepted as plausible, the mind begins exploring secondary consequences and related fears. This escalation amplifies the sense of urgency, driving emotional responses like anxiety and dread, which in turn lead to compulsions as an attempt to reduce the growing fear.

While the narrative may feel most intense in its later stages—where emotional distress and compulsive behaviors take hold—it is the initial phase that sets the entire process in motion. The gap between the initial stimulus and the first seeds of doubt is where the real groundwork for OCD symptoms begins. Once this foundation is established within the inner wheel, the narrative expands, feeding secondary doubts and compulsive responses that define the later stages of the cycle.

Therefore, the elements of the narrative that connect the initial stimulus to the first moments of doubt are the most critical. It is in this early phase of reasoning that obsessional thoughts gain traction, transforming from abstract possibilities into fully formed doubts. Understanding this progression is essential for recognizing how obsessional doubts grow and why they feel so difficult to control. By addressing this foundational stage, we can begin to disrupt the cycle before it spirals into the emotional and compulsive patterns that follow.

Diagram 5.4.
The Bridging Role of Narrative

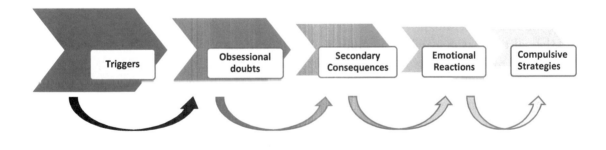

Exercise 5.6.

Creating Obsessional Narratives

This exercise will help you practice constructing an obsessional narrative by using the reasons identified for the obsessional doubts of someone else. Building upon the previous exercise where you identified reasons for two cases, you will now create a detailed obsessional story for the same individual. This practice will enhance your understanding of how the reasons behind obsessional doubts are woven into compelling narratives.

1. **Start with the First Case:**
   - o   Select the first case you previously analyzed in Exercise 5.1.
   - o   Get Form 5.4 ready and write down the name and primary condensed doubt(s) of the person at the top.
2. **Gather All Materials:**
   - o   Retrieve all information available about the case, including the case description in chapter 1 and Appendix B.
   - o   Retrieve the reasons from your answers in Form 5.1 as well as those in Appendix G.
   - o   Review these reasons to ensure you have a comprehensive list.
3. **Write in the First Person:**
   - o   Write the entire narrative in the first person ("I") to make it more compelling.
   - o   Putting yourself in the shoes of the person will help you better understand and convey the emotions and thoughts driving the obsessional doubt.
   - o   Writing out one obsessional narrative is usually sufficient, even if there is more than one primary condensed doubt.
4. **Set the Scene:**
   - o   Describe the context in which the triggers occur for the selected individual.
   - o   Include details about their surroundings, the time of day, who they are with, and any other relevant factors.
   - o   Ensure your description is vivid and detailed to create a clear picture of the scenario.
5. **Develop the Arc of the Story:**
   - o   Use all the reasons you've identified to build a cohesive narrative that connects the initial triggers to the resulting obsessional doubt.
   - o   *Arc of the Story*: This is where the reasons build upon each other, creating a compelling progression that leads up to the primary inference of doubt. The arc shows how various elements come together, lead up to the primary doubt and make it feel plausible and pressing.
   - o   Incorporate the reasons into the storyline, blending abstract facts, past experiences, hearsay, rules, and information from authorities.
   - o   Write in a way that shows how these reasons build upon each other, leading up to the primary inference of doubt and giving it credibility.
   - o   *Important Note*: The arc of the story should make up the majority of the text of the entire narrative (two-thirds or more)
6. **Build the Climax and Describe the Immediate Response:**
   - o   Introduce hypothetical scenarios that illustrate the potential consequences of not addressing the doubt.

- o Make these scenarios vivid and detailed, reflecting the worst-case outcomes the individual imagines.
- o Emphasize the emotions felt during this part of the story, such as fear, anxiety, or panic.
- o Conclude your narrative by detailing the actions or compulsive strategies the individual feels compelled to take to mitigate the perceived threat.
- o The climax and immediate response of the narrative should only make up a short portion of the entire narrative (less than one-third).

7. **Reflect and Record:**
   - o Record the completed narrative in a journal or use Form 5.4.
   - o Take a moment to reflect on how the story unfolds and its impact on the individual's feelings and behaviors.
   - o Consider how similar elements might be at play in your own obsessional narratives.
   - o Consult Appendix H to see how your story compares with the examples listed there.

8. **Expand Your Analysis:**
   - o Follow the same steps for the second case you analyzed in Exercise 5.1 using Form 5.5.
   - o Read and study all the other obsessional narratives listed in Appendix H.
   - o Note any insights or patterns you observe in how obsessional narratives are constructed.

Understanding the Arc and Climax in Obsessional Narratives

When crafting and analyzing obsessional narratives, it's helpful to think of them as stories with a defined arc and climax. The *arc* represents the buildup of events, thoughts, and reasons that lead to the primary obsessional doubt. This includes all the reasoning elements within the narrative of the inner wheel, such as abstract facts, personal experiences, hypothetical scenarios, and past memories.

Often, the narrative begins with the setting and initial trigger, which may include a brief mention of the primary doubt to provide context. However, it is the subsequent progression of reasoning—the weaving together of justifications—that gives the doubt its plausibility and emotional weight. In this way, the primary doubt emerges as the culmination of the reasons, rather than simply existing independently from them.

The *climax* occurs when the primary inference of doubt reaches its full intensity. At this point, all the narrative elements converge, making the doubt feel urgent and compelling. This moment doesn't just reaffirm the doubt—it sets off a cascade of consequences, such as anxiety, compulsive actions, and imagined outcomes, which belong to the outer wheel. The doubt's emotional impact peaks here, propelling the person toward actions meant to resolve or alleviate the perceived threat.

> The distinction between the arc of the story and its climax highlights the difference between the inner wheel and the outer wheel.

Viewing obsessional narratives in terms of their arc and climax provides a clearer structure for understanding how they function. The arc explains how the doubt develops, gaining plausibility and emotional weight over time, while the climax represents the peak of its influence—when the doubt dominates and drives compulsive behavior. Keeping this framework in mind will not only help you construct obsessional stories but also enhance your ability to deconstruct and analyze its mechanics, ultimately paving the way for greater clarity and control.

Form 5.4. First Case: _____

Obsessional Narrative

Condensed Primary Doubt(s):

_____

_____

Form 5.5. Second Case: _____

Obsessional Narrative

Condensed Primary Doubt(s):

_____

_____

_____

_____

_____

_____

_____

_____

_____

_____

_____

_____

_____

_____

_____

_____

_____

Highlight 5.4.
Key Learning Points

Narratives make things real to us by providing context and meaning.

Obsessional doubts are experienced as plausible, because they combine many reasons into a convincing whole.

Obsessional narratives bridge the sensory gap between triggers and obsessional doubt in the OCD outer wheel.

These narratives can make obsessional doubts seem convincing and credible, even without direct evidence.

Writing Down Your Own Story

In the previous section, we explored the obsessional narratives of others, delving into the complex and intricate nature of these stories. By examining such narratives, you can better understand how the mind constructs compelling and often distressing stories that fuel obsessions and compulsions. Now, it is time to shift the focus inward and apply this understanding to your own life.

Writing out your own obsessional narrative is a powerful and transformative exercise. It allows you to externalize and examine the story that drives your OCD. By putting these thoughts into words, you can begin to uncover the patterns and recurring themes that sustain your obsessional thinking. This exercise helps to bring clarity to the automatic and overwhelming nature of these stories, offering a new perspective.

It is important to remember that this process is not about amplifying your fears or giving more weight to your doubts. Instead, it is about recognizing and articulating the story you already tell yourself—the one that fuels your obsessions and intensifies your distress. Writing it down does not make these thoughts more real; rather, it makes them clearer and more manageable by bringing them into focus. If you feel apprehensive about engaging in this process, consider the following strategies:

1. **Realize This Is Not an Exposure Exercise.** It is just to identify and write out your story. You are not expected to accept it or get used to it!
2. **Create a Safe Space:** Ensure you are in a comfortable, private environment where you feel safe to express your thoughts openly.
3. **Set a Time Limit:** Allocate 30–60 minutes per session for writing to avoid feeling overwhelmed. If needed, break the task into multiple sessions to complete it at a comfortable pace.
4. **Practice Self-Compassion:** Remind yourself that this is a non-judgmental exercise aimed at understanding, not criticizing, your thoughts.
5. **Use Supportive Resources:** Have grounding techniques or supportive contacts available if you need to take a break or discuss your feelings during the process.
6. **Let the OCD Speak Freely and Unfiltered.** As you did previously when identifying reasons for your primary doubt, simply allow it to express itself without fighting or debating it.
7. **Stay True to Your Experience.** Keep it real, neither exaggerating nor playing it down.

Exercise 5.7.
My Obsessional Story

1. **Get Ready**
   - o Get Form 5.6 ready or use any other medium that you prefer ((journal, notebook, computer, audio) to record your story.
   - o Write down your condensed primary obsessional doubt(s) that belong together within a single obsessional theme at the top of the form.

2. **Gather Your Reasons:**
   - o Retrieve the reasons from your answers in Form 5.3.
   - o Review these reasons to remind yourself and to get ready for writing your story.

3. **Set the Scene:**
   - o Describe the context in which the triggers occur for you.
   - o Include details about their surroundings, the time of day, who they are with, and any other relevant factors.
   - o Ensure your description is vivid and detailed to create a clear picture of the scenario.

4. **Develop the Arc of the Story:**
   - o *Arc of the Story*: This is where the reasons build upon each other, creating a compelling progression that leads up to the primary inference of doubt.
   - o Incorporate the reasons you identified in Form 5.3 into the storyline, blending facts, past experiences, hearsay, rules, and information from authorities.
   - o Write in a way that shows how these reasons build upon each other, leading up to the primary inference of doubt and giving it credibility.
   - o *Important Note*: The arc of the story should make up the majority of the text of the entire narrative (two-thirds or more).

5. **Describe the Climax and the Immediate Response:**
   - o Conclude the narrative incorporating the feared consequences, emotions and compulsions you identified in Form 3.4 during Exercise 3.3.
   - o *Important Note*: The climax and response should only make up a short portion of the entire narrative (less than one-third).

6. **Reflect and Record:**
   - o Record the completed narrative using Form 5.6 or any other medium.
   - o Take a moment to reflect on how your story unfolds, how it leads up to the obsessional doubt, and eventual impact on your feelings and emotions.
   - o Read the other narratives in Appendix H and see how your own narrative is not really any different from the others.
   - o Recognize that while your own reasons or doubts might be different, your story is built up in the same way as any other.

7. **Multiple Primary Doubts:**
   - o Writing out one obsessional narrative is usually sufficient, even if you have two primary obsessional doubts, unless they belong to entirely different obsessional themes.
   - o If you have condensed primary doubts that require different narratives, or primary doubts in different obsessional themes, write out separate narratives for each of them.
   - o Limit yourself to maximum of three obsessional narratives at a time.

Form 5.6. My Obsessional Story

Condensed Primary Doubt(s):

_____

_____

_____

_____

_____

_____

_____

_____

_____

_____

_____

_____

_____

_____

_____

_____

_____

_____

Creating New Narratives: An Exercise in Imagination

Identifying your own obsessional narrative is an important step towards your recovery, giving you a crucial look under the hood of OCD. You may have even identified and written several of them. Many people with OCD have symptoms across different themes with multiple primary obsessional doubts and stories behind them. If that is the case for you, then there's no need to worry. You are in the majority.

We will revisit these obsessional stories in detail later, but for now, you can set it aside. There is no need to repeatedly go over your obsessional story. For now, it's time to embark on something similar yet fundamentally different: creating a new narrative.

The power of story and narrative is profound, shaping our thoughts, feelings, and behaviors in ways we often don't fully realize. Stories provide a framework through which we interpret our experiences, imbuing events with meaning and guiding our emotional responses. Narratives can inspire and uplift us, offering hope and resilience in the face of challenges, or they can reinforce fears and limiting beliefs, subtly directing our actions and decisions. In this way, the narratives we embrace have the power to transform our lives, for better or worse, by shaping our perceptions, emotions, and ultimately, our actions.

Creating a new narrative can help dislodge the power that an obsessional story holds over you, breaking its automatic hold and allowing you to experience a new perspective. However, it's crucial to approach this correctly. The key is to gently introduce new narratives that offer alternative views, without engaging in a back-and-forth with the obsessive thoughts. This approach allows you to gradually shift your perspective, reducing the influence of the obsessional story and helping you to find a more balanced and freeing way of thinking.

The proper approach to creating a new, non-obsessional story is to treat it as an exercise in imagination first and reasoning second. This involves crafting a completely different narrative on its own terms, independent of the obsessional one. Imagine it like painting: if your previous painting used black and red to represent the obsessional story, you now decide to create a new painting with different colors, like blue and yellow, representing the non-obsessional story.

> Just as OCD uses imagination to fuel doubt, you can harness the same creative power to craft a new, freeing narrative that transforms how you see yourself and your world.

While working on this new painting, you don't constantly compare it to the black and red painting. You don't question whether it is more true or real than the other. Instead, you immerse yourself in creating the new painting on its own terms, without looking over your shoulder at the other.

This is what it means to create and immerse yourself in a new story. You imagine it freely, without constraints. You don't debate its validity or compare it to your obsessional narrative. This perspective, attitude, and approach are essential. By doing so, you can weaken the grip of the obsessional story in an entirely non-compulsive way and open yourself to new, healthier perspectives.

Creating a new narrative is not about rejecting or fighting the old story; it's about exploring an entirely new way of thinking that exists independently of your obsessional doubts. This exercise taps into your creative imagination, enabling you to step away from the confines of your habitual thought patterns. By shifting your focus, you allow yourself to see the world and your experiences through a fresh lens, one that is not dominated by fear or compulsion.

Highlight 5.5.
Key Learning Points

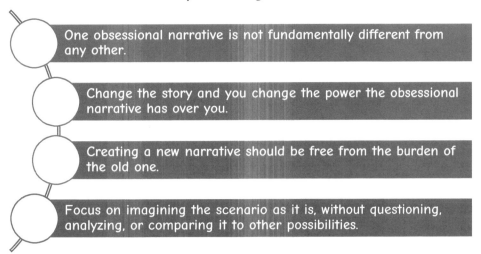

One obsessional narrative is not fundamentally different from any other.

Change the story and you change the power the obsessional narrative has over you.

Creating a new narrative should be free from the burden of the old one.

Focus on imagining the scenario as it is, without questioning, analyzing, or comparing it to other possibilities.

Steps Towards Building Non-Obsessional Narratives

Before writing your own new narrative, it's important to first practice with one or more alternative stories that are neutral to you. This practice helps you to get a good sense of maintaining neutrality and distance, which will serve you well when writing your own new narrative on its terms. The following sections will guide you through this process.

Step 1: Knowing where you want to end up

The first step in creating new and alternative stories is identifying where you want to end up, which should be a place entirely different from your obsessional doubt. Often, this destination is the opposite of the doubt—a contrasting statement. For example, if your doubt is "My hands might be contaminated," the opposite would be "My hands are clean." Similarly, if you doubt that you might have made a mistake, the opposite would be "I performed the task correctly."

It's important to note that in each of these examples, the opposite of the doubt is not phrased as a negation. Instead, it's expressed in the affirmative. This approach helps you avoid falling into the trap of arguing with the OCD. For instance, saying "My hands are not contaminated" can inadvertently reinforce the OCD, as it suggests there's something to prove. On the other hand, saying "My hands are clean" is a self-contained statement that doesn't engage with the OCD's demands for proof.

Determining where you want to end up with an alternative story is often easier than you might think. You may recall practicing this in Chapter 3 (Refer to Exercise 3.1). In that exercise, you were asked to consider the question: "What does this doubt call into question or challenge?" for various obsessional doubts. This question helps you uncover statements that can serve as the foundation for an alternative story, one that stands in direct contrast to the obsessional narrative.

For instance, possible answers to what was called into question or challenged by the obsessional doubt "My food might be poisoned" were (see Appendix A):

- My food is safe to eat.
- The ingredients I used are fresh and clean.
- The meal I prepared is healthy and nourishing.
- I can trust the source of my food.

When reflecting on the obsessional story about poisoning, it's not too difficult to generate additional statements that this doubt challenges. For example:

- The food I am eating will contribute positively to my well-being.
- I am confident in my food preparation and hygiene practices.
- The food I have is free from harmful substances.
- I can enjoy my meals without unnecessary fear or worry.
- I am capable of recognizing unsafe or spoiled food.
- I can trust my judgment and experience in food safety.
- Eating this food will sustain and strengthen me.
- My kitchen is a safe place to prepare and enjoy meals.
- The food I consume supports my health and vitality.
- Eating is a normal, safe, and nourishing part of life.

Any of these statements can serve as a foundation for creating a new, non-obsessional narrative with a completely different conclusion from the original OCD story. However, rather than simply choosing one statement, it's helpful to identify the common thread among them. Just as you summarized your obsessional doubts, you can condense these positive statements into a single, overarching affirmation that captures their collective essence.

"My food is safe, clean, and nourishing, and I can trust the source and preparation"

This single, powerful statement can then serve as the principal foundation for your new, non-obsessional narrative. By grounding your story in this concise affirmation, you are now in the position to create a narrative that is robust, self-sustaining, and entirely separate from the obsessional doubts that previously held sway.

Step 2: Identifying the Building Blocks for the New Story

Once you've determined where you want to end up, the next step is to identify the fundamental building blocks for your new story. Staying with our example, this means gathering any reasons that support the idea that your food is safe, clean, and nourishing. This process mirrors what you did earlier when you wrote down all the reasons supporting your obsessional doubts across various reasoning categories. However, this time, you'll be focusing on reasons that reinforce your new, non-obsessional narrative. For instance, reasons that support this new, positive statement—opposite to the obsessional doubt—might include the following:

Table 5.2.

Potential Reasons Behind a Contrasting Conclusion

Contrasting Conclusion   *"My food is safe, clean, and nourishing, and I can trust the source and preparation"*
Abstract facts and ideas — Things that you know or believe to be true in general.
a. Food safety regulations ensure that food is safely handled and stored properly.   b. Food sustains and nourishes our body.   c. Proper cooking and food handling techniques ensure food is safe to eat.   d. Food packaging often includes safety seals and indicators.   e. Grocery store food supplies are subject to rigorous health and safety regulations.
Personal experience — Your own personal experience, past or present
a. I've had moments of anger or frustration, but I've always maintained control of my actions.   b. I have never acted violently toward anyone, even when upset.   c. In stressful situations, I've always found peaceful solutions without resorting to harm.   d. Friends and family have never expressed concern about my behavior or questioned my self-control.   e. I have a long history of peaceful interactions with others, even in difficult circumstances.
Values, standards and rules — The way of doing things according to an accepted principle.
a. I follow food safety practices, such as washing hands and cleaning surfaces.   b. I adhere to proper cooking temperatures and storage guidelines.   c. I use fresh ingredients and check expiration dates regularly.   d. I use separate cutting boards for raw meat and vegetables to avoid cross-contamination.   e. I generally eat healthy foods.
Authorities — A person, institution or organization that is perceived as important.
a. Government food safety websites provide comprehensive guidelines that I follow.   b. Food safety certifications on products indicate adherence to strict safety standards.   c. Articles from reputable food safety journals support the practices I follow.   d. Food safety certifications on products indicate adherence to strict safety standards.   e. Cooking shows and culinary schools emphasize the importance of food hygiene, which I implement.
Hearsay and news — Information that you got from other people, substantiated or not.
a. Testimonials from others about the reliability of the stores where I buy my groceries.   b. Positive reviews and ratings of the food brands I use.   c. News reports often highlight the safety measures implemented in food production.   d. Colleagues at work also trust the same grocery stores I frequent for quality produce.   e. Friends and family members share similar cooking and food safety habits without issues.
Anything else — Anything that does not fit well in the previous categories
a. Community cooking classes I attend emphasize safety and hygiene, and I apply these practices.   b. I believe in continuous learning and improvement in my cooking skills.   c. I trust the instincts and practices passed down from my family regarding food safety.   d. Food is to be enjoyed.   e. My senses tell me that my food is safe to eat.

As you can see, just as it's possible to generate reasons for an obsessional doubt, it's equally possible to create reasons for a non-obsessional, contrasting conclusion. This means you can construct a narrative that stands entirely apart from the obsessional story. Most importantly, you can do this without directly referencing or arguing with the OCD story. Instead, you build a narrative that supports the contrasting conclusion entirely on its own terms, free from the influence of the obsessional doubts.

Step 3: Writing the New Story

The third step involves bringing your new, non-obsessional narrative to life by writing it out, just as you did with the obsessional story earlier. To craft this alternative story, you'll use similar techniques—such as setting the scene, creating an arc, and developing a coherent narrative. The goal is to create a story that not only supports your contrasting conclusion but also feels vivid and compelling. For instance, a story that supports the new conclusion about food safety, incorporating all the previously identified elements and reasons, might look something like this:

Alternative Narrative

"Why my food is safe, clean, and nourishing, and I can trust the source and my preparation methods."

Whenever I prepare to sit down for a meal, I feel a quiet sense of reassurance wash over me: my food is safe. The world around me supports this confidence. Food safety standards today are more stringent than ever before. Across industries, advancements in protocols and hygiene ensure that the food we consume is handled with care. Every day, millions of people eat out without second thoughts because these basic precautions are in place, and I remind myself that my food is no different.

The grocery store itself is a testament to these precautions. As I stroll through the aisles, the order and cleanliness speak volumes. Shelves are stocked with fresh produce and carefully packaged meats, each item having passed through rigorous quality control before making its way to me. The bright lights and friendly atmosphere fill me with calm, and the simple act of selecting ingredients feels like a small part of a much larger, well-regulated system.

Back in my kitchen, this sense of control continues. The space is warm and inviting, the aroma of fresh ingredients filling the air. I begin my familiar routine—washing vegetables until their colors shine, cooking meat with the practiced ease of someone who knows it will be done to perfection. The rhythmic chopping, the sizzling on the stove, and the bubbling of sauces create a soothing harmony. Each step is purposeful, reinforcing the knowledge that I am doing everything necessary to prepare a safe and nourishing meal.

I think back to all the meals I've made, each one without issue. Time and time again, my cooking practices have proven reliable. Food may not come with tamper-proof seals like medications, but I know the risk is effectively managed through other safety measures—ones I follow consistently. Washing produce, cooking meat thoroughly, and practicing basic hygiene are simple steps that give me peace of mind.

There is more than just my own experience to rely on, though. Experts and authorities make food safety a priority, conducting inspections and enforcing regulations. There are systems in place, like poison control hotlines and product recalls, all designed to protect people. These structures don't just exist in theory; they work effectively, and their existence is a constant reminder that my food is safe.

Friends and family bolster this confidence. We eat the same foods, prepared in similar ways, and none of us have had issues. Supermarkets are filled with products that undergo quality control, and advancements in technology—like pasteurization and refrigeration—further ensure that our food remains safe. Knowing that restaurants are regularly inspected adds another layer of comfort.

As I sit down to eat, I feel a deep sense of appreciation. Each meal becomes more than just an act of nourishment; it's a moment of gratitude for the systems in place that make this meal possible. The flavors, textures, and aromas on my plate are more than just food—they are evidence of safety, care, and attention. The sound of laughter, the clinking of glasses, and the warmth of those around me enrich the experience further, reminding me that food is meant to be shared and enjoyed.

Whether it's a holiday feast or a simple dinner at home, these moments remind me that food is not something to fear. It's something to embrace. The trust I have in the processes that keep food safe allows me to savor each bite fully, to enjoy the connection that meals bring, and to appreciate the effort that goes into every plate. This trust is built on a foundation of experience, expert guidance, and the knowledge that I am part of a system that values safety at every turn.

As you can see, by following the previous steps, it's just as easy to create a non-obsessional story as it is to create an obsessional one. Whether the narrative above resonates with you or not isn't the main concern. For example, you might not enjoy going to supermarkets or cooking, so the story might not resonate with you personally, even if you generally believe your food is safe to eat. The key point is that this narrative is just as valid as the obsessional story, and anyone can create such a story using reasons that feel true to them. The goal is to recognize that the reasoning behind non-obsessional stories can be equally, if not more, plausible once you learn to construct them.

Practicing Alternative Story Creation for Others

The next exercise will ask you to create a non-obsessional narrative for one of the scenarios you previously wrote an obsessional narrative for. Working with a more neutral case first will allow you to develop a strong sense of how to construct an equally compelling alternative narrative without directly referencing or comparing it to the obsessional story. This practice will help you adopt the same approach when crafting your own non-obsessional narrative later on, ensuring that you do so without engaging in comparison or internal debate.

Exercise 5.8.
Crafting Alternative Narratives for Others

1. **Retrieve your Case:**
   - Retrieve all materials relating to one of the cases you previously wrote an obsessional narrative for in Exercise 5.6.
2. **Create a Contrasting Statement:**
   - Ask yourself, what does the primary condensed doubt(s) call into question or challenge?
   - Condense your answers into one or two contrasting statement(s) or conclusion(s) encapsulating their essence.
   - Ensure to phrase the new conclusion(s) in the affirmative without any negation.

3. **Identify Reasons and Record:**
   - Write down the contrasting statement(s) or conclusion(s) at the top of Form 5.7.
   - Reflect on the statement and compile a list of reasons that resonate with you to support the conclusion.
   - Ask yourself questions like:
     - *"Why do I think this statement might be true?"*
     - *"What evidence do I have to support this conclusion?"*
     - *"Why does this statement feel real to me?"*
   - *Note:* Don't worry if you lack immediate insight into the reasons behind a statement. For example, if the contrasting statement is about another's person's character (e.g., "Why I am a peaceful person"), just imagine someone where that conclusion is justified.
   - Examples of contrasting statements and reasons for each case vignette are provided in Appendix I, but try to come up with your own first as much as possible.

4. **Document the Alternative Narrative**
   - Document the alternative narrative in your preferred medium, such as a word processor, journal, audio recording, or Form 5.8.

5. **Set the scene**
   - Begin by describing the surroundings in which the statement is relevant.
   - Include vivid and detailed descriptions of the environment, time of day, who is present, and any other relevant factors to create an engaging picture of the scenario.
   - Write the non-obsessional narrative in the first person ("I") to make it more compelling

6. **Develop the Arc of the Story:**
   - Using the reasons you identified, build the narrative in various contexts, showing how these reasons lead up to the non-obsessional statement or conclusion.
   - Write the reasons and the alternative story in such a way that it does not directly refer back to elements of the OCD story or attempt to dispute these elements.
   - The arc should demonstrate how different elements come together, making the new statement feel plausible and compelling.

7. **Describe the Climax and Immediate Response:**
   - Conclude the narrative by detailing the climax, focusing on the consequences, emotions, and behaviors that follow from the non-obsessional statement.
   - Emphasize positive emotions felt during this part of the story, such as trust, confidence, or peace.
   - Describe the actions taken in line with the new, non-obsessional conclusion.

8. **Reflect:**
   - Take a moment to read and reflect on the alternative narrative. Note any insights and patterns you observe, and how this narrative naturally leads to very different feelings and behaviors compared to the obsessional narrative.
   - Recognize that the contrasting, alternative narrative is at least as valid as the original obsessional narrative.

9. **Optional:**
   - Follow the same steps for the second case in you previously wrote an obsessional narrative for in Exercise 5.5.
   - Read and study all the alternative narratives listed in Appendix J.

Form 5.7.

Reasons Behind a Non-Obsessional Conclusion

Contrasting Conclusion(s)

....

....

Abstract facts and ideas — Things that you know or believe to be true in general.

    a. ....

    b. ....

    c. ....

Personal experience — Your own personal experience, past or present

    a. ....

    b. ....

    c. ....

Values, standards and rules — The way of doing things according to an accepted principle.

    a. ....

    b. ....

    c. ....

Authorities — A person, institution or organization that is perceived as important.

    a. ....

    b. ....

    c. ....

Hearsay and news — Information that you got from other people, substantiated or not.

    a. ....

    b. ....

    c. ....

Anything else — Anything that does not fit well in the previous categories

    a. ....

    b. ....

    c. ....

Form 5.8. Case _____

Alternative Narrative

Contrasting Conclusion(s):

_____

_____

_____

_____

_____

_____

_____

_____

_____

_____

_____

_____

_____

_____

_____

_____

_____

_____

Constructing Your Own Alternative Narrative

Now that you have practiced creating a non-obsessional alternative narrative for someone else, it's time to apply these skills to your own experiences. In this section, you will learn how to construct your own alternative narrative, building on the techniques and insights you gained from the previous exercises. The aim is to take the structure and reasoning you've practiced and tailor it to your specific doubts and personal experiences.

The goal is to create a compelling and positive narrative that stands independent from your obsessional story. This new narrative should reflect a healthier perspective, free from the doubts and fears that typically dominate your thoughts. By developing and immersing yourself in this alternative story, you can begin to shift your focus away from obsessive-compulsive patterns and towards a more balanced and peaceful mindset.

Remember, the key to success in this exercise is to approach it with an open mind and a willingness to engage your imagination. Your new narrative should be crafted on its own terms, without constantly comparing it to or debating with your obsessional story. This exercise is about creating a positive, affirming story that resonates with you and helps you build confidence over time in your new perspective.

Let's dive into the steps to construct your own new, alternative narrative, and begin the journey towards reshaping your thought patterns and reclaiming control over your mind.

Exercise 5.9
Creating Your Own Alternative Narrative

1. **Time, Setting and Attitude:**
   - *Choose the Right Time*: Select a time when your OCD is least active. This will allow you to approach the exercise with the clearest mind possible.
   - *Create a Safe Space*: Ensure you are in a comfortable, private environment where you feel safe to write down and express your thoughts openly.
   - *Focus on Imagination, Not Counterargument*: This exercise is about stretching your imagination in new ways, not about trying to refute your obsessional doubt.
   - *Maintain a Non-Obsessional Perspective*: If you feel OCD starting to protest, hold it at bay and stay focused on your purpose. Take breaks if needed. You don't have to finish the entire story in one sitting; you can add to it over time.

2. **Create a Contrasting Conclusion:**
   - *Retrieve your Condensed Primary Doubts*: Locate the condensed primary obsessional doubt(s) you previously recorded in Form 3.4.
   - *Retrieve your Answers*: Retrieve your answers in Form 3.5 where you identified what your condensed primary doubt calls into question or challenges.
   - *Condense*: Condense your list of what your primary doubts calls into question into one or two contrasting statement(s) or conclusion(s).
   - *Phrase Affirmatively*: Ensure the statement(s) or conclusion(s) is phrased in the affirmative.

3. **Gather Your Reasons:**
   - Write your new contrasting conclusion(s) at the top for Form 5.9.

- o *Compile supporting Reasons:* Compile a list of reasons supporting your new conclusion(s) or statement(s) using the reasoning categorises. Remember, the categories are only there to facilitate identifying reasons. It does not matter whether you categorize them "correctly" or not.
- o *Ask yourself questions:*
  - "Why might this statement be true?
  - "What information might confirm this statement?"
  - "What sort of evidence might underpin this statement?"
  - "What might make this statement real for me?"
  - "Why might I agree with this statement?
  - "Why might this statement seem plausible?
  - "What rationale might back up this statement?
  - "What might corroborate this statement?"
- o *Important Note:* Don't worry if the reasons you come up with don't resonate strongly with you. The obsessional story's hold over you may diminish their usual impact. Don't expect to feel it immediately, nor try to force it.

4. **Write Out the Narrative:**
- o *Set the Scene.* Describe the context in which your new statement is relevant.
  - Use rich, immersive details to make the setting come alive. The richer and more nuanced the details, the more credible the story becomes.
- o *Develop the Arc of the Story.* Using the reasons you identified, create the arc leading up to the new conclusion and climax.
  - Write the reasons and alternative story in a way that does not directly refer back to elements of the OCD story or attempt to dispute these elements. Instead, write the alternative story in its own terms.
  - Ensure the story has a smooth transport, taking you from point A to point B in a credible journey.
- o *Climax and Immediate Response:* Conclude your narrative with the climax, including the emotions and behaviors that follow from your new statement.
  - Personalize the story by centering events around yourself, making the key transition points and meaningful, and touching you emotionally.

5. **Record and Reflect:**
- o *Record the Narrative:* Document the completed narrative in your preferred medium, such as a word processor, journal, audio recording, or Form 5.10.
- o *Reflect on the Impact:* Take a moment reflect on how your new alternative story unfolds and its impact on your feelings and behaviors. Observe any shifts in your perspective, however small, as well as feelings of empowerment and relaxation that may arise.
- o *Recognize its Validity:* Recognize that your new narrative is at least as valid as the original obsessional narrative.

6. **Rinse and Repeat**
- o *Multiple Primary Doubts:* If you have additional condensed primary doubts in different obsessional themes, repeat the process by writing out separate narratives.
- o *Limit to three:* If you have more than three condensed contrasting conclusions, limit yourself to maximum of three alternative narratives.

Form 5.9.
Reasons That Justify My Non-Obsessional Conclusion(s)

Contrasting Conclusion(s)

....

....

Abstract facts and ideas — Things that you know or believe to be true in general.

a. ....

b. ....

c. ....

Personal experience — Your own personal experience, past or present

a. ....

b. ....

c. ....

Values, standards and rules — The way of doing things according to an accepted principle.

a. ....

b. ....

c. ....

Authorities — A person, institution or organization that is perceived as important.

a. ....

b. ....

c. ....

Hearsay and news — Information that you got from other people, substantiated or not.

a. ....

b. ....

c. ....

Anything else — Anything that does not fit well in the previous categories

a. ....

b. ....

c. ....

Form 5.10.
My New Narrative
New Conclusion(s):

Engaging with Your New Narrative

Creating your non-obsessional story is just the first step. This narrative is something you'll continue his narrative will serve as a foundation you'll continue to build upon throughout the exercises in both Volume 1 and Volume 2 of this guide. By regularly engaging with this alternative story, you can gradually reshape your thought patterns, allowing this new perspective to take root and grow stronger over time. While the new narrative might not feel completely authentic at first, consistent immersion— and the gradual dismantling of the obsessional story—will help it resonate more deeply. To reinforce this process, make it a daily practice to engage with your new narrative using the following exercise.

Exercise 5.10.
Engaging with Your New Narrative

1. **Daily Immersion**
   - *Set Aside Time Daily:* Choose a specific time each day to read or listen to each of your new narratives. Make sure it's a time when you can be undisturbed and fully focused.
   - *Duration:* Limit each session to 10-15 minutes.
   - *Create a Comfortable Environment:* Sit in a comfortable, quiet place where you feel safe and relaxed. This will help you fully immerse yourself in the narrative.
   - *Engage Your Senses:* As you read, imagine the sights, sounds, smells, and feelings described in your narrative. Make it as vivid as possible.
   - *Reflect on the Emotions:* Notice how reading the narrative makes you feel. Allow yourself to experience any positive emotions that arise, such as calmness or reassurance.

2. **Visualize:**
   - *Close Your Eyes:* After reading the narrative, replay the entire story in your mind. Close your eyes and visualize the scenes in your mind. Picture yourself in the story, experiencing it as if it were happening in real life.
   - *Use Descriptive Imagery:* Focus on the details in the narrative. Imagine the colors, textures, and sensations described.
   - *Involve All Senses:* Try to include all your senses in the visualization. Hear the sounds, smell the aromas, and feel the textures.

3. **Act As If:**
   - *Suspend disbelief:* Act as if the alternative statement or conclusion is real. Even if you don't fully believe it yet, imagine it as if you do. Just like when watching a movie, temporarily suspend disbelief and allow yourself to fully engage with the new narrative.
   - *Notice the Changes:* Pay attention to any changes in your feelings as you immerse yourself into to the new narrative. Celebrate small victories and shifts in perspective.

4. **Maintain the Proper Attitude:**
   - *Non-Comparative Engagement:* Engage with the new narrative on its own terms. Avoid comparing it with the obsessional story. It is about refocusing your imagination first, allowing proper judgement to naturally follow.
   - *Mindful Practice:* Practice immersing yourself in the new narrative only when you are not actively engaged with OCD. Keep the OCD at a distance during these exercises.

      o *Authenticity Over Conviction:* Understand that the new narrative might not feel authentic initially, but regular engagement will gradually make it feel more real. The goal is not to force belief but to let it naturally become a part of your thought patterns.

      o *Stay Flexible:* If you find yourself unable to maintain the proper attitude, discontinue your practice for the day, and try another time. Alternatively, limit your practice to reading the alternative narrative only for a brief period of time.

5. **Record and Reflect:**

      o *Document Your Experiences:* Keep a journal where you record your daily practice, noting how engaging with the new narrative affects your thoughts and feelings.

      o *Reflect on Progress:* Regularly review your journal entries to observe any patterns, insights, or progress. This can help reinforce the effectiveness of the practice.

Engage with your new narrative daily, but avoid over-practicing. Reading and immersing yourself in the narrative once a day, preferably when you feel most relaxed, is sufficient. If elements from your new narrative arise on their own during moments when the hold of the obsessional doubt seems to lessen, that's a positive sign—allow it to happen organically without comparing the OCD story to the new narrative or trying to determine which is true.

To maintain a healthy approach, ensure that engaging with the new narrative doesn't become another compulsive activity. Practice only when you're feeling calm and can keep OCD at a distance. The goal isn't to prove the obsessional story wrong, as doing so only reinforces its power. Instead, focus on fully experiencing the new narrative on its own terms, embracing this new perspective as a separate, positive outlook rather than a direct rebuttal to the obsessional one.

By consistently practicing and engaging with your new narrative, you will gradually shift your thought patterns and overall mindset. Remember, this exercise is not about immediate transformation, but about allowing the new narrative to take root and grow stronger over time. With patience and persistence, you'll find it easier to live out this new story, reducing the hold of obsessional thoughts and opening yourself up to more positive perspectives, feelings, and behaviors.

Use the training card as a daily reminder and quick reference:

Training Card 5.1.

Engaging With Your New Narrative

1. **Immerse Daily**
    Set aside time daily read or listen to your narrative.

2. **Visualize**
    Vividly visualize the narrative, engaging your senses.

3. **Act "As If"**
    Suspend disbelief and act "as if" it is real.

4. **Maintain the Proper Attitude**
    Engage with the narrative on its own terms, avoiding comparisons.

Reflecting On Your Journey: A Foundation for Change

As we reach the end of *Resolving OCD: Understanding Your Obsessional Experience, Volume 1*, take a moment to recognize how far you've come. Over the course of this journey, you've deepened your understanding of OCD, uncovered the stories that sustain your obsessions, and begun to reshape your imagination. This is no small achievement. You've laid the groundwork for a profound shift, one that empowers you to see OCD not as an undefeatable foe, but as something you can dismantle and overcome.

Through these chapters, you've explored the many different manifestations of OCD and gained insight into its ability to adapt to personal fears and concerns. You've learned to recognize the obsessional sequence within the Outer Wheel—the patterns of thoughts, doubts, and behaviors that perpetuate the cycle of OCD. Perhaps most importantly, you've begun to distinguish everyday doubt from obsessional doubt, an essential skill for loosening OCD's grip on your mind.

This volume has also introduced you to the critical role of stories in sustaining obsessional doubt. You've worked to identify and understand the obsessional narratives that fuel OCD, discovering how they construct a reality that amplifies distress. You've also learned how to create a new, alternative narrative—laying a foundation for freedom and resilience. By doing so, you've begun to shift your perspective, and create space for healthier, freer ways of thinking.

As you move forward, remember that the skills and insights you've developed here are tools you can carry with you, shaping how you approach challenges ahead. This volume marks the beginning of a transformative journey—one that will continue as you deepen your understanding and apply what you've learned to reclaim control over your life. Take pride in how far you've come, and look ahead with optimism for what lies ahead in the next volume.

With each new step, you'll continue to grow stronger, more resilient, and more in control of your life. The work you've done here has laid the groundwork for meaningful change, and the path ahead offers even greater opportunities to strengthen that foundation and move toward freedom and resilience.

Transition to Volume Two: From Awareness to Action

Congratulations on completing *Resolving OCD: Understanding Your Obsessional Experience, Volume One*. Through this first stage of your journey, you've made significant strides in understanding how OCD operates in your life. By identifying your personal obsessional patterns, recognizing the mechanics of obsessional doubt, and practicing reshaping your obsessional narrative, you've not just laid a foundation—you've already begun the process of meaningful change.

But the journey doesn't end here. The insights and strategies you've gained in *Volume One* represent a strong base for continued progress. Now that you have a deeper awareness of the forces driving your OCD and a growing skill set to challenge them, it's time to move forward with even greater confidence. *Volume Two: Advanced Strategies for Overcoming Obsessional Doubt* will guide you through the next stages of recovery, helping you further dismantle the cognitive and emotional barriers that keep obsessional doubt alive.

Looking Ahead to Volume Two

In *Volume Two*, you'll continue exploring *Part 3: The Inner Wheel of OCD*, diving deeper into how reasoning confusion between imagination and reality sustains your obsessions. You'll gain a clearer understanding of how OCD blurs the line between possibility and probability, making fears feel all too real. This exploration will also focus on challenging the fears and doubts tied to your possible self—a crucial element in breaking OCD's hold.

Finally, *Volume Two* will introduce *Part 4: The Doing*, where the emphasis shifts to applying what you've learned. Here, you'll expand on the practices you began in *Volume One*, learning advanced strategies to disrupt the obsessional cycle in real-world settings. From staying out of the OCD bubble to reclaiming your innate ability to effortlessly sense reality, these practical tools will empower you to regain control of your life and build lasting resilience.

The progress you've made in *Volume One* has laid a strong foundation. You've built awareness, developed critical skills, and taken actionable steps toward reducing OCD's influence. Now, let's build on that momentum, deepening your recovery as you continue moving toward greater freedom, confidence, and well-being.

What's Next?

Volume Two: Advanced Strategies for Overcoming Obsessional Doubt is currently in development. Stay tuned for updates on its release by visiting **www.icbt.online**, where you can find the latest news and resources to support your journey.

Once released, *Volume Two* will be available through various online retailers and digital platforms. Availability may vary depending on your region, so check your preferred book outlets for details. Explore these options to continue your journey toward greater freedom from OCD.

Notes and Reflections

Notes and Reflections

Notes and Reflections

Notes and Reflections

Notes and Reflections

Notes and Reflections

Notes and Reflections

Notes and Reflections

Appendices

Form 3.1. Possible Answers
What Do Obsessional Doubts Challenge?

Obsessional Doubt "I might be gay."

- Calls into Question: "I understand my sexual orienation."
- Calls into Question: "I am attracted to the opposite sex."
- Calls into Question: "My past romantic relationships were genuine."
- Calls into Question: "My sexual thoughts and feelings align with my identity."

Obsessional Doubt "My heart might be beating irregular."

- Calls into Question: "My heartbeat is regular and stable."
- Calls into Question: "I can trust my body's signals."
- Calls into Question: "My heart is functioning as it should."
- Calls into Question: "I am safe from a cardiac event."

Obsessional Doubt "What if I live in a virtual world?"

- Calls into Question: "The authenticity of my experiences and surroundings."
- Calls into Question: "The nature of reality and existence."
- Calls into Question: "The validity of relationships and interactions."
- Calls into Question: "The overall meaning and purpose of life."

Obsessional Doubt "Maybe I do not feel enough love my partner."

- Calls into Question: "The strength and signficance of the bond."
- Calls into Question: "My dedication and commitment to the relationship."
- Calls into Question: "The affection and love I feel."
- Calls into Question: "The compatibility of the relationship."

Obsessional Doubt "My food might be poisened"

- Calls into Question: "My food is safe to eat."
- Calls into Question: "The ingredients I used are fresh and clean."
- Calls into Question: "The meal I prepared is healthy and nourishing."
- Calls into Question: "I can trust the source of my food."

APPENDIX B
Form 3.2. Answers
Identifying the Obsessional Sequence in Others.

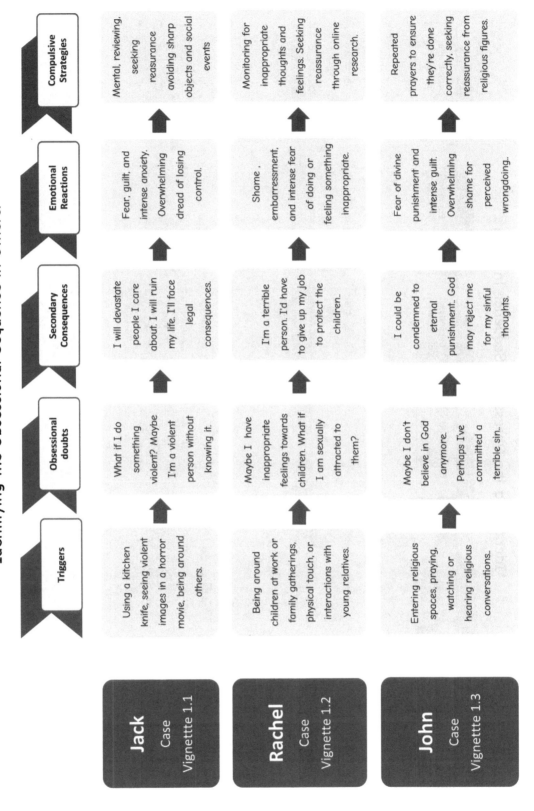

APPENDIX B
Form 3.2. Answers
Identifying the Obsessional Sequence in Others.

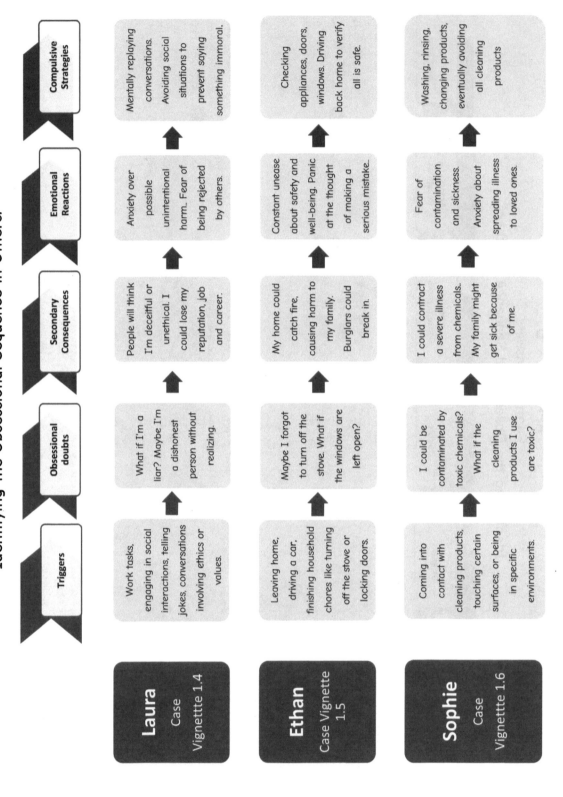

	Triggers	Obsessional doubts	Secondary Consequences	Emotional Reactions	Compulsive Strategies
Laura Case Vignette 1.4	Work tasks, engaging in social interactions, telling jokes, conversations involving ethics or values.	What if I'm a liar? Maybe I'm a dishonest person without realizing.	People will think I'm deceitful or unethical. I could lose my reputation, job and career.	Anxiety over possible unintentional harm. Fear of being rejected by others.	Mentally replaying conversations. Avoiding social situations to prevent saying something immoral.
Ethan Case Vignette 1.5	Leaving home, driving a car, finishing household chores like turning off the stove or locking doors.	Maybe I forgot to turn off the stove. What if the windows are left open?	My home could catch fire, causing harm to my family. Burglars could break in.	Constant unease about safety and well-being. Panic at the thought of making a serious mistake.	Checking appliances, doors, windows. Driving back home to verify all is safe.
Sophie Case Vignette 1.6	Coming into contact with cleaning products, touching certain surfaces, or being in specific environments.	I could be contaminated by toxic chemicals? What if the cleaning products I use are toxic?	I could contract a severe illness from chemicals. My family might get sick because of me.	Fear of contamination and sickness. Anxiety about spreading illness to loved ones.	Washing, rinsing, changing products, eventually avoiding all cleaning products

APPENDIX B
Form 3.2. Answers
Identifying the Obsessional Sequence in Others.

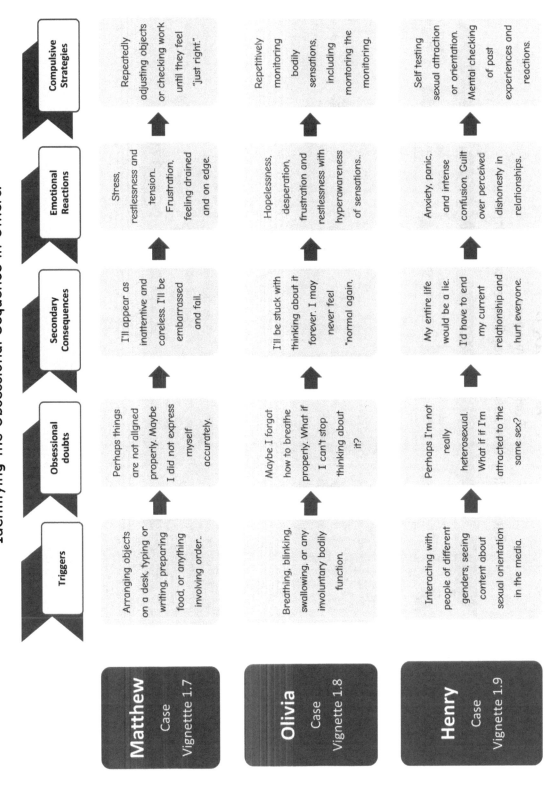

	Triggers	Obsessional doubts	Secondary Consequences	Emotional Reactions	Compulsive Strategies
Matthew Case Vignette 1.7	Arranging objects on a desk, typing or writing, preparing food, or anything involving order.	Perhaps things are not aligned properly. Maybe I did not express myself accurately.	I'll appear as inattentive and careless. I'll be embarrassed and fail.	Stress, restlessness and tension. Frustration, feeling drained and on edge.	Repeatedly adjusting objects or checking work until they feel "just right."
Olivia Case Vignette 1.8	Breathing, blinking, swallowing, or any involuntary bodily function.	Maybe I forgot how to breathe properly. What if I can't stop thinking about it?	I'll be stuck with thinking about it forever. I may never feel "normal again.	Hopelessness, desperation, frustration and restlessness with hyperawareness of sensations.	Repetitively monitoring bodily sensations, including monitoring the monitoring.
Henry Case Vignette 1.9	Interacting with people of different genders, seeing content about sexual orientation in the media.	Perhaps I'm not really heterosexual. What if I'm attracted to the same sex?	My entire life would be a lie. I'd have to end my current relationship and hurt everyone.	Anxiety, panic, and intense confusion. Guilt over perceived dishonesty in relationships.	Self testing sexual attraction or orientation. Mental checking of past experiences and reactions.

APPENDIX B
Form 3.2. Answers
Identifying the Obsessional Sequence in Others.

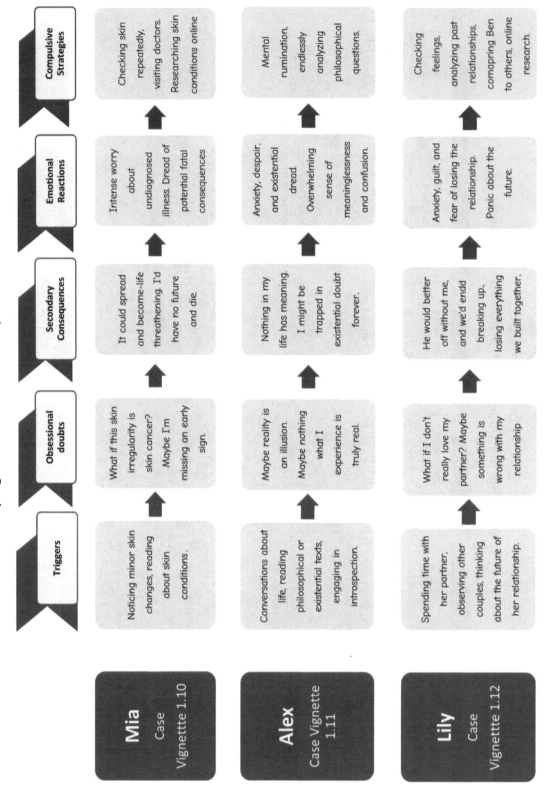

	Triggers	Obsessional doubts	Secondary Consequences	Emotional Reactions	Compulsive Strategies
Mia Case Vignette 1.10	Noticing minor skin changes, reading about skin conditions.	What if this skin irregularity is skin cancer? Maybe I'm missing an early sign.	It could spread and become life threatening. I'd have no future and die.	Intense worry about undiagnosed illness. Dread of potential fatal consequences	Checking skin repeatedly, visiting doctors. Researching skin conditions online
Alex Case Vignette 1.11	Conversations about life, reading philosophical or existential texts, engaging in introspection.	Maybe reality is an illusion. Maybe nothing what I experience is truly real.	Nothing in my life has meaning. I might be trapped in existential doubt forever.	Anxiety, despair, and existential dread. Overwhelming sense of meaninglessness and confusion.	Mental rumination, endlessly analyzing philosophical questions.
Lily Case Vignette 1.12	Spending time with her partner, observing other couples, thinking about the future of her relationship.	What if I don't really love my partner? Maybe something is wrong with my relationship	He would better off without me, and we'd endd breaking up.. losing everything we built together.	Anxiety, guilt, and fear of losing the relationship. Panic about the future.	Checking feelings, analyzing past relationships, comapring Ben to others, online research.

APPENDIX B
Form 3.2. Answers
Identifying the Obsessional Sequence in Others.

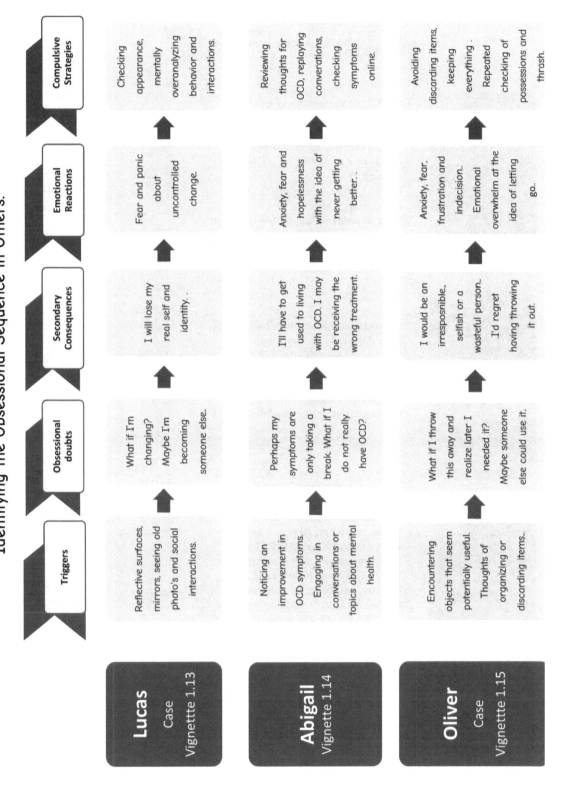

	Triggers	Obsessional doubts	Secondary Consequences	Emotional Reactions	Compulsive Strategies
Lucas Case Vignette 1.13	Reflective surfaces, mirrors, seeing old photo's and social interactions.	What if I'm changing? Maybe I'm becoming someone else.	I will lose my real self and identity.	Fear and panic about uncontrolled change.	Checking appearance, mentally overanalyzing behavior and interactions.
Abigail Vignette 1.14	Noticing an improvement in OCD symptoms. Engaging in conversations or topics about mental health.	Perhaps my symptoms are only taking a break. What if I do not really have OCD?	I'll have to get used to living with OCD. I may be receiving the wrong treatment.	Anxiety, fear and hopelessness with the idea of never getting better.	Reviewing thoughts for OCD, replaying conversations, checking symptoms online.
Oliver Case Vignette 1.15	Encountering objects that seem potentially useful. Thoughts of organizing or discarding items.	What if I throw this away and realize later I needed it? Maybe someone else could use it.	I would be an irresponsible, selfish or a wasteful person. I'd regret having throwing it out.	Anxiety, fear, frustration and indecision. Emotional overwhelm at the idea of letting go.	Avoiding discarding items, keeping everything. Repeated checking of possessions and thrash.

Form 3.3. Answers
Condensing Obsessional Doubts

Primary Obsessional doubts

Condensed Primary Obsessional Doubt(s)

Jack

Case Vignettte 1.1

What if I do something violent?
Maybe I'm a violent person without knowing it.
What if I actually do something violent?
Could I be a dangerous person without realizing it?
I might have already harmed someone and just forgot about it.
What if I suddenly lose control and harm someone?
Am I capable of doing something terrible?

I might be a violent person without knowing it, capable of causing harm at any moment.

Rachel

Case Vignettte 1.2

Maybe I have inappropriate feelings toward the children I work with.
What if I am sexually attracted to them?
What if I'm just fooling myself it is OCD only?
What if I am dangerous to them?
Maybe I am not the person I thought I was.

Maybe I am sexually attracted to children.

John

Case Vignettte 1.3

Perhaps I don't believe in God anymore.
Maybe I've lost my faith.
Waht if I'm not a true believer?
Maybe my prayers dont mean anything.
Waht if God thinks I don't mean it?
Perhaps I've committed a terrible sin.
Maybe I doubted God without realizing.
I could be losing my faith entirely.
What if I'm not living up to God's teachings?
Maybe I already lost my connection to God

Perhaps I don't truly believe in God anymore and have lost my faith.

Form 3.3. Answers
Condensing Obsessional Doubts

| Primary Obsessional doubts | Condensed Primary Obsessional Doubt(s) |

Laura

Case Vignettte 1.4

What if I'm a liar.
Maybe I am a dishonest person without even realizing it.
Did I lie on purpose?
What if I'm hiding something even from myself?
What if I did that on purpose?
Maybe I'm the kind of person who cheats people?
I might be secretly unethical or manipulitive.
Maybe I'm not as moral as I think I am.

I could be a dishonest and unethical person without realizing.

Ethan

Case Vignette 1.5

Maybe I forgot to turn off the stove.
Perhaps the toaster is still on.
Maybe the windows are left open.
What if I left the light on in the bathroom?
Perhaps I don't have everything I need in my wallet.
What if the refrigerator isn't cooling properly?
Maybe the car handbrake isn't engaged.
What if the smoke detector isn't working?
Perhaps my laptop could overheat and catch fire.

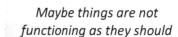

I could have missed something or left something undone

Maybe things are not functioning as they should

Sophie

Case Vignette 1.6

Perhaps I could be contaminated by toxic chemicals.
Maybe the cleaning products I use are toxic.
Could the air still be filled with toxic particles?
Perhaps even these products aren't truly safe.
Maybe these materials contain toxic chemicals.
Could I have spread contaminants from one item to another?
Maybe chemicals are still lingering from the last time I cleaned here.

I could be contaminated by toxic chemicals, both in my surroundings and the environment, that are impossible to avoid or eliminate.

Form 3.3. Answers
Condensing Obsessional Doubts

Primary Obsessional doubts

Condensed Primary Obsessional Doubt(s)

Mathew

Case Vignettte 1.7

Maybe the papers aren't lined up properly.
What if the lines aren't perfectly straight?
Maybe the books on the self aren't evenly spaced.
Maybe I did explain that clearly enough.
What if I haven't chopped the vegetables evenly.
Perhaps the books have shifted slightly since I last checked.
Perhaps my hair is not symmetrical enough on both sides.
Perhaps my shirt cuffs are uneven.
Perhaps something is still wrong with how I left things.

Things might not be aligned or arranged correctly.

Maybe I've missed something or made a mistake somehere.

Olivia

Case Vignette 1.8

Maybe my breathing is too shallow or irregular.
Perhaps I'll forget how to breathe, blink, or swallow properly.
What if I cannot stop monitoring my bodily functions?
Perhaps my body won't function properly unless I control it.
I may be unable to focus on anything else than my bodily sensations.
Maybe my body will betray me in public or professional situations.

Perhaps things haven't been placed right, or done right, or well enough.

Henry

Case Vignette 1.9

Perhaps I'm not really heterosexual What if I'm attracted to the same sex? Maybe I've been lying to myself about my sexuality all along.
Maybe I have been in denial all these years.
What if I'm just pretending?
Maybe I'm giving off signals that make others think I'm gay.
What if I'm lying to myself and everyone around me?

Maybe I'm really gay and have been lying to myself

Form 3.3. Answers
Condensing Obsessional Doubts

Primary Obsessional doubts		Condensed Primary Obsessional Doubt(s)

Mia

Case

Vignettte 1.10

What if this mole is skin cancer?
Is it changing shape?
Has it gotten bigger?
Maybe it's darker than before.
Waht if it's spreading.
Maybe the doctor missed something.
What if did not point out the right mole?
Perhaps I missed something important in the articles.
Perhaps the cancer is spreading and I'm not noticing.
What if I miss something important and it's too late to treat?

I might have skin cancer, and I'm not catching it in time.

Alex

Case

Vignette 1.11

Maybe reality is an illusion.
Maybe nothing I experience is truly real.
How do I know this is real?
What if none of this exists?
Is this actually happening, or is it all in my mind?
What if life has no meaning?
What if everything I believe is an illusion?
What if I'm trapped in a simulation?
What if nothing exists when I fall asleep?

Maybe reality is an illusion, and nothing I experience is truly real.

Lily

Case

Vignette 1.12

What if I don't really love him?
What if this isn't real love?
Maybe I am not atrracted to him
Perhaps we're not compatible.
Maybe I'm just pretending to love him?
Do I feel happy enough?
Do I feel connected enough?
Was my love stronger before?
Are these feelings enough?
Is there somehting wrong with my relationshop?
Maybe I'm not happy enough.

Maybe my feelings for him aren't real, and we don;t belong together.

Form 3.3. Answers
Condensing Obsessional Doubts

Primary Obsessional doubts	Condensed Primary Obsessional Doubt(s)

Lucas

Case Vignettte 1.13

Maybe I'm changing.
What if I'm turning into someone else.
Perhaps I don't look the same as I did before.
Perhaps I no longer look the same? Or maybe I'm slowly turning into someone unrecognizable?
What if I'm turning into someone lazy?
What if my thoughts and behaviors are not really mine?
Maybe I'm adopting traits from people around me.
What if media or conversations are influencing my identity?

Maybe I'm changing into someone else.

Abigail

Case Vignette 1.14

Maybe this improvement is a trap.
Perhaps my OCD will come back even stronger.
What if I don't actually have OCD?
Maybe I have convinced myself I have OCD as an excuse.
Maybe I'm not trying hard enough to get better.
What if my orginal symptoms are coming back?
Maybe my OCD will shift its focus to something else.
Maybe my OCD is different from everyone else's.

Maybe my OCD is coming back.

What if I don't really have OCD.

Oliver

Case Vignette 1.15

Perhaps I'll need this later.
Maybe I won't be able to replace it when I need it.
What if getting rid of this prevents me from being prepared for future emergencies?
What if it turns out to be important after all?
If I throw this away, I might be losing a piece of myself.
Maybe someone else could use it.
What if it turns out to be irraplaceble?

Maybe getting rid of anything is a mistake.

Scenario 4.2: The Dog Spa

A. What is the primary doubt and the feared consequences in this scenario?

The primary doubt is, "How do I know they will treat my dog well?" or "What if they won't take good care of him?" This doubt leads to several secondary consequences: Sarah fears that his dog might be traumatized if treated badly, leaving her to deal with the emotional aftermath. She worries about the potential guilt and responsibility for choosing the wrong spa and the safety and well-being of her dog.

1. Is there any concrete evidence in the senses for the doubt in the here-and-now?

No, there is no concrete evidence for the doubt. Sarah has no tangible evidence that the new dog spa is either good or bad. Her concern arises from the lack of prior experience with their services, but nothing else.

2. Does the doubt occur in an appropriate context?

Yes, the doubt occurs in an appropriate context. Given that Sarah is dealing with a new and unknown service provider for her dog's grooming, it is reasonable for her to have concerns and seek reassurance about the spa's quality and care.

3. Is the doubt based on a real uncertainty?

Yes, the doubt is based on real uncertainty. Sarah genuinely lacks information about the new dog spa's quality of service and their treatment of pets, making her concerns valid and based on a real lack of information.

4. Does acting on the doubt help to resolve it?

Yes, acting on the doubt by researching the new dog spa can help to resolve it. Reading reviews, checking ratings, and possibly even visiting the spa beforehand can provide Sarah with more information, alleviating her concerns and allowing her to make an informed decision. Contacting the spa directly and asking questions can also offer reassurance. The extent to which anyone continues to worry after gaining more information varies from person to person and depends on individual risk tolerance and the ability to tolerate true uncertainty. This does not automatically make her doubt obsessional. Ultimately, with more information, her anxiety about the dog spa is likely to subside.

5. Is the doubt rooted in common sense?

Yes, the doubt is rooted in common sense. It is logical for Sarah to want to ensure that the new spa will take good care of her dog. Her actions to gather more information and seek reassurance are reasonable and appropriate for the situation.

B. Considering all of your answers, is the doubt obsessional?

Given the scenario and all the answers, the doubt about the new dog spa is an everyday doubt. While there was no direct evidence for the doubt, this alone is not always sufficient to determine if the doubt is obsessional or typical. Obsessional doubts exclusively occur without direct evidence, but so can everyday doubts occasionally. In this case, the doubt was based on real uncertainty, occurred in context, and was resolvable. In the end, the anxiety regarding trying a new place subsided. Depending on the amount of information needed and the extent to which worry persists, it can also be considered an exaggerated doubt, influenced by a low tolerance for risk and uncertainty. However, this pattern does not automatically make it obsessional. Even exaggerated worries usually subside over time with more information, whereas obsessional doubts are typically immune to additional information.

Form 4.3. Answers
Scenario 4.3: Asbestos Contamination

A. **What is the primary doubt and the feared consequences in this scenario?**

The primary obsessional doubt in Mark's scenario is, "What if I do something in my everyday activities that would disturb the asbestos so that it is released?" This thought causes him significant anxiety as he fears the potential health risks associated with asbestos exposure. The secondary consequences of this doubt include a pervasive fear of serious health problems, leading him to avoid certain rooms and areas in the house.

1. **Is there any concrete evidence in the senses for the doubt in the here-and-now?**

No, there is no concrete evidence in the here-and-now to suggest that asbestos fibers are being released. In fact, multiple inspections have confirmed that the asbestos is safely sealed and poses no health risk if undisturbed.

2. **Does the doubt occur in an appropriate context?**

No, the doubt occurs in situations that do not represent any real disturbance. His doubt would be in context if, for example, there were visible signs of damage to the asbestos-containing materials, such as crumbling floorboards or walls, which could reasonably lead to concerns about asbestos exposure. However, none of this the case here.

3. **Is the doubt based on a real uncertainty?**

No, the doubt is not based on real uncertainty. The house has been inspected multiple times and declared safe. There is no lack of information or any need for more information.

4. **Does acting on the doubt help to resolve it?**

No, acting on the doubt by researching asbestos, repeatedly checking the house, calling professionals, and wearing protective gear does not resolve it. Mark's anxiety persists despite his exhaustive efforts and negative test results.

5. **Is the doubt rooted in common sense?**

No, while it is reasonable to worry about asbestos when moving into an old house, Mark's doubts centers around doubts about how it might be disturbed despite everything. His behavior goes beyond what is necessary and is not rooted in common sense. Mark would likely recognize this if he would temporarily step back out of the cycle.

B. *Considering all of your answers, is the doubt obsessional?*

In Mark's scenario, the doubt about asbestos contamination is obsessional rather than typical. There is no concrete evidence for his doubt, it occurs out of context, and it is not based on real uncertainty. There is no lack of information, and any new information fails to resolve the doubt. All together, this indicates his doubt is obsessional rather than an everyday doubt.

Form 4.4. Answers
Scenario 4.4: The Perfect Presentation

A. *What is the primary doubt and the feared consequences in this scenario?*

The primary doubt of Alex is that he might do poorly in his presentation. The secondary consequences of the doubt are that this would damage his professional reputation and lead to lost opportunities.

1. *Is there any concrete evidence in the senses for the doubt in the here-and-now?*

There is no concrete evidence in the here-and-now to suggest that Alex will do poorly. However, there is no tangible evidence either that the audience will find his presentation engaging.

2. *Does the doubt occur in an appropriate context?*

The doubt occurs in an appropriate context. It is typical to feel nervous and seek reassurance when preparing for a significant event like a major presentation.

3. *Is the doubt based on a real uncertainty?*

The doubt is based on a real uncertainty. Public speaking can be unpredictable, and it is natural to worry about performance. Also, the doubt does not relate to the present, but to the future. The future is inherently uncertain.

4. *Does acting on the doubt help to resolve it?*

Acting on the doubt by rehearsing the presentation, seeking feedback, and researching public speaking tips helps to resolve it. These actions provide Alex with more confidence and reassurance. However, because the doubt is focused on a future event, some anxiety may persist until the presentation is complete.

5. *Is the doubt rooted in common sense?*

The doubt is rooted in common sense. It is logical to want to ensure a successful presentation and to take steps to prepare thoroughly. Alex's actions are driven by a rational desire to perform well and make a positive impression.

B. *Considering all of your answers, is the doubt obsessional?*

There is no direct evidence for the doubt, but this does not automatically make the doubt obsessional. To determine if it is an everyday doubt, the context of the doubt needs to be taken into consideration. Alex's actions to prepare and seek feedback are appropriate given the context and are aimed at ensuring a successful presentation. The doubt is also based on real uncertainty given it deals with the future, *which is inherently uncertain. In fact, for a doubt to be obsessional, it typically must be focused on the here-and-now. The extent to which a person handles such natural uncertainties differs; for instance, poor handling of such uncertainties or overestimating the likelihood of negative events might lead to a panic attack or a public speaking phobia. However, such reactions still do not make the doubt obsessional.*

Form 4.5. Answers
Scenario 4.5: A Question of Sexual Identity

A. What is the primary doubt and the feared consequences in this scenario?

The primary doubt of Natalie in this scenario is: "What if I am not really bisexual?"

1. Is there any concrete evidence in the senses for the doubt in the here-and-now?

There is no concrete evidence in the here-and-now to support the doubt that Natalie might be exclusively heterosexual or gay instead of bisexual. In fact, her current attractions and relationships with both men and women affirm her bisexual identity. The doubt goes directly against her inner and outer senses. She feels genuine attraction to people of both genders. Her inner senses—her feelings and emotions—consistently validate her bisexuality, and her outer senses—her interactions and experiences—confirm this as well. This persistent doubt lacks any tangible basis and contradicts the reality she perceives through both her internal experiences and external interactions.

2. Does the doubt occur in an appropriate context?

No, the doubt occurs out of context. Her actual personal relationships and self-reflection do not require scrutiny given that her genuine feelings and experiences already naturally affirm her identity.

3. Is the doubt based on a real uncertainty?

The doubt is not based on a real uncertainty. Natalie's inner and outer senses already provide her with all the information she needs regarding her sexual orientation, grounded in her emotions and attractions towards both men and women. Real uncertainties arise from a lack of information or true ambivalence, which is not the case here.

4. Does acting on the doubt help to resolve it?

Acting on the doubt by over-analyzing her past relationships and interactions does not resolve it. The repetitive questioning and analysis indicate that the doubt is not being alleviated and persists despite everything. Each analysis provides temporary relief but does not truly address the fact that the underlying doubt arose without direct evidence to start with. Consequently, new information fails to have any real effect.

5. Is the doubt rooted in common sense?

The doubt is not based on common sense. Common sense would prompt Natalie to trust her consistent feelings and experiences as a bisexual person. Her continued worry and over-analysis are driven by fear rather than logical assessment. Common sense would conclude that her genuine attraction to both men and women is a clear indicator of her bisexual orientation.

B. *Considering all of your answers, is the doubt obsessional?*
Natalie's doubts about her sexual orientation are obsessional rather than typical because they persist despite her genuine and consistent experiences of attraction to both men and women. These doubts lack concrete evidence and arise from an unfounded fear rather than real uncertainty or ambiguity about her sexual orientation. Her inner senses—her feelings and emotional responses—consistently validate her bisexuality, as she experiences genuine attraction and emotional connections with both men and women. This inner sensory evidence, combined with her outward experiences and relationships, provides a clear and consistent affirmation of her bisexual identity. Yet, the obsessional doubts persist, leading her to repeatedly question her identity, analyze past relationships, and seek excessive reassurance from friends and partners. No resolution is ever achieved because the obsessional doubt excludes direct evidence from the start. This persistent questioning and the inability to find closure despite clear evidence indicates the presence of an obsessional doubt.

Form 4.6. Answers
Scenario 4.6: Haunted by Memories

A. *What is the primary doubt and the feared consequences in this scenario?*
In Sam's scenario, the primary doubts are centered around the accuracy of his memory documentation: "What if I forgot an important detail?", "What if my memory of this event isn't exactly right?", and "What if these photos don't represent the memory accurately?" The secondary feared consequences of these doubts include losing touch with important moments of his life and distorting his understanding of his past.

1. *Is there any concrete evidence in the senses for the doubt in the here-and-now?*
No, there is no concrete evidence in the here-and-now to suggest that Sam's memories are inaccurately recorded. The doubt is solely based on the possibility of not memorizing or documenting something correctly, despite his meticulous efforts.

2. *Does the doubt occur in an appropriate context?*
No, the doubt occurs out of context. Sam is not recording memories and events as part of a profession where such meticulous accuracy might be necessary, such as a historian or a court reporter. In those professions, precise documentation is critical and justified. In Sam's case, he is documenting personal memories for his own recollection, which does not require the same level of scrutiny. The measures he takes to ensure accuracy are therefore out of context given his personal situation.

3. *Is the doubt based on a real uncertainty?*
The doubt is not based on real uncertainty. The information needed to resolve the doubt is already available—his detailed journal entries and photos. The doubt arises from questioning the accuracy of these records rather than a lack of information.

4. Does acting on the doubt help to resolve it?

Acting on the doubt by rewriting journal entries and rearranging photos does not help to resolve it. Despite his exhaustive efforts, Sam's doubt and anxiety persist, indicating that his actions are not effective in addressing his concern.

5. Is the doubt rooted in common sense?

No, while it is logical to want accurate records of memories, the measures Sam takes to ensure accuracy are unreasonable. His behavior goes beyond what is necessary for accurate documentation and is not rooted in common sense. Sam would probably readily agree with this if he takes a moment to distance himself from his actions. Yet, he is likely unable to stop his compulsions regardless.

B. Considering all of your answers, is the doubt obsessional?

In Sam's scenario, the doubt about the accuracy of his memories is obsessional rather than typical. The doubt persists despite detailed and comprehensive documentation, occurs inappropriately out of context as his meticulous records should naturally eliminate such concerns, is not based on real uncertainty, is not resolved through his exhaustive efforts, and lacks a foundation in common sense. These factors indicate that his doubt is characteristic of obsessional thinking.

Form 4.7. Answers
Scenario 4.7: Health Scare

A. What is the primary doubt and the feared consequences in this scenario?

In David's scenario, the primary doubt is centered around the idea that he might have a serious gastrointestinal condition.

1. Is there any concrete evidence in the senses for the doubt in the here-and-now?

Yes, the concern occurs with tangible and concrete evidence of the doubt. David noticed an unusual and persistent abdominal discomfort, which justifies the need for medical evaluation and subsequent worry. This is a reasonable and everyday doubt based on tangible evidence.

2. Does the doubt occur in an appropriate context?

Yes, the doubt occurs in an appropriate context. David's concern about a gastrointestinal condition is based on persistent abdominal discomfort, which is a reasonable context for seeking medical advice. In contrast, if David were to have the same doubt about serious health issues every time he felt mild and temporary indigestion or bloating, this doubt would occur out of context.

3. Is the doubt based on a real uncertainty?

Yes, the doubt is based on real uncertainty. Until the ultrasound results are completed, there is an unknown factor regarding the cause of David's discomfort. While David experiences significant distress, this does not make the doubt obsessional. The level of anxiety from real uncertainty varies with an individual's ability to manage perceived threats; the extent of worry does not automatically indicate whether the doubt is obsessional.

4. *Does acting on the doubt help to resolve it?*

Yes, acting on the doubt by consulting his doctor, undergoing an ultrasound, and following up helps to resolve it. Once the tests confirm that there are no concerning findings, David's anxiety is alleviated.

5. *Is the doubt rooted in common sense?*

Yes, the doubt is rooted in common sense. Experiencing persistent abdominal discomfort warrants concern and justifies seeking medical attention. It is logical and prudent to investigate potential causes when tangible symptoms persist and are unexplained. Consulting with healthcare professionals and undergoing recommended tests are reasonable steps to ensure one's health. This common-sense approach contrasts with obsessional doubts that repeat and persist despite evidence and reassurance.

B. *Considering all of your answers, is the doubt obsessional?*

In this scenario, David's doubt about having a serious gastrointestinal condition is an everyday doubt. It is based on concrete evidence of experiencing persistent discomfort and occurs in an appropriate context. The doubt is rooted in real uncertainty about his health, which is resolved through medical investigation and professional reassurance. Unlike an obsessional doubt, David's concern is reasonable and alleviated by taking appropriate action and obtaining clear medical information.

Form 4.8 Answers
Scenario 4.8: Church Service

A. *What is the primary doubt and the feared consequences in this scenario?*

The primary doubt of Emily in this scenario is: "What if I am a blasphemer?" The feared consequences of Emily's doubt include judgment and condemnation from her religious community and a sense of spiritual failure.

1. *Is there any concrete evidence in the senses for the doubt in the here-and-now?*

There is no concrete evidence in the here-and-now to support the doubt that Emily is a blasphemer. There is no direct evidence she did anything wrong in the moments leading to the doubt. As she becomes immersed in this doubt, it is accompanied by intrusive thoughts and images related to blasphemy, but this is something entirely different from a real act of blasphemy with motivated intent. The occurrence of these intrusive thoughts and images can make it seem to Emily as though her inner senses provide concrete evidence for the doubt, but there was no such evidence in her inner senses initially. Any intrusive images or thoughts are merely expressions of her fear of blasphemy and do not reflect real, intentional blasphemous actions. They are byproducts of her obsessional doubt.

2. *Does the doubt occur in an appropriate context?*

The doubt that Emily might be blasphemer occurs completely out of context. She was actively participating in the church service, fully engaged in her worship, which indicates her sincere devotion. The context of her actions—praying, singing hymns, and focusing on the service—provides no basis for her having any inclination towards blasphemy. Therefore, the doubt that she might blaspheme was inappropriate for the context in which it arose.

3. Is the doubt based on a real uncertainty?

The doubt is not based on a real uncertainty. Real uncertainty arises from a lack of information or true ambiguity. Before the obsessional doubt arose, Emily was fully engaged in the service, focused on worship, and committed to her faith. Emily already has all the certainty she needs, given her sincere devotion and intentions. Her fear is not rooted in any actual uncertainty regarding her piety or intentions.

4. Does acting on the doubt help to resolve it?

Acting on the doubt by repeatedly reviewing her thoughts and actions does not resolve it. The repetitive mental checking indicates that the doubt is not being alleviated and persists despite clear evidence. Each review provides temporary relief but does not address the underlying obsessional doubt.

5. Is the doubt rooted in common sense?

The doubt is not based on common sense. Common sense would prompt Emily to trust her awareness and knowledge of her own behavior. Her continued worry and mental checking are driven by an irrational fear rather than logical assessment. Common sense would conclude that since she is aware of her actions and has no intention of blaspheming, there is no need for further mental review. Her obsessional doubt dismisses this evidence, leading to unnecessary anxiety and guilt.

B. Considering all of your answers, is the doubt obsessional?

Emily's doubt is obsessional because it lacks concrete evidence, occurs out of context, and persists despite efforts to resolve it. Her fear of having blasphemed arises even though she has not done anything disrespectful. Any images or thoughts related to blasphemy that arise from this fear do not provide direct evidence for it; they are merely byproducts of her obsessional doubt. The doubt is also not based on real uncertainty, as her actions and thoughts are consistent with her faith. Furthermore, her repetitive mental reviewing and seeking reassurance do not alleviate her anxiety. This irrational and disproportionate doubt, driven by an unfounded fear, typifies obsessional thinking.

Worse than Worry
Scenario 4.2. Obsessional Version of "The Dog Spa"

Sarah's dog is overdue for a grooming. Unfortunately, the dog spa she normally goes to went out of business, so she has to find a new one. After checking online, Sarah finds a spa nearby that has good reviews and comes highly recommended. She books an appointment, but despite the positive feedback, Sarah becomes increasingly anxious as the appointment approaches. "What if they don't treat my dog well?" she worries, even though there is no evidence to suggest this might be the case.

As the day of the appointment nears, Sarah's worry intensifies. She begins to imagine worst-case scenarios where her dog is mistreated or traumatized. These fears become so vivid that Sarah finds it hard to focus on anything else. She starts re-reading the reviews multiple times, obsessing over even the slightest neutral or vaguely negative comment. A persistent thought nags at her: "What if I missed something important while reading the reviews or researching online?"

Despite visiting the spa and initially feeling reassured by the staff and the facility, Sarah's anxiety does not subside. She starts calling the spa repeatedly, asking detailed questions about their procedures and staff qualifications. She even drives by the spa several times to observe from outside, hoping to catch a glimpse of how they handle other pets. Despite these actions, the thought that she might have overlooked a crucial piece of information while researching keeps gnawing at her.

The night before the appointment, Sarah hardly sleeps, consumed by worry. She spends hours online, researching alternative spas and reading articles about pet grooming mishaps. Her anxiety only grows, fueled by the hypothetical scenarios she envisions. On the day of the grooming, she arrives at the spa early and waits anxiously, constantly checking her watch and texting friends for reassurance.

Even after the grooming session, Sarah continues to worry. She meticulously checks her dog for any signs of trauma or mistreatment, repeatedly asking the staff if everything went well. Despite their reassurances and her dog appearing perfectly fine, the doubt persists. Sarah continues to feel anxious, trapped in a cycle of worry and seeking reassurance, plagued by the thought that she might have missed something important during her research.

Why is this an obsessional scenario?

Like in the non-obsessional scenario, Sarah's initial doubt about her dog possibly being mistreated is an everyday doubt, stemming from real uncertainty due to the lack of information about the new dog spa. However, what makes this scenario obsessional is the subsequent doubt that emerges: Sarah begins to doubt that she might have missed something important during her research. There is no actual evidence for this new doubt; it occurs out of context and is therefore unresolvable. Sarah's anxiety does not subside but instead builds up, even to the point where she continues to worry after her dog has been to the spa with no indication of harm. This persistent, irrational, and contextually inappropriate doubt characterizes obsessional thinking, contrasting with the initial reasonable concern that was based on real uncertainty. It exemplifies how everyday or excessive worrying can sometimes interact with obsessional doubt, yet they represent distinct processes.

Reasonable Precautions
Scenario 4.3: Non-Obsessional Version of "Asbestos Contamination"

Mark recently moved into an older house and learned that asbestos was commonly used in building materials during the time his house was constructed. The home inspector informed him that there is asbestos in some of the building materials but assured him that there are no health risks since it is sealed behind floorboards and in good condition.

The inspector emphasized that there is nothing to worry about as long as the asbestos is left undisturbed. Despite this reassurance, Mark becomes slightly concerned about the possibility of contamination. He starts thinking, "If the asbestos is disturbed, there might be a risk of contamination."

This thought prompts Mark to take several precautions. He avoids unnecessary renovations and ensures that any repairs are done by professionals who are aware of the asbestos and know how to handle it safely. He also occasionally checks the condition of the floorboards and walls. He feels reassured by the professional inspections and takes comfort in knowing that as long as the asbestos remains undisturbed, there is no risk.

Mark does some research on asbestos to better understand it but focuses on credible sources that emphasize safety measures rather than sensational horror stories. He makes sure to follow the recommended guidelines for living in a house with asbestos-containing materials. Mark feels confident that by following these guidelines, he is protecting himself and his family.

Why is this a non-obsessional scenario?

In this scenario, Mark's concern about asbestos contamination if it is disturbed, is an everyday doubt. It is grounded in concrete evidence and information directly relevant to the present situation. The risk of contamination if the asbestos is disturbed represents a real uncertainty, which can be addressed by obtaining more information and taking precautions in situations where there are concrete and visible disturbances. This contrasts with the obsessional scenario, where Mark worried about the possibility of disturbance without any tangible evidence. Overall, Mark's concern about contamination in this scenario reflects an everyday and reasonable doubt.

Endless Preparation
Scenario 4.4: Obsessional Version of "The Perfect Presentation"

Alex is preparing for an important presentation at work. Although he has already prepared thoroughly, he becomes increasingly anxious about the possibility of not being sufficiently prepared. Despite having all his materials organized and rehearsing multiple times, he starts thinking, "What if I'm not prepared enough?" This doubt begins to dominate his thoughts.

Alex starts repeatedly going over his presentation, even though he has already received positive feedback from colleagues. He spends hours rechecking his slides, rewriting his notes, and rehearsing his speech. He begins to worry about minute details, such as the exact wording of his slides and the order of his bullet points, fearing that any small error could ruin the presentation. He fears that not being adequately prepared might lead to a series of negative consequences: not being able to answer questions, making a fool of himself in front of his colleagues, damaging his professional reputation, and ultimately harming his career prospects.

To calm his anxiety, Alex repeatedly asks his colleagues for feedback, even after they assure him that his presentation is excellent. He also spends an excessive amount of time researching best practices for presentations, looking for anything he might have overlooked. Despite this, his doubt persists, making it difficult for him to focus on other tasks.

The night before the presentation, Alex barely sleeps. He stays up late, constantly tweaking his slides and notes. He even considers canceling the presentation, fearing that he is not fully prepared. On the day of the presentation, his anxiety is at its peak. He goes through his materials one last time, but the doubt remains.

Why is this an obsessional scenario?

There is no concrete evidence suggesting that Alex has not prepared enough. In fact, he has prepared thoroughly and received positive feedback. While it is possible that a presentation could go badly, these are real uncertainties about the future. It can make anyone feel nervous about a presentation, especially when one overestimates the likelihood of things going wrong or when having difficulty dealing with these uncertainties. However, this is not what makes the scenario obsessional. What makes this scenario obsessional is that Alex already has certainty regarding his thorough preparation, yet he doubts this without any direct evidence. Moreover, these doubts occur out of context in situations unrelated to giving a good presentation. As a result, additional preparation does not help to resolve the doubt and lessen his anxiety. It's a bottomless pit of preparation during which his anxiety can only further increase.

Natalie's Path to Self-Discovery
Scenario 4.5: Non-Obsessional Version of "A Question of Sexual Identity"

Natalie, a woman who has identified as bisexual for many years, has recently started questioning her sexual orientation. She has been in relationships with both men and women, but over the past year, she has noticed a shift in her attractions. She realizes she has not felt a genuine attraction to men in quite some time, and her emotional and physical interest has been exclusively toward women.

During a conversation with her therapist, Natalie shares these changes. "I've been wondering if I might actually be gay, not bisexual," she says. This thought feels unsettling, as she has always believed her bisexual identity was a core part of who she is. Natalie is curious but cautious, wanting to understand these feelings without invalidating her past experiences.

Her therapist encourages Natalie to reflect on her feelings in the present. As part of this process, Natalie notices how her emotional and physical connections with women currently feel deeper and more fulfilling. This realization emerges naturally as part of her self-exploration, rather than through exhaustive analysis of her past.

Natalie also shares her thoughts with a few close friends, choosing people she knows will listen with empathy. These conversations help Natalie affirm what she already senses: her feelings are valid, and her identity can evolve over time. Her friends remind her that discovering herself is about honoring the truth of her present.

As Natalie continues her introspective journey, she begins to accept that her recent lack of attraction to men and her stronger connections with women are genuine reflections of her current self. Through journaling and supportive conversations, Natalie feels empowered to embrace the possibility that she might identify as gay. She also acknowledges that the process of understanding herself fully is not one of complete certainty. Instead, she finds comfort in knowing that uncertainty is a part of her journey and something she can live with as she continues to grow.

Although the process was initially accompanied by confusion and anxiety, Natalie begins to feel a growing sense of peace. She recognizes that her understanding of herself is evolving, and each step brings her closer to what feels authentic. For Natalie, this is an ongoing process, and she feels a deepening clarity with every moment of reflection and connection.

Why is this a non-obsessional scenario?

In this non-obsessional scenario, Natalie's doubts about her sexual orientation arise from real changes in her attractions and feelings. Her actions—such as reflecting on her emotions, journaling, and speaking with trusted friends—are appropriate and aimed at understanding her evolving identity. These actions are rooted in genuine experiences and self-awareness, not in compulsive analysis or reasoning.

While Natalie feels some anxiety due to the personal significance of her sexual orientation, her concerns are grounded in real, tangible uncertainty and genuine experiences. She approaches her feelings with curiosity and openness, recognizing the evolving nature of her attractions and avoiding the trap of overanalyzing her past.

As Natalie continues her journey, her anxiety subsides, and she begins to feel more at peace. While she is not entirely certain about her identity, she is able to embrace this uncertainty as a natural part of her process of self-discovery. This reflects a healthy, grounded approach to understanding and accepting her evolving sexual orientation.

Critical Precision
Scenario 4.6: Non-Obsessional Version of "Haunted by Memories"

Sam, an experienced intelligence officer, has been assigned a high-stakes mission involving the capture of a notorious terrorist leader. The mission's success hinges on the precise and accurate documentation of intelligence reports, which will be used to plan and execute the operation. Any error could lead to catastrophic consequences, including the potential loss of lives.

As Sam reviews the intelligence reports, he notices a discrepancy in the timing of a critical event. The report indicates that the target was seen at two different locations simultaneously. This discrepancy immediately raises a red flag. "What if there's an error in the data?" Sam thinks. This doubt is not just a minor concern but a critical issue that needs to be addressed to ensure the operation's success.

Understanding the gravity of the situation, Sam decides to re-examine the surveillance footage and cross-reference it with satellite images and eyewitness accounts. He spends several hours meticulously going through the data, ensuring that every piece of information is accurate.

Throughout the process, Sam feels a mix of anxiety and determination. He understands that the accuracy of his report is crucial. "If I miss anything, it could jeopardize the entire mission," he reminds himself. The weight of responsibility is immense, but Sam knows that his diligence can make the difference between success and failure.

Finally, after an exhaustive review, Sam identifies the source of the discrepancy: a timestamp error in one of the surveillance videos. He corrects the mistake and updates the report with the verified information. Feeling confident about the accuracy of the data, Sam prepares for the final briefing with the operation team.

Why is this a non-obsessional scenario?

In Sam's scenario, the doubt about the accuracy of the intelligence report is typical rather than obsessional. The doubt is based on concrete evidence, occurs in an appropriate context given the nature of his job, is rooted in real uncertainty, is resolved through meticulous verification, and is grounded in common sense. These factors indicate that his doubt is rational and necessary, characteristic of the critical precision required in his role as an intelligence officer.

Digestive Doubts
Scenario 4.7: Obsessional Version of "Health Scare"

David, a 35-year-old man, comes across an article online about gastrointestinal cancers. The article lists several symptoms, including persistent abdominal pain, unexplained bloating, and changes in bowel habits. Although David hasn't experienced severe issues with his digestion, he recently noticed occasional discomfort in his abdomen after meals. This discomfort starts to consume his thoughts, making him anxious about the possibility of having a serious health condition.

The idea that he could have cancer begins to dominate his mind. He schedules an appointment with his primary care physician, who performs an examination and reassures David that his symptoms are likely due to mild indigestion or dietary choices. Despite this reassurance, David insists on undergoing a series of diagnostic tests to rule out cancer completely.

After receiving test results showing no evidence of any abnormalities, David's anxiety intensifies. He starts thinking, "What if the tests missed something? What if it's too early for anything to show up?" These thoughts spiral into a pervasive fear that refuses to abate.

David begins obsessively researching gastrointestinal cancers and their symptoms. He spends hours reading medical forums and horror stories about misdiagnoses. He starts scrutinizing every minor sensation in his abdomen, interpreting normal digestive functions as potential warning signs of cancer. He frequently presses on his stomach, trying to detect lumps or areas of tenderness, and becomes hyper-aware of any subtle changes in his body.

To soothe his growing anxiety, David repeatedly seeks reassurance from his doctor and even consults multiple specialists. Despite all of them confirming that there is no evidence of cancer, his doubts persist, making it increasingly hard for him to focus on work or social activities.

David's fear escalates to the point where he avoids certain foods and activities, believing they might exacerbate his symptoms or cause further harm. He keeps detailed records of every sensation and digestive change he notices, constantly analyzing and revisiting his logs for patterns that might indicate illness. Despite all the medical evidence and reassurance pointing to his good health, David cannot shake the overwhelming fear that something is seriously wrong.

Why is this a non-obsessional scenario?

In this scenario, David's doubt about having gastrointestinal cancer is obsessional rather than an everyday doubt. His concern persists despite mild symptoms and multiple medical assurances of good health. This doubt occurs out of context, as there are no significant signs like severe pain or unexplained weight loss to justify his worry. Despite thorough evaluations and reassurances, David continues to monitor his body obsessively and seek unnecessary tests, with no resolution to his anxiety. The lack of concrete evidence and the out-of-context nature of his doubt clearly distinguish it as obsessional rather than a typical, resolvable concern.

Navigating Values and Real Uncertainty
Scenario 4.8: Non-Obsessional Version of "Church Service"

Emily, a devoutly religious person, is attending a church service. During a moment of intense frustration earlier in the day, she had a slip of the tongue and accidentally said a word that could be considered blasphemous. This incident has been weighing heavily on her mind.

As she participates in the service, the memory of her words resurfaces, and she begins to worry: "What if what I said was truly blasphemous?" This thought causes her significant distress because she values her faith deeply and strives to live according to its principles.

Emily is concerned that her words might have been disrespectful to her faith, and she fears judgment from her religious community and from a higher power. Throughout the service, Emily feels a mix of guilt and anxiety. She mentally reviews the incident, trying to remember exactly what she said and the context in which she said it. She reassures herself that she did not intend to be disrespectful, but the doubt persists, making it difficult for her to focus on the service.

After the service, Emily approaches her pastor and explains what happened. Her pastor listens attentively and tells her that it was indeed a blasphemous word, but also reminds her that faith is about intention and growth, and that she can seek forgiveness and move forward. He also reminds her of her genuine commitment to her faith and the fact that everyone makes mistakes. This conversation helps Emily feel more at ease, knowing that she can address her mistake and continue to grow in her faith.

Why is this a non-obsessional scenario?

In this alternate scenario with Emily, the doubt about whether she said something blasphemous is an everyday doubt rather than an obsessional doubt. The doubt is based on concrete evidence and arises in an appropriate context during a moment of intense frustration. It is also rooted in real uncertainty, which can be resolved through seeking guidance from her pastor. These factors indicate that her doubt is rational and grounded in common sense, reflecting the behavior of someone genuinely concerned about aligning their actions with their values while addressing a potential mistake. Additionally, her doubt is based on her inner senses, as she really did have a slip of the tongue when highly frustrated, which adds validity to her concern and makes it an everyday, resolvable doubt.

On the Hamster Wheel
Form 4.14: Crafting Obsessions: "Going Through My Exercise Routine"

John always prided himself on his consistent exercise routine. Every morning, he would wake up at 6 AM and head to the gym. However, over time, his routine began to be overshadowed by doubts. It started subtly. After completing his workout, John would find himself questioning whether he had done enough to stay in shape. He would think, "Did I really push myself hard enough today?" This doubt gnawed at him, despite feeling exhausted and knowing he followed his usual routine.

Soon, the doubts became more persistent. John started checking the time constantly during his workout. He would repeatedly glance at the clock, worrying that he hadn't spent enough time on each exercise. Even if his watch showed the usual hour-long session, he couldn't shake the feeling that he needed to do more. His workout routine turned into a series of endless, repetitive actions. John meticulously counted his reps and sets, doubting his memory and recounting several times. "Did I do ten push-ups or only nine?" This thought would linger, prompting him to do extra reps just to be sure. The need for certainty led him to prolong his sessions, turning what was once a one-hour routine into a two-hour ordeal.

John's obsession extended beyond counting. He began avoiding exercises he wasn't confident about, sticking only to those he felt he could perform perfectly. Even then, he would often redo sets, fearing he hadn't executed them correctly. The thought, "Was that squat deep enough??" would prompt him to repeat the exercise. His quest for the perfect workout led him down rabbit holes of online research. John became the Sherlock Holmes of fitness routines, piecing together clues from various fitness blogs. Each new discovery led to a complete overhaul of his plan, spawning even more doubt.

John's social life began to suffer. Invitations from friends were declined because he needed to fit in extra workouts. He avoided activities that might interfere with his exercise schedule, all the while feeling trapped in a cycle of doubt and compulsion, much like a hamster running endlessly on its wheel. Despite his increased efforts, John never felt satisfied. The reassurance he sought was always just out of reach, replaced by new doubts and more stringent routines. His once-enjoyable exercise regimen had become a source of anxiety, and yet he felt compelled to continue, unable to break free from the hamster wheel of his obsessional doubts.

Pizzagate
Form 4.14: Crafting Obsessions: "Making my Favorite Meal"

Hannah loved making her favorite pizza every Friday night. It was a tradition she looked forward to all week. However, over time, her joy began to be overshadowed by obsessional doubts, primarily the fear of accidentally poisoning someone with her cooking. It started subtly. After kneading the dough and spreading the sauce, Hannah would find herself wondering if the ingredients were fresh enough. She would think, "What if the cheese isn't safe to eat?" This doubt gnawed at her, despite knowing she had purchased the ingredients just the day before.

Soon, the doubts became more persistent. Hannah started double-checking the expiration dates on every single ingredient—not once, but multiple times. Even if the dates clearly indicated the items were fresh, she couldn't shake the feeling that something might still be wrong. Each time, she carefully examined every item, doubting her memory and re-checking over and over. "Did I rinse the vegetables properly?" This thought would stick, prompting her to rinse them repeatedly, just to be sure.

Hannah's obsession extended beyond checking ingredients. She began avoiding certain toppings she didn't feel confident using, sticking only to those she believed were unquestionably safe. Even then, she would often repeat steps, worrying they weren't done correctly. "Did I cook the sausage enough?" would prompt her to put it back on the stove, even if it was already overdone. Her quest for the perfect, safe pizza led her into endless online research. Hannah became obsessed with food safety tips, scouring countless blogs for advice. Each new discovery led her to question her methods even further, sparking additional doubts. She'd joke to herself, "Maybe I should start a blog: Confessions of a Paranoid Pizzaiolo."

Hannah's social life started to take a hit. Friends would suggest pizza nights, but she often declined, saying she needed extra time to prepare. ""Sorry, can't make it tonight, I'm having a culinary crisis," she'd joke, though her friends knew there was some truth to it. Hosting friends felt like purposely trying to poison someone. She began to worry, "Maybe I really do have something to confess. Am I a killer without even knowing it?"

Form 5.1. Case of Jack (Vignette 1.1)
Potential Reasons Behind Jack's Obsessional Doubts

Condensed Primary Doubt(s)
"I might be a violent person without knowing it, capable of causing harm at any moment."

Abstract facts and ideas — Things that you know or believe to be true in general.

a. Everyone has a capacity for violence under certain circumstances.
b. The mind can harbor unconscious desires that we are completely unaware of.
c. It is possible to do something terrible without remembering it.

Personal experience — Your own personal experience, past or present

a. I've lost my temper before; what if it escalates?
b. I once accidentally struck someone's fingers with a hammer while we were working on a project.
c. I once had a very vivid dream about hurting someone, and it felt disturbingly real.

Values, standards and rules — The way of doing things according to an accepted principle.

a. It's always better to be cautious about one's own potential for harmful behavior.
b. If you suspect you could be a threat, it's responsible to take preventive measures.
c. People can be unpredictable, so it's wise to remain vigilant about one's own behavior.

Authorities — A person, institution or organization that is perceived as important.

a. Experts say that some mental health issues can go unnoticed for years.
b. Therapists say that unresolved childhood issues can manifest as violence in adulthood.
c. I read that even people who seem gentle can have hidden aggressive tendencies.

Hearsay and news — Information that you got from other people, substantiated or not.

a. I heard stories and news reports about people who seemed perfectly normal but had sudden violent outbursts.
b. There was an article about a well-liked teacher who was arrested for assault, shocking everyone who knew them.
c. Someone told me about a distant family member who had a hidden violent streak

Anything else — Anything that does not fit well in the previous categories

a. Why would I be thinking about violence if I'm not violent?
b. Sometimes I feel a strange sense of detachment, like I'm not in control of my own actions.
c. I've noticed a pattern where I'm more irritable when I'm tired, and I fear this could lead to something worse.

Form 5.1. Case of Rachel (Vignette 1.2)
Potential reasons behind Rachel's Obsessional doubts

Condensed Primary Doubt(s)
"Maybe I am sexually attracted to children."

Abstract facts and ideas — Things that you know or believe to be true in general.

a. Some people have hidden feelings or tendencies they are unaware of until later in life.
b. Unwanted intrusive thoughts can feel like they reveal something deeper about a person.
c. Psychology suggests that people sometimes misinterpret their own feelings or sensations, leading to doubt.

Personal experience — Your own personal experience, past or present

a. Sometimes, when I interact with children, I feel a sensation or reaction that makes me question myself.
b. There have been moments where I second-guessed whether my actions, like a smile or touch, were entirely appropriate.
c. I very much enjoy my work and spending time with children.

Values, standards and rules — The way of doing things according to an accepted principle.

a. I believe that it's essential to maintain control over my thoughts and feelings to ensure I am a good person.
b. I hold myself to high moral standards and feel deeply ashamed if I believe I've fallen short.
c. It's my responsibility as a teacher to protect the children in my care.

Authorities — A person, institution or organization that is perceived as important.

a. I've read that some people hide inappropriate tendencies for years without realizing it.
b. Experts say that inappropriate feelings can sometimes manifest in subtle or unexpected ways.
c. A famous psychologist once said that we many desires hidden in the unconscious.

Hearsay and news — Information that you got from other people, substantiated or not.

a. Media often covers stories of individuals who appeared normal but were later revealed to have hidden tendencies.
b. I've heard people discuss how others misinterpret their feelings or don't realize the implications of their thoughts.
c. I've read an online discussion about inappropriate thoughts about children and what they might mean.

Anything else — Anything that does not fit well in the previous categories

a. The very fact that I keep questioning my thoughts makes me feel like something must be wrong.
b. The intensity and persistence of these doubts make them feel like they must have a real basis.
c. My emotional reactions, like guilt and shame, make it seem as though my thoughts reflect something true about me.

Form 5.1. Case of John (Vignette 1.3)
Potential reasons behind John's Obsessional doubts

Condensed Primary Doubt(s)
"Perhaps I don't truly believe in God anymore and have lost my faith."

Abstract facts and ideas — Things that you know or believe to be true in general.

a. People can lose their faith even after years of being devout.
b. Spiritual crises are common and are often signs of weakening or loss of belief.
c. Doubt could indicate a lack of true belief.

Personal experience — Your own personal experience, past or present

a. I've experienced moments where I felt disconnected during spiritual practices.
b. There was a period in my life I did not believe in anything.
c. Some family members close to me have lost their faith.

Values, standards and rules — The way of doing things according to an accepted principle.

a. I want to ensue having a strong and unwavering connection to God.
b. It's important for me to be faithful and not question God.
c. I want to do everything I can to remain faithful.

Authorities — A person, institution or organization that is perceived as important.

a. Religious teachings frequently emphasize the importance of faith.
b. It is said that even the most faithful people can lose their faith.
c. Religious scholars often talk about how prolonged questioning can erode belief.

Hearsay and news — Information that you got from other people, substantiated or not.

a. I saw on a religious TV program that some people lose their faith when they stop feeling God's presence.
b. A friend mentioned how someone they knew lost their faith after a period of intense questioning.
c. I saw on the news that faith is declining across the country.

Anything else — Anything that does not fit well in the previous categories

a. A strong faith means trusting without constant questioning, but I question everything now.
b. Faith should provide clear guidance in life, and if it doesn't, maybe it's not real anymore.
c. Losing faith can catch you by surprise.

Form 5.1. Case of Laura (Vignette 1.4)
Potential reasons behind Laura's Obsessional doubts

Condensed Primary Doubt(s)
"I could be a dishonest and unethical person without realizing."

Abstract facts and ideas — Things that you know or believe to be true in general.

a. People sometimes lie or act unethically without realizing it, especially in subtle situations.
b. Small, unintentional actions can reflect deeper character flaws that might not be obvious.
c. Dishonesty isn't always deliberate; people can deceive others without fully intending to.

Personal experience — Your own personal experience, past or present

a. I forgot to credit a colleague on a project, which made me wonder if I am more careless or dishonest than I realized.
b. There have been times when I felt uncertain about whether I was entirely truthful in my words.
c. I once accidentally overcharged a client, which left me questioning my intentions and ethics.

Values, standards and rules — The way of doing things according to an accepted principle.

a. I hold myself to high standards of honesty.
b. If I can't guarantee 100% honesty, then maybe I'm not as ethical as I think I am.
c. A truly moral person should be able to avoid even the appearance of dishonesty at all times.

Authorities — A person, institution or organization that is perceived as important.

a. Ethical guidelines at work emphasize the importance of transparency, and any mistake could be seen as dishonesty.
b. I've read that good character is about consistency; even a small lapse could indicate a lack of integrity.
c. Moral and ethical teachings often warn that self-deception can lead people to act immorally without being aware of it.

Hearsay and news — Information that you got from other people, substantiated or not.

a. I've heard stories about seemingly honest people who were later exposed as dishonest.
b. Friends and family sometimes mention that everyone is capable of mistakes, but it makes me wonder if these mistakes reveal something deeper.
c. I saw a news story about someone who unknowingly committed fraud, which made me worry that I might also act unethically without realizing it.

Anything else — Anything that does not fit well in the previous categories

a. If I'm constantly doubting myself, it might be because there's something I'm missing about my own behavior.
b. My intense need for validation from others makes me worry that I'm not trustworthy on my own.
c. The fact that I keep questioning my own honesty could mean there's truth to my doubts.

Form 5.1. Case of Ethan (Vignette 1.5)
Potential reasons behind Ethan's Obsessional doubts

> ### Condensed Primary Doubt(s)
> *"I could have missed something or left something undone."*
> *"Maybe things are not functioning as they should."*

Abstract facts and ideas — Things that you know or believe to be true in general.

a. It's possible to overlook small details or make mistakes without realizing it.
b. Safety measures and appliances can fail unexpectedly, even if they appear to be functioning.
c. Just because something seems secure doesn't mean it is; unexpected failures can happen at any time.

Personal experience — Your own personal experience, past or present

a. I've left things on before, like lights or the stove, and had to return home to turn them off.
b. There have been times when I didn't fully remember whether I had locked the door or turned off an appliance.
c. Once, I thought something was properly secured, but it wasn't, which made me more cautious afterward.

Values, standards and rules — The way of doing things according to an accepted principle.
a. I believe in being thorough and responsible, especially with tasks that involve safety.
b. Any small lapse in checking could have serious consequences, so it's better to be safe than sorry.
c. True responsibility means ensuring things are in order, even if it takes extra time.

Authorities — A person, institution or organization that is perceived as important.

a. Safety guidelines often emphasize the importance of double-checking to prevent accidents.
b. Articles I've read recommend checking appliances and doors carefully, as accidents can happen when they're overlooked.
c. Instructions on devices often advise confirming they're off or unplugged to avoid malfunctions or hazards.

Hearsay and news — Information that you got from other people, substantiated or not.
a. I've heard stories about house fires and accidents caused by small oversights, like leaving something on.
b. News reports frequently cover incidents where a minor oversight led to larger issues, such as electrical fires.
c. Friends or family have mentioned times they forgot to turn something off, which caused them worry later.

Anything else — Anything that does not fit well in the previous categories
a. The fact that I keep questioning myself might mean I'm missing something important each time.
b. My frequent need to check could be a signal that things aren't working as they should.
c. Constant doubt about whether things are in order could mean I need to improve my attention to detail.

Form 5.1. Case of Sophie (Vignette 1.6)
Potential reasons behind Sophie's Obsessional doubts

> ### Condensed Primary Doubt(s)
> *"I could be contaminated by toxic chemicals, both in my surroundings and the environment, that are impossible to avoid or eliminate."*

Abstract facts and ideas — Things that you know or believe to be true in general.

a. Many common products contain chemicals that can be harmful with prolonged exposure.
b. Research often highlights the potential dangers of synthetic materials and chemicals in everyday items.
c. Toxic substances can linger on surfaces and in the air, potentially spreading to other areas.

Personal experience — Your own personal experience, past or present

a. I've experienced times when I felt a strong reaction or sensitivity to certain cleaning products.
b. There was a time I accidentally spilled a strong-smelling product in my bag, and the smell lingered on everything for days, even after cleaning it.
c. I once noticed that after touching something sticky, it felt like I kept finding residue on different things I touched throughout the day, even after I thought I'd cleaned my hands.

Values, standards and rules — The way of doing things according to an accepted principle.

a. I believe in keeping my environment safe and uncontaminated for myself and others.
b. I feel responsible for making sure I'm not exposing anyone to potentially harmful chemicals.
c. I value cleanliness and thoroughness, and any uncertainty around toxins feels like a failure to protect those values.

Authorities — A person, institution or organization that is perceived as important.

a. Experts often warn about the risks of long-term exposure to certain household chemicals.
b. Many environmental organizations caution against the widespread use of chemical-based products, recommending limited exposure.
c. Many chemical products come with health warnings.

Hearsay and news — Information that you got from other people, substantiated or not.

a. I've seen news stories about people experiencing serious health issues from chemical exposure.
b. I read an article on the harmful effects of household cleaners, which made me question what's truly safe.
c. I heard about cases where people unknowingly spread contaminants, causing harm to others.

Anything else — Anything that does not fit well in the previous categories

a. The more I read about toxins, the harder it feels to keep my environment truly safe from them.
b. The constant possibility of missing contaminants makes me fear that I'm unable to protect myself or others effectively.
c. Even when I've done my best to clean, I sometimes still notice lingering odors or stains, which makes me wonder if other substances I can't see are still present.

Form 5.1. Case of Matthew (Vignette 1.7)
Potential reasons behind Matthew's Obsessional doubts

Condensed Primary Doubt(s)
"Perhaps things haven't been placed right, or done right, or well enough."

Abstract facts and ideas — Things that you know or believe to be true in general.

a. Small misalignments can impact the overall balance and harmony of a design or environment.
b. Mistakes, even minor ones, can lead to larger issues if left unchecked.
c. Precision is essential in many fields to achieve quality and prevent errors.

Personal experience — Your own personal experience, past or present

a. I've made minor mistakes in projects before, which were only noticed later and required extra time to correct.
b. There have been times when I felt something was off but couldn't pinpoint it until I spent extra time reviewing it.
c. My attention to detail is often praised, which makes me worry that I'll let people down if something isn't perfect.

Values, standards and rules — The way of doing things according to an accepted principle.

a. I believe that a job should be done well.
b. Accuracy and symmetry reflect high standards and professionalism, especially in architecture.
c. Maintaining order and alignment in my environment helps me feel grounded and in control.

Authorities — A person, institution or organization that is perceived as important.

a. My training in architecture emphasized precision and attention to detail, as even minor mistakes can affect the entire structure.
b. Experts in design stress that even slight misalignments can disrupt the aesthetics and balance of a space.
c. Professional standards in architecture and design uphold that perfection and symmetry are fundamental to quality work.

Hearsay and news — Information that you got from other people, substantiated or not.

a. I've heard colleagues talk about how clients and supervisors notice even small mistakes in our line of work.
b. I read an article that discussed the importance of alignment and order in creating pleasing and functional spaces.
c. Friends have mentioned that first impressions, even with something small like a desk setup, can influence people's perceptions.

Anything else — Anything that does not fit well in the previous categories

a. When I feel something is out of place, it creates a sense of discomfort that's hard to ignore.
b. I worry that if I don't double-check things, I'll overlook something that could affect my work or surroundings.
c. The urge to make sure everything is perfect feels instinctual, as if it's the only way to truly feel at ease.

Form 5.1. Case of Olivia (Vignette 1.8)
Potential reasons behind Olivia's Obsessional doubts

Condensed Primary Doubt(s)
"Perhaps my body is not performing as it should."
"Perhaps I will lose control over my attention and mind."

Abstract facts and ideas — Things that you know or believe to be true in general.

a. The body can sometimes malfunction or act unpredictably without clear signs.
b. The mind can fixate on certain sensations, creating difficulty in focusing elsewhere.
c. It's possible to become overly aware of the functions of body and mind.

Personal experience — Your own personal experience, past or present

a. I've noticed that sometimes my breathing feels shallow, which makes me wonder if it's functioning properly.
b. I've experienced times when I couldn't stop thinking about certain sensations, making me feel as though my body wasn't acting normally.
c. A past experience where I felt I had lost control over my mind makes me worry it could happen again, leaving me feeling vulnerable.

Values, standards and rules — The way of doing things according to an accepted principle.

a. I value being in control of my mind and body and believe it's important to maintain that control.
b. Self-awareness helps to avoid bad habits that might otherwise go unnoticed.
c. I value self-awareness and attentiveness to my body's functioning to avoid developing unnoticed habits that might impact my well-being.

Authorities — A person, institution or organization that is perceived as important.

a. Health experts often suggest that monitoring body signals is essential to detect early signs of issues.
b. Some people need to actively control their breathing or swallowing due to specific health conditions.
c. Mental health professionals acknowledge that certain sensations can become highly fixated, making it difficult to focus elsewhere.

Hearsay and news — Information that you got from other people, substantiated or not.

a. I've heard stories of people who needed to focus on breathing or other bodily functions to maintain their health.
b. News articles on health sometimes emphasize that being attentive to bodily sensations is beneficial for long-term well-being.
c. I read about a story of a person with hiccups for years unable to concentrate on anything else.

Anything else — Anything that does not fit well in the previous categories

a. The more I notice a bodily sensation, the harder it is to let go of it, making me feel like something might be wrong.
b. The fact that I repeatedly think about these functions makes me feel like there may be a deeper issue with how my body or mind is performing.
c. My strong urge to control my mind and bodily sensations makes me wonder if I'm missing something important about my own functioning.

Form 5.1. Case of Henry (Vignette 1.9)
Potential reasons behind Henry's Obsessional doubts

Condensed Primary Doubt(s)
"Maybe I'm really gay and have been lying to myself."

Abstract facts and ideas — Things that you know or believe to be true in general.

a. People can discover hidden aspects of themselves later in life, which makes me wonder if my true sexuality could be one of them.
b. It's possible for people to be in denial about their sexual orientation without realizing it, as I've read or heard before.
c. Attraction isn't always clear-cut, and I could be misinterpreting or suppressing my own feelings without being aware of it.

Personal experience — Your own personal experience, past or present

a. In the past, I've questioned my feelings in relationships, which makes me wonder if I was ignoring something deeper.
b. I've had sexual experiences with the same sex when growing up and exploring sexuality.
c. When I'm with my girlfriend, I sometimes feel distant or distracted, which makes me wonder if my lack of engagement is a sign of suppressed attraction elsewhere.

Values, standards and rules — The way of doing things according to an accepted principle.

a. It feels wrong if I'm hiding part of my identity.
b. I believe relationships should be based on genuine attraction.
c. Authenticity in relationships is important to me.

Authorities — A person, institution or organization that is perceived as important.

a. Mental health professionals and media sources often discuss "coming out later in life," which makes me question if that could apply to me.
b. I've read articles where people talked about being in denial about their orientation for years, which makes me worry that I could be suppressing something.
c. Sexuality is frequently portrayed as fluid, which makes me feel that perhaps my understanding of myself could shift in unexpected ways.

Hearsay and news — Information that you got from other people, substantiated or not.

a. I've heard of other people who didn't realize their orientation until later, which makes me worry I might be in a similar situation.
b. Friends have mentioned how common it is to question one's sexuality, which makes me think my doubts could be significant.
c. I once saw a story on social media about someone coming out after years of dating the opposite sex, which makes me worry that I might have a hidden orientation as well.

Anything else — Anything that does not fit well in the previous categories

a. The fact that these thoughts won't go away makes me feel that they must be telling me something important about my true self.
b. If I notice myself analyzing my reactions around men more than women, it feels like there might be something hidden I'm not fully acknowledging.
c. I've been surrounded by heterosexual norms and assumptions, which makes me question if my self-identity has been shaped more by expectation than by genuine self-awareness.

Form 5.1. Case of Mia (Vignette 1.10)
Potential reasons behind Mia's Obsessional doubts

Condensed Primary Doubt(s)
"I might have skin cancer, and I'm not catching it in time."

Abstract facts and ideas — Things that you know or believe to be true in general.

a. Skin cancer can develop quietly and without noticeable symptoms,
b. Early detection is often crucial in treating cancer effectively.
c. Early signs of skin issues are visible and noticeable, and a consistent routine of awareness allows for early detection without excessive vigilance.

Personal experience — Your own personal experience, past or present

a. I once ignored a health symptom that later needed medical treatment,
b. When I've let small concerns go unchecked, it sometimes made them worse
c. When I was younger, a family member had a health condition that went undiagnosed for some time, ultimately resulting in a tragic outcome

Values, standards and rules — The way of doing things according to an accepted principle.

a. I value being proactive with my health and believe it's better to catch something early than to regret not taking it seriously.
b. Taking responsibility for my own well-being is important to me, and I feel it's my duty to monitor any changes that could indicate a health risk.
c. I believe good self-care includes being aware of my body, so I see it as essential to notice any early warning signs of disease.

Authorities — A person, institution or organization that is perceived as important.

a. Skin cancer awareness campaigns emphasize regular self-checks and paying attention to new or changing moles,
b. I've seen public health messages that stress the risks of skin cancer.
c. Medical articles often mention the dangers of melanoma.

Hearsay and news — Information that you got from other people, substantiated or not.

a. I've heard stories of people who ignored a mole or skin spot that turned out to be cancerous.
b. A friend mentioned the need of being extra careful with moles or skin spots,
c. I once read a story about someone who didn't notice skin cancer until it was advanced.

Anything else — Anything that does not fit well in the previous categories

a. The urge I feel to keep checking my skin makes me think there's an important reason I'm not letting it go.
b. Being cautious feels protective, almost like an instinct to guard against any unseen risks that could affect my health.
c. Being aware of my body's signals feels essential to staying in tune with my well-being, especially when health can change without notice.

Form 5.1. Case of Alex (Vignette 1.11)
Potential reasons behind Alex' Obsessional doubts

Condensed Primary Doubt(s)
"Maybe reality is an illusion, and nothing I experience is truly real."

Abstract facts and ideas — Things that you know or believe to be true in general.

a. Reality is a philosophical concept that has been questioned by thinkers for centuries.
b. The concept of reality being a simulation is a well-known topic in scientific and philosophical discussions.
c. In nature, humans and animals perceive only fragments of reality, as different species experience distinct spectrums of light and sound.

Personal experience — Your own personal experience, past or present

a. I sometimes experience vivid dreams that feel entirely real, and waking up from them feels like shifting between worlds
b. I've had moments where I felt disconnected from people I'm close to, almost as if I'm watching them from a distance rather than truly connecting.
c. There are times when familiar places suddenly feel strange, even though I know I've been there many times.

Values, standards and rules — The way of doing things according to an accepted principle.

a. I value understanding truth and reality deeply.
b. Being in control of my understanding of the world is important to me.
c. I believe that clarity and truth are essential to leading a meaningful life.

Authorities — A person, institution or organization that is perceived as important.

a. Philosophers like Descartes questioned the nature of existence.
b. Prominent scientists have speculated about simulation theory, suggesting it's possible that reality could be a simulation.
c. Spiritual and philosophical traditions often question the material world.

Hearsay and news — Information that you got from other people, substantiated or not.

a. I've read online discussions where people share similar doubts about reality.
b. Movies and media often explore the idea of simulated or false realities.
c. I once heard about a person who had a similar existential crisis, and they described feeling like reality was slipping away.

Anything else — Anything that does not fit well in the previous categories

a. My intense feeling of disconnection and detachment seems like a "sign" that reality might be an illusion.
b. I sometimes feel like the world's complexity is too immense to comprehend, which makes me question whether the reality I perceive is just a simplified version of something far more complicated.
c. The fact that people have different versions of reality might mean that my perception of reality will later be disproven.

Form 5.1. Case of Lily (Vignette 1.12)
Potential reasons behind Lily's Obsessional doubts

Condensed Primary Doubt(s)
"Maybe my feelings for him aren't real, and we don't belong together."

Abstract facts and ideas — Things that you know or believe to be true in general.

a. Feelings in relationships can sometimes be complex and difficult to interpret.
b. People can be in relationships that don't feel right without initially realizing it.
c. Compatibility isn't always clear-cut and can be harder to identify, especially when trying to assess long-term suitability.

Personal experience — Your own personal experience, past or present

a. In past relationships, I've sometimes questioned my feelings.
b. I've had moments in previous relationships where doubts led to eventual breakups.
c. In my current relationship, I sometimes feel uncertain or detached.

Values, standards and rules — The way of doing things according to an accepted principle.

a. I value authenticity in relationships, and I feel I need to understand my feelings fully to be true to both myself and my partner.
b. I believe that love should come with clarity and feel effortless in its connection.
c. I hold myself to high standards of commitment.

Authorities — A person, institution or organization that is perceived as important.

a. Psychologists talk about how doubts can be indicators of incompatibility.
b. I've read that signs of a lasting relationship include feeling a deep, intuitive connection.
c. A scientific article reported that attachment issues can sometimes indicate that a person isn't in the right relationship.

Hearsay and news — Information that you got from other people, substantiated or not.

a. I've heard people say that "you just know" when it's the right person.
b. Friends have told me about their own breakups that started with similar doubts.
c. I've seen social media posts about relationships where people talk about feeling deeply assured about their partners.

Anything else — Anything that does not fit well in the previous categories

a. I would feel more aligned with my feelings if I loved my partner
b. Perhaps I've learned to believe I love my partner without truly understanding what love feels like.
c. If I loved him, I wouldn't experience this level of doubt.

Form 5.1. Case of Lucas (Vignette 1.13)
Potential reasons behind Lucas's Obsessional doubts

Condensed Primary Doubt(s)
"Maybe I'm changing into someone else."

Abstract facts and ideas — Things that you know or believe to be true in general.

a. People can change without realizing it, often influenced by their environment or the people around them.
b. There's research suggesting that personality and identity are fluid, meaning change is not only possible but likely over time.
c. Genetics and age can alter appearance in unexpected ways, sometimes making people look different from how they've looked before.

Personal experience — Your own personal experience, past or present

a. I've noticed that after spending time with certain friends, I sometimes adopt some of their expressions or habits, even unintentionally.
b. Sometimes, I've caught a glimpse of myself in the mirror and felt that my face looked unfamiliar, as though it were morphing subtly.
c. I don't look the same as I did several years ago.

Values, standards and rules — The way of doing things according to an accepted principle.

a. I believe that it's essential to stay true to oneself and avoid outside influences that might distort one's identity.
b. Authenticity is important to me, and I feel uneasy at the thought of unknowingly becoming someone I don't recognize.
c. I value personal integrity and feel it's my responsibility to maintain control over my identity and personality.

Authorities — A person, institution or organization that is perceived as important.

a. Scientists say that subtle changes in our bodies and appearance happen continuously at levels beyond our immediate awareness,
b. There are studies that suggest that prolonged exposure to certain environments or people can influence a person's traits and personality.
c. Experts on media discuss how repeated exposure to media can subconsciously shape beliefs, behaviors, and even our identity.

Hearsay and news — Information that you got from other people, substantiated or not.

a. I've heard people talk about "losing themselves" when they're around certain groups, as if their identity weakens over time.
b. Friends have mentioned that spending too much time on social media can change a person's beliefs and personality.
c. I once read a story about someone who started to resemble a close friend so much that they began to question their own identity.

Anything else — Anything that does not fit well in the previous categories

a. There are continuous small changes in how I feel or act.
b. If I was not changing, it would be easier to recognize myself each time I check.
c. People may have an energy or aura around them influencing others.

Form 5.1. Case of Abigail (Vignette 1.14)
Potential reasons behind Abilgail's Obsessional doubts

Condensed Primary Doubt(s)
"Maybe my OCD is coming back." *"What if I don't really have OCD."*

Abstract facts and ideas — Things that you know or believe to be true in general.

a. Some mental health issues can resemble OCD, which makes me wonder if my diagnosis was correct.
b. There are cases where people misattribute their symptoms to the wrong condition.
c. Stress can act as a trigger for OCD symptoms to resurface.

Personal experience — Your own personal experience, past or present

a. In the past, I've experienced brief periods of relief, only to have my symptoms return worse than before.
b. I've had moments when my symptoms felt different or inconsistent with what I've read about OCD, which makes me question whether I truly have it.
c. There have been moments when a new obsession and compulsion appeared.

Values, standards and rules — The way of doing things according to an accepted principle.

a. I believe it's my responsibility to stay vigilant for signs of relapse, as early intervention is key.
b. I value control over my mental health and feel that not noticing early signs of OCD's return would be failing myself.
c. I value honesty and feel that misidentifying my condition would mean I've been dishonest with myself and my therapist.

Authorities — A person, institution or organization that is perceived as important.

a. OCD is often described as a chronic condition that can fluctuate in intensity over time.
b. Articles I've come across highlight that relapse is common among individuals with OCD.
c. Some therapists emphasize that OCD can sometimes resemble other disorders.

Hearsay and news — Information that you got from other people, substantiated or not.

a. I've read that OCD can seem to improve temporarily, only to come back even stronger later on.
b. I've seen online discussions where people questioned their diagnosis, and it turned out they were misdiagnosed.
c. I've heard people say their OCD symptoms returned unexpectedly, even after years of improvement.

Anything else — Anything that does not fit well in the previous categories

a. Periods of calm can be unnatural, like a deceptive silence before the storm.
b. The amount of effort I put into getting better might mean things could easily unravel.
c. Getting better is too good to be true.

Form 5.1. Case of Oliver (Vignette 1.15)
Potential reasons behind Oliver's Obsessional doubts

Contrasting Conclusion
"Maybe getting rid of anything is a mistake.""

Abstract facts and ideas — Things that you know or believe to be true in general.

a. Certain items have hidden value that isn't immediately obvious but becomes important later.
b. You can't always predict when something seemingly insignificant will become useful.
c. In emergencies, having extra resources could make all the difference.

Personal experience — Your own personal experience, past or present

a. I've regretted throwing something away in the past when I ended up needing it later.
b. There have been times when I found new uses for things I thought were useless.
c. I've had moments when rediscovering an old item brought back meaningful memories or emotions.

Values, standards and rules — The way of doing things according to an accepted principle.

a. I value being prepared and feel responsible for keeping items that might serve a purpose in the future.
b. I believe that being wasteful is wrong, especially when others could use what I'm considering discarding.
c. I feel that maintaining connections to the past through objects is an important part of honoring my identity.

Authorities — A person, institution or organization that is perceived as important.

a. Experts on sustainability emphasize the importance of reusing and repurposing items rather than discarding them.
b. Documentaries about frugal living or sustainability often highlight the value of repurposing and holding onto items for future use.
c. Experts in emergency preparedness emphasize the importance of being resourceful and having essential items on hand, which makes discarding items feel risky.

Hearsay and news — Information that you got from other people, substantiated or not.

a. I've heard stories of people regretting throwing out sentimental or valuable possessions.
b. I once saw a news report of how someone discovered a valuable and historical items among their belongings.
c. Friends have told me about moments when they needed something they had just discarded.

Anything else — Anything that does not fit well in the previous categories

a. Each item I own feels tied to a part of my identity or a specific memory, making it feel irreplaceable.
b. Discarding something feels like losing control, as though I might regret the decision forever.
c. Holding onto things provides a sense of security, like I'm safeguarding against an uncertain future.

Obsessional Narrative 5.1. Case of Jack (Vignette 1.1)

"I might be a violent person without knowing it, capable of causing harm at any moment."

It's a quiet evening, and I'm cooking dinner alone in my apartment. I'm chopping vegetables with a large knife, just like I always do. But then, as I pause for a moment, I notice the sharpness of the blade glinting under the kitchen light, and suddenly, it hits me—this is the exact kind of knife people use in horror movies to commit violent acts. And that's when the thought intrudes, almost out of nowhere: What if I do something violent? What if I lose control?

I try to shake it off, but the thought clings to me like a shadow. I've heard before that everyone has a capacity for violence under certain circumstances. It's just part of being human. People snap, right? Even normal people, people who seem perfectly calm, have these sudden outbursts. I remember reading about that well-liked teacher who was arrested for assault—no one expected it, no one saw it coming. What if that's me? What if there's something inside me waiting to explode?

And then I start thinking about other things I've heard—that the mind can harbor unconscious desires that we're not even aware of. Maybe there's some hidden part of me that could hurt someone, and I just don't know it yet. After all, it's possible to do something terrible and not even remember it, isn't it? What if I've already done something violent and just can't recall it?

My mind drifts to the times when I've lost my temper. I've been angry before—who hasn't? But there was that one time, during a small argument, when I felt the anger rise so quickly, it scared me. It was like I couldn't control it, and for a moment, I wondered how much worse it could get. What if next time, I can't stop myself? And there was that day when I accidentally hit my friend's fingers with a hammer while we were working on a project. I didn't mean to, but the way they cried out in pain made me feel awful. If I can cause that kind of pain without even thinking, what else might I do without realizing it?

I start questioning everything I've learned. I know that people can be unpredictable, and it's always better to be cautious. If there's even a chance that I could be dangerous, then I have a responsibility to stop it, don't I? After all, experts say mental health issues can go unnoticed for years—what if I have something, some condition, that I don't even know about yet? Maybe unresolved issues from my past are building up inside me, ready to come out in violent ways. Therapists always talk about how unresolved childhood problems can lead to aggression in adulthood. Could that be happening to me?

Then there's the news. I can't help but remember all those stories about people who seemed perfectly fine—until they weren't. One day, they were ordinary, calm individuals, and the next, they were on the front page for doing something horrific. If it could happen to them, it could happen to me, right? I'm just like anyone else.

I've also noticed that when I get tired, I feel irritable. Sometimes it's so intense that I snap at people without meaning to. What if one day, when I'm exhausted, I snap in a way that's much worse? What if I act out violently without even realizing it until it's too late?

The thought sends a chill down my spine. What if I'm not as in control as I think? What if one day, I pick up a knife or any sharp object and just...snap? I can picture it clearly—hurting someone, someone I care about, and not being able to stop myself. The thought of causing someone that kind of pain, the kind that lingers not just physically but emotionally, is unbearable. I see the faces of my family, my friends, all shocked and horrified. What would I say to them after? How could I live with myself? The shame, the guilt, the thought of being locked up for the rest of my life for something I couldn't stop—it all plays out vividly in my mind. Would they ever forgive me? Would I lose everything? My freedom, my relationships, my career? I'd become the violent criminal I fear, shunned by everyone I care about.

I can't let that happen. I can't take the chance. So, I do what I have to do. I stop using knives entirely. I avoid situations where I might be close to someone with a sharp object. I stay away from crowded places, where the urge to push someone could strike without warning. And when I do have to use a sharp tool at work, I'm constantly checking myself, making sure I'm holding it the right way, ensuring I don't slip up. If I start to feel overwhelmed, I step away, wash my hands, and remind myself that I need to stay in control. I perform these rituals to "cleanse" myself of the thoughts, but no matter what I do, the fear remains. The doubt lingers.

Obsessional Narrative 5.1. Case of Rachel (Vignette 1.2)
"Maybe I am sexually attracted to children"

It all began with a deeper question that I never thought I'd have to ask: "Do I really know who I am?" I've always thought of myself as compassionate, nurturing, and someone who genuinely enjoys being around children. But over time, that certainty started to waver. I came across a discussion once, saying that people sometimes have hidden aspects of themselves that only reveal themselves later in life. The idea unsettled me. What if there's something about me I don't fully understand? That thought lingered, growing stronger until it took on a shape I couldn't ignore: "What if my thoughts or feelings about children are unnatural?"

I tried to tell myself that the question was absurd, but once it was there, it felt impossible to dismiss. I've read that psychology often suggests people misinterpret their own sensations or feelings, and I started to wonder if I was doing the same. My mind kept replaying interactions at work—an innocent smile, a kind touch, a fleeting moment of warmth—and twisting them into something that felt darker. What if these were signs of something I didn't want to admit? The idea consumed me, making me question every aspect of my interactions.

At work, my doubts started to take over. Every time a child hugged me or I bent down to tie their shoe, I found myself second-guessing my actions. Did I linger too long? Was my touch appropriate? Sometimes, I'd feel a fleeting sensation—a warmth or a reaction that felt entirely normal—but my mind wouldn't let it rest. Instead, I'd think, "What if this means something about me?" I've read stories of people who seemed completely normal but were later found to have hidden tendencies. Could I be like them? That thought terrifies me.

I've always believed it's essential to maintain control over my thoughts and feelings, to ensure I'm a good person. I hold myself to high moral standards and feel deeply ashamed whenever I think I might fall short. These doubts feel like proof that I've already failed, that I'm not the person I thought I was. The shame is overwhelming. How can I continue working with children when I can't even trust my own instincts? The thought of unintentionally harming them—emotionally, mentally, or otherwise—haunts me. It's my responsibility as a teacher to protect them, and these doubts make me feel like I'm failing in the worst possible way.

The more I think about it, the more these doubts feel persistent and intense, as if they must mean something. I've read about intrusive thoughts and how they sometimes reveal deeper truths about a person. What if that's what's happening to me? What if I've been lying to myself this entire time? That question plays on a loop in my mind, leaving me terrified to even be around children.

Outside of work, the doubts follow me. At family gatherings, I avoid hugging my nieces and nephews, afraid that my thoughts might betray me. Even innocent moments—like a smile or a playful interaction— feel loaded with uncertainty. I find myself avoiding situations where I might need to interact with children altogether, isolating myself out of fear. This isn't who I want to be, but I don't know how to stop.

At home, the doubts affect my relationship with my partner. I find myself analyzing every intimate moment, questioning whether my feelings or reactions are "normal." I test myself constantly, searching for reassurance, but no matter how hard I try, the doubts remain. I've spent hours researching, reading articles and forum posts, trying to find proof that my thoughts don't mean anything. But the more I search, the more confused I become. For every reassuring answer, there's another one that deepens my fear. I've read discussions about inappropriate thoughts and how people misinterpret them, but I can't help wondering: what if I'm fooling myself?

The guilt and shame have become unbearable. How can I explain these thoughts to anyone without them judging me? How can I continue working with children when I can't even trust myself? Every interaction feels tainted by doubt, and every attempt to reassure myself feels hollow. I feel trapped, unable to escape the relentless question: "What if I've been wrong about who I am all along?"

Obsessional Narrative 5.3. Case of John (Vignette 1.3)

"Perhaps I don't truly believe in God anymore and have lost my faith."

Every time I sit down to pray, a familiar doubt creeps into my mind: What if I don't truly believe in God anymore? It's usually in the morning, after I've woken up and am sitting in my quiet room, preparing to begin my daily prayer. The sun shines through the window, casting soft light on my Bible. Everything appears normal, but the doubt still lingers. Have I lost my faith? I wonder.

I know that people can lose their faith, even after being devout for many years. Faith is not something guaranteed, and spiritual crises are common. These crises are often seen as signs of a deeper loss of belief, and I can't help but think that's what I'm experiencing. I've heard religious teachings warn that true faith should be unwavering, but mine feels shaky, filled with doubt. Doesn't that mean I might no longer truly believe?

I remember times when I felt deeply connected during spiritual practices, but lately, I've experienced moments where I feel nothing. I sit through prayers and worship, but it's as if I'm just going through the motions. I recall a period in my life when I didn't believe in anything. Could it be that I'm returning to that place of disbelief? I think about family members who have lost their faith; if it can happen to them, why not me?

Faith is important to me. I've always believed that having a strong and unwavering connection to God is essential, but now I'm not so sure if I have that anymore. The idea of losing my faith terrifies me. It's something I've always valued, something I want to hold onto, but the more I question, the more it feels like it's slipping away. I've always held myself to the standard that faith should be constant, but with these doubts creeping in, am I failing to live up to that?

Religious authorities often emphasize how critical it is to remain faithful, but they also warn that even the most devout people can lose their belief. I've read religious scholars who say that prolonged questioning can erode one's faith, and I've been questioning everything for so long now. What if these doubts are a sign that I've already lost my connection to God?

I've heard stories about people who once believed but, after years of doubt, lost their faith entirely. I saw on a religious TV program that some people stop feeling God's presence and eventually drift away from their belief. Even a friend told me how someone they knew lost their faith after a long period of intense questioning, just like I'm going through now. And recently, the news has been filled with reports about declining faith across the country. Is it happening to me, too?

I question everything now. I used to trust that my faith would guide me, that I wouldn't need to doubt. But now I find myself wondering constantly: Is my faith real? If faith is supposed to bring clarity, why do I feel so confused? I always believed that faith should be a guiding light, something that makes me feel secure. But what if my doubts mean that my faith was never real in the first place? Could I be losing my faith without even realizing it?

The fear of losing my faith is overwhelming. I imagine what it would be like if I truly lost my belief. I would feel spiritually lost, like I no longer had a purpose. What if I'm already disconnected from God, and I'm just going through the motions, fooling myself? The thought of living without God's grace fills me with dread. It feels like my life would lose all meaning if I lost my faith.

To deal with these doubts, I find myself repeating prayers over and over, hoping to feel that connection again. I seek reassurance from my spiritual advisor, asking the same questions about my spiritual state, but nothing seems to calm my mind. I've started avoiding worship gatherings because I'm afraid that others will see through me and realize I'm not as faithful as I used to be. I obsess over my religious practices, trying to perfect them in the hopes that it will bring back the certainty I've lost. But nothing works—the doubts persist, and the fear of losing my faith continues to grow stronger.

Obsessional Narrative 5.4. Case of Laura (Vignette 1.4)

"I could be a dishonest and unethical person without realizing."

It's another day at the office, and I'm going over a report I prepared for a client. As I review it, a thought begins to creep in: Did I make sure everything I wrote was entirely accurate? I suddenly remember the incident six months ago when I accidentally forgot to credit a colleague for their contribution. Even though it seemed like a minor oversight at the time, the memory still haunts me. What if it wasn't just a mistake? What if that's part of who I am—someone who doesn't always acknowledge others fairly? If my colleagues ever thought I was lying or hiding something, they might lose their trust in me.

I know people sometimes deceive others without fully realizing it, and that thought makes me uneasy. I wonder: Could I be doing the same thing? Dishonesty isn't always intentional; it can be subtle, slipping into conversations or actions without notice. Even good people sometimes lie or act unethically without realizing it. What if that's happening to me? I think about how even small actions can reveal hidden flaws, and that worries me. Could I be the kind of person who fails to live up to my own standards without even knowing it?

Throughout the day, my mind keeps returning to that mistake with my colleague, replaying the moment over and over. There was also the time I mistakenly overcharged a client. It was corrected quickly, but I remember the shame I felt afterward. Could I have done that on purpose? If I can't even trust my own actions, how can I be sure that I'm as honest as I want to believe? Then there are moments I remember when I've felt disconnected from my own words, wondering if I exaggerated or misrepresented something. What if that's a sign of deeper dishonesty?

As I go through my interactions with colleagues, I begin to question everything I say. If I make even a minor error or accidentally leave something out, I feel this rush of anxiety. I know that true integrity is about maintaining high standards consistently, and even a small lapse could indicate a lack of character. If I can't be sure of every word, maybe that means I'm hiding something from myself. What if I'm not as honest as I believe myself to be? The idea that I could lose respect at work terrifies me. I try to shake off these doubts, but they keep creeping back in.

The standards I hold myself to are high—I believe in being honest and fair in everything I do. But if I can't guarantee that I'm always truthful, maybe I'm not as ethical as I think I am. I start to wonder if a truly moral person would struggle this much to be sure of their actions. The guidelines at work emphasize transparency, and I wonder if I'm failing to live up to that. I remember reading that good character is about consistency, and any inconsistency could mean I'm not truly trustworthy.

By the time I get home, the doubts have intensified. I sit down, mentally replaying every conversation, every email, every interaction from the day. I wonder if my constant need to check and recheck is a sign that I'm not trustworthy. If I were really a person of integrity, wouldn't I be able to trust myself more? I think back to stories I've heard of people who seemed honest but later turned out to be hiding something. Could I be like that, unknowingly acting in ways that betray my values?

And then there's my family—they've always believed that I'm a person of integrity. But what if I've been misleading them all along? Friends sometimes say that everyone makes mistakes, but I can't shake the thought that my mistakes might reveal something deeper. I even remember a news story about someone who unknowingly committed fraud, and it terrifies me to think that I could act unethically without even being aware of it.

The weight of these thoughts fills me with dread. If I'm constantly doubting myself, maybe there's a reason. What if I'm not as moral as I believe, and these doubts are just the beginning of uncovering an uncomfortable truth about myself? I start to imagine the consequences: If my colleagues or clients suspected I was unethical, I could lose my job. My reputation, something I've worked so hard to build, could be shattered. I could lose the trust of those I care about. The thought of becoming known as someone who's dishonest is unbearable—it feels like my entire life could fall apart.

I try to reassure myself, going over my actions again and again, but nothing seems to calm the doubt. I feel like I'm trapped in this endless cycle of questioning, unable to find any relief. The fear that I might be hiding something dishonest, even from myself, is overwhelming. It's as if I'm standing on the edge of a cliff, staring down into a version of myself I don't recognize, but can't escape.

Obsessional Narrative 5.5. Case of Ethan (Vignette 1.5)
"I could have missed something or left something undone."
"Maybe things are not functioning as they should."

Every morning, as I prepare to leave my apartment, I'm overtaken by a familiar feeling of unease. Just as I reach for the door, a thought hits me: What if I forgot to turn off the stove? I know I checked it before, but there's a nagging sensation that something is wrong. I can't ignore it, so I head back to the kitchen, carefully inspecting each burner. I run my hand over the surface to make sure it's cool. Finally, I feel a hint of relief—but it's fleeting.

I make my way back to the door, but the doubts creep in again. Did I check the toaster? I wasn't even using it, but what if it somehow got left on? I return to unplug it, just in case. And as I near the exit again, the worries evolve: What if I left the windows open? What if a draft blows something over, causing an accident? Each time, I circle back through my apartment, scanning each room, looking for signs of anything left undone. I remember stories of accidents caused by tiny mistakes, and the thought of leaving something unaddressed feels unbearable. No matter how many times I check, there's always another detail that could be wrong.

Once I finally step outside, I can't shake the feeling that I missed something crucial. What if I left the bathroom light on? What if I forgot my wallet or ID? These are small things, but I know that even a minor oversight could have consequences. If I truly held myself to the high standards I believe in, wouldn't I be able to avoid these lapses altogether? My mind races, picturing worst-case scenarios where something goes horribly wrong because of my oversight.

At work, my mind drifts back to my morning routine. Did I close the fridge properly? Is my food going to spoil? I can't stop myself from replaying every step I took before leaving. No matter how hard I try to concentrate, the doubts linger in the background, a constant reminder that something might not be right. It's exhausting, mentally retracing my actions, but I don't feel safe until I've convinced myself that everything was done properly. Even though I check, the fact that these doubts keep coming back makes me wonder if I'm somehow missing something each time.

Driving home, my worries take on a new form. I check the handbrake at every stoplight, tugging on it repeatedly to make sure it's secure. What if it wasn't fully engaged? I imagine my car rolling backward or causing an accident, all because of a careless mistake. Every stop feels like a test, and I can't relax until I've confirmed everything is as it should be. But as soon as I arrive home, new doubts surface.

In the evenings, I try to unwind, but the same fears creep back in. What if the smoke detector isn't working? What if it malfunctioned since the last time I checked? I climb up, press the test button, and listen for the beep, feeling a temporary relief when it sounds. But minutes later, the doubt returns. What if something went wrong in that brief moment? I know that smoke detectors and appliances can sometimes fail without warning, so I feel compelled to check again. The more I check, the more it feels like I'm chasing a sense of certainty that I can never reach.

Before bed, I go through my nightly routine of locking the doors and checking the windows, feeling each handle and deadbolt to make sure everything is secure. But once I'm in bed, I start to doubt whether I truly locked everything. What if I missed something? What if someone could enter because of my mistake? I get up, sometimes two or three times, repeating the same checks until I'm too exhausted to do it anymore.

Each day feels like a test I'm destined to fail. No matter how careful I am, there's always the possibility that something was left undone. My frequent doubts make me feel as if I'm overlooking something crucial each time. I imagine the worst happening because of a small oversight—a fire from an appliance, an unlocked door, or a forgotten item. I can't escape the fear that my constant need to check means I'm somehow missing something vital every time. It's a cycle that leaves me drained, anxious, and uncertain, unable to find peace in any aspect of my life.

Obsessional Narrative 5.6. Case of Sophie (Vignette 1.6)

"I could be contaminated by toxic chemicals that are impossible to avoid or eliminate."
"I might be spreading dangerous contaminants, harming myself or others."

Every day, as I move through my routine, I'm reminded of the invisible risks that seem to be everywhere. The world feels filled with potential hazards—chemicals in the air, surfaces that might carry toxins, and products that claim to be safe but hide ingredients I don't fully understand. I try to feel reassured by the labels on things I buy, but doubt always seems to creep in. I can't help but remember reading about the harmful effects of common household products. It makes me wonder: How can I be sure I'm truly safe?

Mt many common products contain chemicals that can be harmful with prolonged exposure. It's like a shadow of doubt hanging over everything I touch. When I spray cleaner on the countertops, a thought immediately takes hold: What if the chemicals in this product are dangerous? I try to remind myself that it's a product I've used before, but the uncertainty lingers. I wonder if I'm exposing myself to something that might accumulate in my system over time, something invisible but harmful. Research often emphasizes how synthetic materials can release dangerous chemicals, and it makes me question every surface, every product I come in contact with.

I do my best to avoid contact with these products, wearing gloves and even a mask, but it's hard to feel truly safe. The air feels thick after cleaning, and I can't help but think that toxic particles might still be lingering, spreading invisibly to other parts of my apartment. I try to air out the rooms, but the thought stays with me: Maybe I'm breathing in something harmful right now, and I just don't realize it. Even after I've aired everything out, there's always that lingering doubt.

I remember once spilling a strong-smelling product in my bag, and even after cleaning it multiple times, the smell clung to everything. It makes me think: If a simple spill can leave traces for days, what if chemicals from these products stick around just as stubbornly, even when I think everything is clean? I feel a sense of responsibility to protect myself and others from these invisible threats. It's important to keep my environment uncontaminated, but I'm not sure I'm doing enough.

Even my own experiences make me doubt my effectiveness. I've noticed how even after touching something sticky, it seemed like the residue kept transferring onto other things, no matter how well I thought I'd washed my hands. When I'm at work, handling decorations and materials, I start to worry: What if this material contains something toxic? I picture chemicals lingering on my skin and spreading to everything I touch. Sometimes I wash my hands multiple times, but that feeling of residue stays with me. I worry that I might be carrying these particles with me, accidentally contaminating my workspace and, worse, the people around me.

It's hard to ignore all the warnings I've read from health and safety authorities about the importance of reducing exposure to synthetic chemicals. Articles and news stories often highlight the risks, with examples of people who developed serious health issues due to toxic exposure. And with so many environmental organizations advocating for limited use of chemical-based products, I wonder if I'm doing enough to avoid harm. I worry that no matter how careful I am, these toxic substances might be present in places I'd never suspect.

The more I try to stay informed, the harder it feels to keep everything safe. The constant updates and information about toxic exposure make it seem like these risks are everywhere, harder to control than I'd ever imagined. I sometimes notice strange odors or faint stains that make me wonder if something harmful might still be there, unseen and unchecked. And as I read more about the dangers of everyday products, I feel like I'm constantly missing something. It's like no matter what I do, there could be something I've overlooked, some risk I haven't managed to prevent.

I think about my family and friends, and a wave of guilt washes over me. What if I'm the reason someone else gets sick? I can't bear the thought of unknowingly causing harm to the people I care about. Even after changing clothes and scrubbing my hands, I worry that contaminants might still cling to me, that I might spread something dangerous just by being near them. It's exhausting, trying to be so careful, but the thought of someone else suffering because of me is too much to ignore.

When I go shopping, the doubt follows me. I scrutinize each product, searching for labels that say "chemical-free" or "organic," hoping that they'll offer some reassurance. But even when I find these labels, I question their validity. What if "chemical-free" doesn't really mean safe? Fruits and vegetables, things that should feel wholesome, start to seem like potential hazards because of pesticide residue. Even after washing them, I worry that traces might still remain.

No matter how many precautions I take, the fear never fully leaves me. Each day brings new information that makes me question if I'm truly safe. The more I learn, the more it seems like no amount of effort will ever eliminate these invisible contaminants. I worry that these toxins are everywhere, and no amount of scrubbing or avoidance will be enough. The possibility that I'm missing something dangerous weighs on me constantly. I feel trapped, wondering if I'll ever be able to feel safe in my own space again. Even in moments of rest, that thought returns: Maybe I'll never be free from this fear.

The more I try to protect myself, the more I feel like I'm failing. It's as if no level of cleanliness is enough, and every action seems to carry some risk of contamination. The anxiety grows stronger, leaving me exhausted and isolated, yet the fear of toxic chemicals remains constant, influencing every decision I make.

Obsessional Narrative 5.7. Case of Matthew (Vignette 1.7)
"Perhaps things haven't been placed right, or done right, or well enough."

I often start my day with a quiet sense of unease, a feeling that things around me might not be quite as they should be. At first glance, my surroundings seem orderly, but there's an underlying tension that I can't shake, an urge to make sure everything is exactly in place. I've always valued balance and precision, especially in my work as an architect. In my field, even slight misalignments or unnoticed details could theoretically impact the quality of a project, and I've heard countless times that precision and accuracy are the hallmarks of good design.

When I sit at my desk, I feel the urge to go over every aspect of my work, even when I know I've checked it before. Small misalignments, I've learned, can disrupt the flow of a design or affect the harmony of a structure, creating an impact that's hard to ignore. I think about the standards emphasized in my training—standards that stress how even the slightest deviation could lead to a ripple effect, affecting the stability or the aesthetics of an entire project.

At home, this mindset follows me. I'll stand in my living room, looking around, and feel the need to adjust various items to ensure they're arranged just right. I know that maintaining an ordered and balanced environment is part of creating a harmonious space, one that feels grounded and complete. But sometimes, I feel as though achieving that balance requires a constant series of small adjustments, as if the sense of order can only be preserved through careful attention. I'll shift a book slightly or adjust a cushion, not because I see something off, but because it feels necessary to make sure everything is as it should be.

This need for precision doesn't just apply to physical arrangements but also extends to my work and interactions. I know that in architecture, missing a single detail can alter the functionality or aesthetic balance of a design. I've read about clients who notice even the smallest inconsistencies in their projects, and I worry that if I let something slip, it could compromise my work or create dissatisfaction. When I'm working on a draft, I go over each line, each measurement, making sure every element feels aligned, symmetrical, and precise. Even though I know I've done the work thoroughly, I can't resist double-checking to make sure everything holds up to the standards I've come to expect.

As I move through my day, the doubts continue to resurface. I wonder if my work might have a detail that's less than ideal, or if there's something in my environment that isn't balanced. I think back to moments when others have praised my attention to detail, and I feel the weight of maintaining that level of precision, especially knowing that even small adjustments, when made thoughtfully, can enhance the overall feel of a space or a project. My profession, I remind myself, is one where balance and symmetry play a key role, where clients and colleagues often expect meticulous attention to detail. Letting go of that expectation feels impossible, as if the quality of my work depends on maintaining that heightened awareness.

Even in social settings, the same thoughts linger. When I'm out with friends, I'll find myself adjusting a glass or repositioning my silverware, feeling an urge to keep things orderly and balanced. It's as though the way things are arranged reflects my own care and attentiveness, and I worry that others might see a lack of alignment as a sign of carelessness. This sense of responsibility isn't something I can ignore—it feels tied to my values, to the idea that well-maintained spaces create a certain kind of respect and order. I've read articles that discuss how alignment in design affects first impressions, and I wonder if the same applies to personal interactions as well.

In moments of self-reflection, I worry about the consequences of not keeping up with these adjustments. I imagine my work being scrutinized, with someone pointing out an inconsistency I failed to notice. I picture clients, supervisors, or colleagues losing confidence in my abilities, questioning my dedication. I fear that even the smallest overlooked detail could impact their perception of me, making them wonder if I'm truly committed to the quality I claim to value. And at home, I envision a growing sense of disorder, as though without my intervention, my surroundings would somehow become chaotic, lacking the balance that brings a sense of calm.

These thoughts weigh heavily on me. The pressure to maintain order and alignment, to avoid even the smallest perceived flaw, feels constant. I find myself checking, arranging, and adjusting, always seeking that elusive moment when everything finally feels "right." Yet, as much as I try, the doubt remains, leaving me with a persistent feeling that something more could be done to ensure the order I strive to create.

Obsessional Narrative 5.8. Case of Olivia (Vignette 1.8)

"Perhaps my body is not performing as it should."
"Perhaps I will lose control over my attention and mind."

Lately, I've become increasingly aware of sensations in my body, as if my mind has turned inward, constantly monitoring my own functions. I used to trust that my body would just work as it should, but now, I feel like I can't be certain of that. I've heard that the body can sometimes act unpredictably without showing obvious signs, and this possibility makes me question if everything is really functioning as it should. What if I'm overlooking something important that's affecting how my body works?

I often find myself fixating on my breathing. Sometimes it feels shallow or uneven, and I wonder if that's a sign that something isn't right. I've read that if the body doesn't perform correctly, even minor issues can have serious consequences over time. This makes me worry that my body might not be working as efficiently as I assume. The more I think about it, the more I worry that without my constant awareness, something might go wrong without me realizing it. If I stop paying attention, who's to say my body won't fail me?

It's possible, I know, to become overly aware of bodily functions and lose the ability to trust them. This thought keeps coming back: What if my body isn't performing as it should? It's as if each time I try to ignore these sensations, my mind pulls me right back to them, making me feel as though I'm losing control. I find myself unable to stop thinking about my breathing, blinking, or even my heartbeat, as though any lapse in attention could result in something going wrong. The idea that I could lose control over my focus makes it even harder to let go.

Even when I'm around other people, I notice my mind drifting back to these sensations, no matter how hard I try to focus elsewhere. I've had moments in the past when I felt trapped by certain thoughts, unable to shift my attention, and I worry it could happen again. Each time I try to direct my focus elsewhere, it feels like my mind drags me back to monitoring my own body, as if it has its own agenda. I'm haunted by the fear that I might lose control over my attention and get stuck in this loop.

This fear of losing control over my attention is growing stronger. I know it's possible for people to become stuck in certain patterns of thought, and I fear that's exactly what's happening to me. If my mind fixates on my bodily sensations indefinitely, how will I ever focus on anything else? Each day, it seems harder to shake off this hyper-awareness, and I start to doubt my own ability to let go. The thought that I might be trapped in this self-monitoring state for the rest of my life fills me with dread.

I've heard of people who become so focused on certain sensations that they can't experience anything beyond them. This scares me, as I can feel myself slipping into that pattern. If I'm always monitoring my breathing, blinking, or heart rate, how will I be able to concentrate on my work, engage with friends, or even enjoy simple moments of relaxation? My body feels like a puzzle I can't solve, and the harder I try, the more trapped I feel. The more I notice these sensations, the harder it becomes to let go of them, as if something isn't quite right.

Even when I try to reassure myself, the doubts creep back in, stronger each time. Each time I tell myself everything is fine, my mind counters with a new "what if." What if my body isn't performing correctly? What if I can't stop monitoring these functions? These doubts build upon each other, creating a relentless cycle that leaves me feeling as if I'm losing control.

The fear that perhaps my body is not performing as it should and that perhaps I will lose control over my attention and mind becomes overwhelming. I can't shake the feeling that if I let my guard down, I'll be trapped in this monitoring forever, unable to experience life normally again.

Even at night, there's no escape. I lie awake, aware of my breathing and heartbeat, terrified that if I don't concentrate, something might go wrong with my body. At the same time, I worry that I'll never stop monitoring these sensations, that I'll never be able to let my mind simply rest. The fear that I could lose all sense of control over both my bodily functions and my ability to focus on anything else keeps me feeling trapped, caught in a relentless cycle of vigilance and anxiety.

Obsessional Narrative 5.9. Case of Henry (Vignette 1.9)
"Maybe I'm really gay and have been lying to myself."

It's a quiet Saturday afternoon, and I'm sitting on the couch, scrolling through my social media feed while my girlfriend, Sarah, is in the kitchen making lunch. The apartment feels calm, but underlying this peace is a persistent question that's been gnawing at me: "What if I'm not really heterosexual? What if I've been lying to myself all along?" I've heard stories of people who've discovered hidden aspects of themselves later in life, and I can't help but wonder if that could be my situation. If others have hidden or denied parts of themselves without knowing, isn't it possible I could be doing the same?

The doubt follows me everywhere. I find myself revisiting memories, analyzing past interactions, replaying conversations with friends, and looking for signs that I might have missed. There were moments in my teenage years when I had fleeting explorations with the same sex—at the time, I thought nothing of them, but now they loom large, like clues to a hidden truth I failed to recognize. I know people sometimes misinterpret their own feelings, so what if I've been overlooking signs all along? My mind keeps going back to these moments, convinced there must be something buried there, waiting to be acknowledged.

Being around Sarah only intensifies my anxiety. Sometimes, I feel a distance between us, a sense that my attraction is less intense than it should be. Could this be a sign that I'm not truly attracted to her? Authenticity in relationships is essential to me, and if I'm pretending on any level, I feel an obligation to uncover the truth, no matter how painful. Attraction isn't always clear-cut, and I wonder if I've misinterpreted or even suppressed my own feelings. The thought gnaws at me—what if my relationship with her is based on something that isn't entirely genuine? I worry I might be misleading her, and even myself.

Desperate for clarity, I've begun "testing" myself, exposing myself to images of men and gauging my reaction. Every article or story I read suggests that denial about sexual orientation is possible, and I start to wonder: am I in denial? Do I feel something when I see these images? Am I attracted to them? When I don't feel anything, I feel a brief relief—but the questions always return. Perhaps I'm overlooking a subtle feeling, or maybe I don't know myself as well as I think. I've heard of people realizing their orientation later in life, and I can't shake the feeling that maybe that's happening to me.

At work, this doubt creeps in as well. In meetings or interactions with male colleagues, I feel hyper-aware of every glance, every small gesture, and I analyze how I feel in those moments. People can sometimes sense things about others that they don't realize themselves—what if my colleagues see something in me that I can't see? When I interact with men, I worry that I might be giving off "signals" without realizing it, making others question my orientation. It's exhausting to stay vigilant, but I can't ignore the possibility that something could be "off" about my interactions.

Every interaction seems to be laced with doubt, and even my time alone doesn't offer relief. People can suppress or ignore their true feelings for years, and the idea that I could be doing the same keeps haunting me. Even with friends, I worry about whether I'm expressing myself genuinely, fearing that any lapse could be a sign of something hidden. In moments of desperation, I seek out stories and forums online, hoping to find validation or clarity. I've read countless personal accounts where people finally "realized" their orientation later in life. Could I be one of those people?

The consequences feel overwhelming. If I've been living a lie, then every aspect of my life—my relationship, my friendships, my self-perception—has been built on a false foundation. The thought of telling Sarah, of revealing doubts I can barely accept myself, fills me with guilt and fear. If I am truly hiding a part of myself, then I've betrayed her trust, as well as my own. It would mean dismantling our relationship, hurting her in a way I can't bear to imagine. The guilt of potentially deceiving everyone I care about weighs on me, making me feel as though I'm trapped in a cycle of confusion and shame.

This guilt, this overwhelming need to uncover "the truth," pushes me to keep testing, analyzing, and seeking reassurance. But every answer I find only leads to more questions, and the doubt digs in deeper. I feel more alone, more disconnected from the person I thought I was, and the life I thought I had built.

Obsessional Narrative 5.10. Case of Mia (Vignette 1.10)
"I might have skin cancer, and I'm not catching it in time."

I'm in my bathroom, staring at the mole on my arm again. It's small, but it's been on my mind all day. I know skin cancer can develop quietly, without noticeable symptoms, just like I've read online. What if this mole is one of those cases? I can't just ignore it—too many times, I've read about how melanoma can be aggressive if left unchecked.

It's not just the mole, though. There are so many spots on my skin—moles, freckles, blemishes—and any one of them could be dangerous. I remember ignoring a health symptom once, thinking it was nothing, but it eventually led to treatment. That experience left a mark on me, a reminder that brushing things off could lead to something serious. Now, when I look at this mole, that memory surfaces, telling me I need to pay attention, to check, to be sure. This time, I can't afford to be complacent.

I think back to my aunt. She had a health issue that went undiagnosed for a while, and by the time it was addressed, it was too late. She passed away, and the thought of that happening to me is terrifying. I know I'm healthy, but I also know that cancer doesn't always show itself until it's advanced. Early detection is key, everyone says that. My mind keeps circling back to one worry: I might have skin cancer, and I'm not catching it in time.

I value being proactive with my health—it's one of my core principles. It feels irresponsible not to check on these things, especially when so many stories and campaigns emphasize the importance of vigilance. I can't help but think of the responsibility I owe myself, and even my family, to stay on top of my health. They'd expect me to be responsible, to avoid any regrets down the line. It's like there's a duty to notice any warning signs as soon as they appear.

The last time I visited my doctor, he said my moles were benign. But doctors can make mistakes, and maybe he didn't look closely enough. What if he missed something? Or what if I forgot to mention the right mole? Every time I replay that appointment in my mind, I feel like there's a part of the conversation that's slipping through my memory, a tiny detail I might have overlooked. I can't shake the feeling that I didn't ask enough questions or point out the exact spot I meant to. What if the reassurance I got wasn't thorough enough?

I've seen enough public health messages and skin cancer awareness ads to know that a missed diagnosis is all it takes for a life to change drastically. They always talk about how early intervention saves lives, and that thought presses on me every time I look at my skin. I just read an article yesterday that mentioned the dangers of melanoma. It could be spreading as I stand here, looking in the mirror. And if that's true, if the cancer is advancing and I'm not noticing, I might not find out until it's too late.

The urge I feel to keep checking my skin feels very real, almost as if there must be something to it. It's like a force that keeps pushing me to look closer, to take pictures, to search for answers online. I've ignored my body's signals before, and I don't want to make that mistake again. The urge to check feels like a necessary precaution, like an instinct I shouldn't ignore.

At night, I lay awake, thinking about my future, wondering if I'll be one of those people who has a diagnosis come out of nowhere, ending my plans, my dreams, my time with loved ones. I imagine myself in hospital rooms, surrounded by doctors, feeling the life I've built slip away because I didn't pay close enough attention. I picture my family, devastated, wondering how this could have happened. The unbearable thought of dying fills me with dread. I can't shake the idea that my future might be cut short, that my life could be ending right now, all because I missed a small but crucial detail.

Obsessional Narrative 5.11. Case of Alex (Vignette 1.11)
"Maybe reality is an illusion, and nothing I experience is truly real."

One evening, after reading an article about simulation theory, I found myself lying in bed, replaying the ideas in my mind. The article discussed how reality might be a highly advanced simulation – a concept I'd heard before, but this time, it lingered. What if reality as I know it isn't real? Scientists, philosophers, even well-known spiritual traditions have questioned the very nature of existence. With so many respected authorities delving into this idea, who's to say they aren't right?

The thought grew more unsettling, and I began to feel as if my life was framed by hidden layers I couldn't see. It felt as though there was something just beyond my reach, something more complex than I could comprehend. If my senses are so limited – if I can only perceive a fraction of the light and sound spectrums, while animals experience other layers of reality – then perhaps everything I'm experiencing is only a narrow slice of something far more complex. The reality I know might just be a filtered, incomplete version of what truly exists.

As I lay there, memories surfaced of times when reality itself had seemed strange or dreamlike. I recalled vivid dreams that felt entirely real, where waking up was like switching from one world to another. In those moments, the line between dream and reality was thin; now, it feels as if that line could dissolve entirely. These experiences that I used to dismiss now seem like evidence – proof that my perception of reality is fragile and, maybe, illusory.

The thought spiraled, and I started to question everything. How do I know any of this is real? Even during ordinary moments, I've had flashes where the world around me feels slightly "off" – familiar places suddenly seem strange, people I know feel distant, almost as if I'm watching from a distance rather than truly being present. These moments of detachment, while unsettling, now feel like hints that reality might indeed be an illusion.

My values make it even harder to let go of these thoughts. I value understanding truth and reality deeply; being connected to what's real has always felt essential to leading a meaningful life. But if reality itself is uncertain, then what happens to that meaning? If I can't know what's real, how can I trust anything in my life? It feels like everything I've built – my relationships, my achievements, my memories – could just be part of an elaborate mirage.

Then there's the unsettling idea that others have shared similar feelings. Online, I've read forums where people share their own doubts about reality. Movies, media, and even respected authorities raise questions about simulations, alternate realities, and false worlds. The more I read, the more I wonder if I'm experiencing something beyond mere doubt – as if reality itself could unravel at any moment.

The cycle feels endless. Each time I try to brush off these thoughts, more questions flood my mind. What if I'm just trapped in this loop forever, always questioning but never finding solid ground? I worry that I'll live out my days searching for answers, never able to trust the world around me. If I can't find reassurance, then my life might be consumed by these doubts – and without clarity, I'm afraid I'll never find peace. The more I think about it, the more it feels like reality is slipping away, leaving me lost in an unending search for truth that might never come.

Obsessional Narrative 5.12. Case of Lily (Vignette 1.12)
"Maybe my feelings for him aren't real, and we don't belong together."

I keep coming back to this thought: Maybe my feelings for Ben aren't real. The possibility that my love for him might not be genuine fills me with dread. People talk about love feeling natural, about having an inner certainty, and yet here I am, questioning whether my feelings are enough. What if I'm only pretending to love him? What if I'm forcing something that isn't truly there? These doubts leave me wondering if we're even compatible. If I can't know my feelings with certainty, what does that say about us as a couple?

I know that long-term relationships don't require constant intense feelings. I've heard others say that love often manifests as a steady, comforting presence and that it's natural for the initial "spark" to calm down over time. But even knowing this, I can't stop questioning what I actually feel. If I truly loved him, shouldn't I feel more certain? Instead, these doubts leave me feeling as if I'm performing, as though I'm forcing something that isn't really there.

Despite how caring and supportive Ben is, I can't shake the doubt that something might be missing. I often feel warm and safe with him, but the absence of those intense "in love" feelings makes me wonder: Am I really in love, or am I just settling? I find myself comparing our relationship to stories of others who talk about a "deep, intuitive connection" that they say defines true love. If I don't feel that with Ben, what does that mean about us as a couple? The more I question my own feelings, the more anxious and uncertain I become.

I examine every interaction we have, trying to understand what I actually feel. When we hug, it feels good, but almost immediately, I find myself wondering, Is this feeling enough? If my heart doesn't skip a beat every time I see him, does that mean my feelings aren't real? Each small moment between us is an opportunity for self-analysis, but I never find the reassurance I'm looking for. Instead, every hug, kiss, and conversation becomes another test, and with each test, my doubts grow stronger.

Thinking about the future feels overwhelming. If I continue to doubt my feelings like this, does it mean that I should end things with Ben? Would breaking up give me clarity? But the thought of leaving him fills me with dread. I'd be walking away from someone who cares about me deeply, someone who's been there for me through so much. Still, if I stay, am I trapping him in a relationship that's built on uncertain feelings? I find myself going in circles, afraid of staying, but terrified of leaving, unable to imagine my life either way without fear and regret.

Then there are the memories of past relationships. I remember the thrill and intensity of first dates and short-lived romances, and I wonder if I should feel that same intensity with Ben all the time. I find myself looking for signs that my attachment to him is flawed, that my current feelings don't measure up to some ideal of love. Even though I know love can look different in different relationships, the absence of that intense excitement leaves me feeling like there's something wrong with what we have.

Each time I try to reassure myself, I only open up more questions. If I loved him, would I be doubting like this? The cycle feels endless, and the harder I try to feel certain, the more distant that certainty becomes. I'm left wondering if I'll ever be able to know my true feelings or if I'm destined to feel this uncertainty forever.

Obsessional Narrative 5.13. Case of Lucas (Vignette 1.13)
"Maybe I'm changing into someone else."

Lately, I can't stop thinking that I might be changing into someone else. Every time I look in the mirror, I'm hit with the fear that I no longer recognize my own face. Sometimes, I catch my reflection and it feels foreign, like I'm looking at someone who isn't quite me. They say people can change without realizing it, and I can't shake the feeling that subtle, unnoticeable shifts might be happening to me too. What if, without realizing it, I'm gradually transforming into someone I'd never want to be?

I think back to how easily I seem to pick up little traits from people I spend time with, often without intending to. A friend once joked that I was "starting to act just like him," and even though it was a harmless comment, it made me wonder. If I'm absorbing these small habits, what's stopping me from absorbing even more, deeper changes? And if I can't recognize these shifts in real time, how will I know when they're happening? Maybe my personality, even my values, are constantly being influenced in ways I can't control.

I've read that media, too, can influence a person's beliefs and personality. Scientists and psychologists mention how prolonged exposure to certain environments can subtly reshape who we are. If I'm not careful, could even the movies I watch or the books I read affect my identity? Each time I consume something, it feels like another layer of control is slipping away, as though every outside influence is tugging at my sense of self. I know it sounds irrational, but I can't help wondering if these things are reshaping me bit by bit.

Every now and then, when I'm around certain people, I notice myself taking on their tone or expressions. It's like I can't help but absorb their way of thinking or reacting. It's unsettling to think that simply being near someone could alter who I am. I've even heard people say that certain individuals have an "energy" that can influence those around them, without anyone being aware. Maybe I'm being molded by the personalities and attitudes of those around me, gradually changing into a version of myself that I don't want to become.

The fear isn't just about my personality, though. Even physically, I don't look exactly as I did a few years ago. Every small shift in my appearance, even a slight change in the way I see myself in the mirror, feels like proof that my face, my body, and everything about me is shifting. I've read that as we age, genetics cause subtle, constant changes that make us look different from how we did in the past. But what if this is more than just normal aging? What if my face is slowly morphing into someone else's face, and one day, I'll look in the mirror and won't see myself at all?

Sometimes, it feels like even the little things I do no longer feel completely mine. I wonder, are these thoughts, these reactions, truly mine? Or have they been shaped by others, by the media, by everything around me? I know I value authenticity deeply, yet it feels like I'm losing control over my own identity, like I'm watching myself from a distance as my personality shifts without my permission. I fear that if I lose my grasp on who I am, I'll wake up one day and feel like a stranger in my own skin.

I can't stop checking myself to make sure I'm still "me." Every time I pass a mirror, I feel compelled to look, to check if anything has changed. I compare recent photos of myself, searching for differences that might mean I'm becoming someone else. Each time I find even the slightest difference, it sends me into a spiral, convinced that the transformation has already begun. I've even started avoiding looking at photos from a few years back because I'm afraid that they'll show how much I've already changed, how far I am from who I used to be.

If I continue down this path, I'm afraid I'll lose my real self entirely. If I can't hold onto my identity, what will be left of me? The thought fills me with a sense of dread and helplessness. I imagine a future where I've lost my connection to who I am, where my personality and appearance have completely morphed into someone unrecognizable. If that happens, I don't know how I'll go on. I'll be living as a stranger, disconnected from myself, unable to find any comfort in my own skin.

Obsessional Narrative 5.14. *Case of Abigail (Vignette 1.14)*
"Maybe my OCD is coming back."
"What if I don't really have OCD?"

For as long as I can remember, OCD has been a part of my life. The rituals, the endless checking, the constant doubts—I've lived with it for years. But recently, things seemed to change. My symptoms started to ease. The compulsion to wash my hands multiple times a day faded, and the intrusive thoughts that used to dominate my mind became quieter. At first, I felt a brief sense of relief, but almost immediately, the questions began. Maybe this improvement means my OCD is coming back even worse. I've read that stress can trigger relapses, and with so much going on in my life, I can't help but wonder if I'm standing at the edge of something I can't see yet.

The silence of calm feels unnatural, almost deceptive, like the quiet before a storm. I've read articles saying that relapse is common for those with OCD, and that improvement can mask underlying problems that haven't really gone away. What if my progress isn't real but is just a temporary lull? I've experienced this before: brief moments of relief only to have my symptoms come back stronger and harder to control. That memory haunts me, making it impossible to trust any improvement. The better I feel, the more I wonder if I'm letting my guard down, and with that thought comes guilt. If I miss the signs, wouldn't that mean I failed to stay vigilant and let myself slip back into old patterns?

These thoughts lead to an even darker question: What if I don't actually have OCD? If I've been misdiagnosed, everything I've done to manage my symptoms could have been for the wrong condition. I know there are disorders that resemble OCD, and I've read stories of people whose symptoms were misattributed to the wrong issue. Some of my symptoms have felt inconsistent or different from what I've read about OCD, which makes me wonder: Did I misinterpret my own experiences? What if my struggles were something else all along—something worse?

I can't ignore the fact that my diagnosis was based on my reporting. If I got something wrong or missed something important, could that mean I've misled my therapist? The idea of being dishonest with myself or others fills me with shame. I value honesty and integrity, and I feel it's my responsibility to understand my own condition. But if I don't have OCD, what does that say about everything I've done in therapy? Could I have wasted years focusing on the wrong problem?

These doubts lead me to compulsions I can't control. I replay conversations with my therapist, dissecting every word, looking for proof that my diagnosis was correct. Online, I search endlessly, reading about OCD symptoms, comparing them to my own experiences, and scrolling through forums where others question their diagnoses. I've seen stories of people whose symptoms seemed to match mine, only to find out later they were misdiagnosed. Could I be one of them? The more I search for answers, the more questions I uncover, and the doubts only grow louder.

In my quiet moments, the fear is most intense. If I don't have OCD, then what's wrong with me? Could it be something worse, something that could take over completely? If my OCD is coming back, what if I never recover, and I'm left trapped in this endless cycle of doubt and uncertainty? Every time I think I'm making progress, the fear that it's all an illusion keeps pulling me back. Getting better almost feels too good to be true, as if improvement is just setting me up for a greater fall.

I try to convince myself that my progress is real, but the more I think about it, the more it feels fragile, like something that could unravel at any moment. My mind races with questions I can't answer, and I'm left wondering if I'll ever find the clarity I desperately need. If my OCD is returning—or if I never had it at all—what does that mean for my future? These doubts leave me stuck in a cycle of endless self-monitoring and fear, unable to trust my own mind or the progress I thought I had made.

Obsessional Narrative 5.15. Case of Oliver (Vignette 1.15)
"Maybe getting rid of anything is a mistake."

Every time I try to declutter, I'm flooded with the same thought: What if I'm making a mistake? It's not just a small hesitation—it feels like a critical decision, one that could have irreversible consequences. I've read that even seemingly useless objects can later gain value, and I can't shake the idea that the very thing I throw away today might turn out to be essential tomorrow. What if something I discard becomes rare or important? I know that human judgment is flawed—how can I trust myself to know what I'll need in the future?

I've seen this happen before. There was a time I threw away an old stack of magazines, thinking I'd never look at them again, only to discover later that they had an article I needed for a project. The memory still stings. Another time, I discarded a broken gadget, only to realize it could have been repaired and repurposed. I've had enough experiences like this to convince me that keeping everything is the safer option. The regret of needing something I've thrown away feels unbearable, and I can't let it happen again.

But it's not just about practicality. Each object I own feels connected to a specific memory or moment in my life. An old t-shirt isn't just fabric—it's a reminder of the concert where I bought it. A broken coffee mug is tied to a morning spent with friends. Discarding these things feels like erasing parts of myself, like I'm letting go of pieces of my identity. I value those connections deeply; they make me who I am.

Even when I try to rationalize, the doubt creeps in. What if someone else could have used this? Throwing it away feels selfish, as though I'm wasting something that might have helped another person. I've read articles emphasizing the importance of sustainability and reuse, and I can't ignore the guilt of contributing to waste. If I throw something away and later realize it could have been useful, wouldn't that mean I've failed—not just myself, but also the planet?

These thoughts make it impossible to let go of anything. I've heard stories about people finding treasures among what they almost discarded, and I can't stop wondering if I might have something valuable hidden in my piles of belongings. Even old receipts and scraps of paper feel like they might matter someday, if only I could figure out how. The idea of letting go feels like closing a door on possibilities I can't yet foresee.

When I look at the clutter, I know it's overwhelming. My friends stopped visiting long ago, and I barely use most of my apartment because there's nowhere to sit or move. But every time I try to throw something away, the same fear takes over: What if I need this later? What if this item turns out to be irreplaceable? I've read stories about people regretting similar decisions, and I can't stop myself from imagining the same outcome for me. Even when I do manage to discard something, I often find myself retrieving it later, the doubt pulling me back to the same cycle.

The thought of losing something essential feels like losing control. If I make a mistake, it feels like I'll have failed in my responsibility to be prepared for the future. Every item I keep gives me a small sense of security, like I'm safeguarding against an uncertain world. The clutter is stifling, but it feels safer than the alternative. Letting go would mean opening myself up to regret, vulnerability, and the possibility of losing parts of myself that I can never get back.

This fear consumes me. It's not just about the objects themselves—it's about what they represent: safety, identity, responsibility, and preparation. If I make the wrong decision, I'll not only lose an item but also a part of my sense of control. The weight of these possibilities keeps me stuck, endlessly circling through the same decisions, unable to move forward.

Form 5.1. Case of Jack (Vignette 1.1)
Potential Reasons Behind a Contrasting Conclusion

Contrasting Conclusion
"I am a peaceful person that is in control of himself"

Abstract facts and ideas — Things that you know or believe to be true in general.

a. Violent behavior is often the result of extreme circumstances, and I have never been in such situations.
b. My daily routine and life decisions are generally peaceful and well-considered.
c. People who truly lose control often exhibit warning signs over time, which I do not display.

Personal experience — Your own personal experience, past or present

a. I have never acted violently toward anyone, even when upset.
b. Friends and family have never expressed concern about my behavior or questioned my self-control.
c. I have a long history of peaceful interactions with others, even in difficult circumstances.

Values, standards and rules — The way of doing things according to an accepted principle.

a. I value kindness and peaceful behavior, and I actively practice it in my life.
b. I follow personal guidelines to remain calm and composed, even when frustrated.
c. I have always been committed to non-violence, which is a fundamental principle in my life.

Authorities — A person, institution or organization that is perceived as important.

a. Research shows that individuals who reflect on their actions are less likely to behave impulsively.
b. Studies indicate that individuals who value self-control, like myself, tend to consistently act in line with those values.
c. Research shows that individuals who have consistently displayed peaceful behavior in the past are likely to continue doing so in the future.

Hearsay and news — Information that you got from other people, substantiated or not.

a. People often describe me as thoughtful and compassionate.
b. I've heard from others that they appreciate my peaceful approach to handling stressful situations.
c. I once watched a documentary that explored how people's true character is revealed in their consistent actions over time, and it resonated with how I live my life.

Anything else — Anything that does not fit well in the previous categories

a. My professional life as a graphic designer involves creativity and expression, not aggression.
b. My actions consistently reflect a desire to nurture and care for others.
c. I enjoy peaceful, relaxing activities like reading and spending time outdoors.

Form 5.2. Case of Rachel (Vignette 1.2)
Potential Reasons Behind a Contrasting Conclusion

Contrasting Conclusion
"I have healthy and natural feelings towards children"

Abstract facts and ideas — Things that you know or believe to be true in general.

a. Healthy feelings are consistent with a nurturing role, as seen in most caretakers and educators.
b. Intrusive thoughts are a well-known phenomenon that does not reflect a person's true intentions or character.
c. Genuine warmth and care for children are normal in those who dedicate their lives to teaching or caregiving.

Personal experience — Your own personal experience, past or present

a. My interactions with children are guided by a genuine desire to support and care for them, as shown by their positive responses to me.
b. I've received feedback from parents and colleagues praising my ability to connect with children in a healthy and supportive way.
c. My past experiences have shown that my instincts and intentions are always focused on the well-being of the children I work with.

Values, standards and rules — The way of doing things according to an accepted principle.

a. I deeply value the responsibility of creating a safe, caring, and supportive environment for the children in my care.
b. My moral standards guide my thoughts and actions, ensuring that I prioritize the well-being of others.
c. Protecting and nurturing children is a principle that I take seriously.

Authorities — A person, institution or organization that is perceived as important.

a. Organizations supporting teachers highlight the natural role of educators in fostering trust and safety for children.
b. Research into effective teaching practices highlights that warmth and care are essential to building trust and helping children thrive.
c. Ethical teaching guidelines from respected education boards highlight the importance of empathy and care in working with young children.

Hearsay and news — Information that you got from other people, substantiated or not.

a. Friends and colleagues have often commented on how much children enjoy being around me and how positively they respond to my teaching style.
b. I've heard from parents that their children feel safe and cared for in my classroom, which reflects the kind of environment I create.
c. Articles about teaching often describe the natural bond between educators and their students as a cornerstone of effective education.

Anything else — Anything that does not fit well in the previous categories

a. The intrusive thoughts I experience are driven by OCD, not reality.
b. My consistent ability to maintain professional boundaries and prioritize children's well-being demonstrates my healthy approach to caregiving.
c. The emotional rewards I feel from seeing children thrive under my care reflect a natural and healthy connection.

Form 5.3. Case of John (Vignette 1.3)
Potential Reasons Behind a Contrasting Conclusion

Contrasting Conclusion *"I am a faithful person who truly believes in God."*

Abstract facts and ideas — Things that you know or believe to be true in general.

a. Faith provides a moral compass and direction in life, and I follow that path daily.
b. Being committed to prayer, worship, and service to others is a sign of genuine faith.
c. Believers who live by the teachings of their faith are evidence of their genuine belief.

Personal experience — Your own personal experience, past or present

a. I have felt deeply connected to God many times in prayer and worship.
b. I've consistently relied on my faith for guidance during difficult times.
c. I've experienced peace and comfort through my faith on numerous occasions.

Values, standards and rules — The way of doing things according to an accepted principle.

a. I value living a life guided by faith and prioritize my spiritual growth.
b. My faith is the foundation of my values and decisions.
c. I make a conscious effort to further deepen my relationship with God.

Authorities — A person, institution or organization that is perceived as important.

a. My spiritual mentors have always encouraged me in my journey, affirming my faith.
b. Religious leaders emphasize that commitment to prayer and worship is a sign of true belief.
c. Scriptures reinforce that living by God's word is proof of genuine faith.

Hearsay and news — Information that you got from other people, substantiated or not.

a. I've heard religious programs where faithful people describe lives of devotion similar to mine.
b. Friends and family members have often spoken of my deep faith and commitment to God.
c. People close to me view me as a spiritual role model, reflecting their belief in my strong faith.

Anything else — Anything that does not fit well in the previous categories

a. My daily life is centered around my faith and devotion to God.
b. My faith is reflected in my actions, choices, and relationships with others.
c. I find fulfillment and meaning in my religious practices.

Form 5.2. Case of Laura (Vignette 1.4)
Potential Reasons Behind a Contrasting Conclusion

Contrasting Conclusion *"I am an honest and ethical person"*

Abstract facts and ideas — Things that you know or believe to be true in general.

a. Integrity is about owning up to mistakes and correcting them.
b. Ethical people are not perfect; they strive to do the right thing.
c. Honesty and integrity are shown through a person's overall intentions and actions over time.

Personal experience — Your own personal experience, past or present

a. I have always felt a deep sense of responsibility in my work, especially when it comes to being honest with clients and colleagues.
b. When I made mistakes in the past, I corrected them, which reflects my commitment to integrity.
c. Friends and colleagues have trusted me for years, often coming to me for guidance because they see me as a person of integrity.

Values, standards and rules — The way of doing things according to an accepted principle.

a. I value honesty and fairness, and I try to make choices that align with these principles in all areas of my life.
b. My high ethical standards are a reflection of my values, not just habits or routines.
c. I consciously work to ensure my actions are transparent and fair, upholding my commitment to integrity.

Authorities — A person, institution or organization that is perceived as important.

a. Ethical teachings and workplace guidelines emphasize that integrity involves effort, not perfection.
b. Mentors and supervisors have complimented me on my honesty and conscientiousness in my professional role.
c. Research shows that honest individuals tend to correct mistakes quickly, as I do, rather than hide them.

Hearsay and news — Information that you got from other people, substantiated or not.

a. I've heard from colleagues that they appreciate my honesty, often remarking on how careful I am with details.
b. Friends have told me they see me as a trustworthy and reliable person, which reflects my commitment to being truthful.
c. I know people whose actions I respect, and I try to model the same integrity I admire in others.

Anything else — Anything that does not fit well in the previous categories

a. My work and personal life are both guided by a strong sense of ethics.
b. My actions reflect my desire to be fair and honest, even when it's difficult.
c. I feel fulfilled by my commitment to integrity, knowing it aligns with who I am at my core.

Form 5.2. Case of Ethan (Vignette 1.5)
Potential Reasons Behind a Contrasting Conclusion

> **Contrasting Conclusion**
> *"I am thorough and attentive in my actions, ensuring that things are in order."*
> *"The things around me are functioning as expected and are reliable."*

Abstract facts and ideas — Things that you know or believe to be true in general.

a. Most appliances and systems are designed to work reliably and safely with occasional checks.
b. Small, reasonable actions help keep things in good order without needing constant attention.
c. When used as intended, daily-use items tend to function consistently and without issue.

Personal experience — Your own personal experience, past or present

a. My belongings and appliances have generally worked smoothly over time.
b. In my experience, once I check things, they tend to stay secure, allowing me to trust my initial efforts.
c. I've noticed that when I follow normal checking routines, things tend to work as they should.

Values, standards and rules — The way of doing things according to an accepted principle.

a. I value a sensible approach to care and safety, which gives me confidence in my actions.
b. My standard of checking things once aligns with my sense of responsibility without needing to go overboard.
c. My commitment to reasonable care allows me to feel prepared and reassured in my environment.

Authorities — A person, institution or organization that is perceived as important.

a. Manufacturers build in safeguards, and experts suggest that moderate, routine checks are enough for safety.
b. Safety guidelines emphasize using items as intended and following basic precautions, which supports my approach.
c. Industry standards recommend periodic maintenance without over-checking, making me feel secure in my habits.

Hearsay and news — Information that you got from other people, substantiated or not.

a. Friends and family trust their appliances to work as expected, which shows that most things are dependable
b. I've heard from others that household items rarely fail when used properly.
c. Media often highlight that everyday safety habits are enough to keep things functioning smoothly.

Anything else — Anything that does not fit well in the previous categories

a. I can feel comfortable knowing that my routines support a well-maintained home and workspace.
b. My approach balances attentiveness with trust in the reliability of my environment.
c. I find reassurance in knowing that most things work as intended when handled reasonably.

Form 5.2. Case of Sophie (Vignette 1.6)
Potential Reasons Behind a Contrasting Conclusion

Contrasting Conclusion
"My environment and the products I use are safe, supporting the well-being of myself and others."

Abstract facts and ideas — Things that you know or believe to be true in general.

a. Household products are rigorously tested to ensure they meet health and safety standards, particularly for everyday use.
b. Most cleaning products, when used as directed, are designed to be safe and effective without posing health risks.
c. Healthy environments are created by balanced, reasonable habits rather than excessive avoidance or worry.

Personal experience — Your own personal experience, past or present

a. I have used many common household products without issue, and they have helped me maintain a clean and pleasant living space.
b. I have successfully maintained a healthy home with regular, simple routines, which shows my environment is manageable and safe.
c. Friends and family visit my home regularly and have never expressed concerns about its safety.

Values, standards and rules — The way of doing things according to an accepted principle.

a. My commitment to maintaining a healthy environment aligns with my values of care and responsibility.
b. Following basic cleaning and health guidelines allows me to maintain a safe home without excessive effort.
c. I value a balanced approach to cleanliness that supports a peaceful, sustainable environment for myself and others.

Authorities — A person, institution or organization that is perceived as important.

a. Health and safety experts emphasize that household products are safe when used as directed.
b. Environmental and health agencies have strict regulations that ensure household items and cleaning products are safe for consumer use.
c. Scientific studies show that everyday exposure to household products poses minimal risk when used responsibly.

Hearsay and news — Information that you got from other people, substantiated or not.

a. I've heard others talk about their experiences with similar products and environments, which have supported their health and comfort without issue.
b. Friends and family have shared positive stories about creating safe, healthy spaces using everyday products.
c. News articles and sources frequently reassure that household products are safe under normal usage conditions, offering added peace of mind.

Anything else — Anything that does not fit well in the previous categories

a. I feel reassured knowing that my routines promote a healthy, safe space for myself and others.
b. My environment supports my well-being, and the practices I follow are reasonable and effective.
c. Knowing that I have a well-maintained, healthy space allows me to enjoy my surroundings with confidence.

Form 5.2. Case of Matthew (Vignette 1.7)
Potential Reasons Behind a Contrasting Conclusion

Contrasting Conclusion
"Things are placed well enough, done right, and adequately complete for their purpose."

Abstract facts and ideas — Things that you know or believe to be true in general.

a. In design and daily life, alignment and arrangement follow logical task requirements and are complete when these needs are met.
b. A well-arranged environment or completed task doesn't require additional checking to maintain its function or quality.
c. Everyday tasks, whether personal or professional, generally have a natural endpoint at which they meet their purpose effectively.

Personal experience — Your own personal experience, past or present

a. My work has consistently met professional standards, which shows my attention to detail is effective without additional adjustments.
b. Once I arrange my environment to a reasonable standard, it usually stays in good order and serves its function.
c. Colleagues and clients are consistently satisfied with my projects, showing that my first efforts are accurate and complete.

Values, standards and rules — The way of doing things according to an accepted principle.

a. I value clarity and efficiency, which allow me to trust my initial work and arrangements.
b. My goal is to balance accuracy with the demands of each task, allowing me to focus on what each requires without overextending.
c. I appreciate environments that are functional and comfortable, rather than requiring perfect alignment in every detail.

Authorities — A person, institution or organization that is perceived as important.

a. Architectural training emphasizes that designs are functional and meet standards without constant re-adjustment.
b. Experts in design and architecture acknowledge that minor variances don't impact the utility or quality of a space.
c. Professional guidelines encourage thoughtful but efficient work, trusting that initial efforts are reliable when completed to standard.

Hearsay and news — Information that you got from other people, substantiated or not.

a. Colleagues often mention that trusted work doesn't require endless adjustments.
b. Friends and family share how they enjoy environments that feel balanced when aligned with their intended function.
c. Articles often highlight that a well-done job usually meets needs without requiring ongoing changes.

Anything else — Anything that does not fit well in the previous categories

a. I feel reassured knowing that my initial attention to tasks supports their quality and reliability.
b. My spaces and projects are naturally aligned with my values and professional skills, and they feel complete once finished.
c. I am comfortable knowing that my work and surroundings are effective as they are, supporting my goals and well-being.

Form 5.2. Case of Olivia (Vignette 1.8)
Potential Reasons Behind a Contrasting Conclusion

Contrasting Conclusion
"My body performs its natural functions effectively," *"I am in control of my attention and can direct my focus as I choose."*

Abstract facts and ideas — Things that you know or believe to be true in general.

a. The body's natural functions, like breathing and blinking, are regulated automatically and don't require conscious effort to perform well.
b. Human bodies are designed to manage basic functions smoothly without needing active monitoring.
c. Mental focus is flexible; attention can shift naturally as needed.

Personal experience — Your own personal experience, past or present

a. I've noticed that when I stop thinking about breathing or blinking, my body continues performing these functions on its own.
b. When I've shifted my attention to something engaging, I've seen how my body performs automatically without conscious effort.
c. I've had days where I could focus on tasks and conversations without fixating on my body, which reinforces my control over my attention.

Values, standards and rules — The way of doing things according to an accepted principle.

a. A healthy relationship with my body involves understanding that natural functions are reliable and self-regulating.
b. I believe that a flexible mind allows me to shift my focus as needed, and I value this natural adaptability.
c. I practice engaging fully in activities, which supports my focus on what truly matters in the moment.

Authorities — A person, institution or organization that is perceived as important.

a. Medical professionals affirm that bodily functions like breathing, blinking, and swallowing are automatic processes we don't need to control consciously.
b. Neuroscientists indicate that the brain's attention systems are resilient and capable of refocusing on new tasks when given the opportunity to do so.
c. Scientific studies show that the body's automatic systems are designed to function without conscious effort, even under varied conditions.

Hearsay and news — Information that you got from other people, substantiated or not.

a. Articles I've read mention that bodily functions are reliable without attention, offering a natural sense of stability.
b. Conversations with others reinforce that allowing natural processes to work independently leads to a sense of calm and engagement with life.
c. People around me seem able to focus on activities without worrying about their bodily sensations, showing that bodily trust is achievable and effective.

Anything else — Anything that does not fit well in the previous categories

a. I feel reassured knowing my body is dependable, freeing my attention for things that enrich my life.
b. Knowing my mind and body is self-regulating allows me to feel grounded and confident as I move through my day.
c. In situations where I get distracted from monitoring, I'm reassured to notice that my body and mind have continued to function reliably on their own.

Form 5.2. Case of Henry (Vignette 1.9)
Potential Reasons Behind a Contrasting Conclusion

Contrasting Conclusion
"My sexuality aligns with my heterosexual identity, and I am authentically connected to who I truly am."

Abstract facts and ideas — Things that you know or believe to be true in general.

a. I know that sexuality is often stable and consistent once a person understands their own preferences.
b. Being true to myself includes acknowledging my consistent attraction to women, which has always felt natural and genuine.
c. A person's long-standing attractions and relationships are often clear indicators of their authentic sexual identity.

Personal experience — Your own personal experience, past or present

a. My past relationships and interactions with women have always felt authentic and fulfilling.
b. My relationship with my girlfriend is meaningful to me, reflecting my natural attraction and emotional connection with her.
c. In everyday life, I feel comfortable and connected in my relationship, which reinforces my sense of stability in my orientation.

Values, standards and rules — The way of doing things according to an accepted principle.

a. I value understanding myself honestly, and I feel my history and experiences align naturally with my heterosexual identity.
b. In relationships, I value sincerity, and the emotional bond I feel with my girlfriend feels genuine.
c. Integrity in relationships matters to me, and I seek meaningful connections that resonate with who I am.

Authorities — A person, institution or organization that is perceived as important.

a. Psychological research suggests that individuals typically understand their orientation based on enduring patterns and connections.
b. Trusted resources in sexuality studies indicate that natural, long-standing relationships often reflect authentic orientation.
c. Experts highlight that consistent attraction patterns and meaningful relationships support a person's understanding of their identity.

Hearsay and news — Information that you got from other people, substantiated or not.

a. Friends who know me well see the genuine happiness I find in my relationship, which they recognize as natural and sincere.
b. Many people I know have described feeling secure in their relationships, emphasizing that orientation feels more like a part of one's core than something that fluctuates.
c. Media often highlight stories of individuals who embrace and feel grounded in their orientation based on a lifetime of consistent feelings and relationships, which aligns with my own journey.

Anything else — Anything that does not fit well in the previous categories

a. There is a consistent pattern that aligns with my heterosexual identity.
b. When I think about the future, When I think about the future, the thought of being with anyone other than my girlfriend feels deeply upsetting.
c. I feel no desire or meaningful connection on any deep level toward a same-sex relationship.

Form 5.2. Case of Mia (Vignette 1.10)
Potential Reasons Behind a Contrasting Conclusion

Condensed Primary Doubt(s)
"My skin is healthy, and I am aware of its natural changes."

Abstract facts and ideas — Things that you know or believe to be true in general.

a. Routine skin changes are common and natural, especially with age or exposure to everyday elements.
b. Skin health is generally stable with consistent care, like using sunscreen and following a basic skincare routine.
c. Early signs of skin issues are visible and noticeable, and a consistent routine of awareness allows for early detection without excessive vigilance.

Personal experience — Your own personal experience, past or present

a. I've had minor concerns about skin changes before, but each time, they were resolved without issue.
b. I've always noticed changes in my skin on time, and when I've consulted a doctor, they were deemed harmless.
c. During past check-ups, doctors have reassured me that my skin is healthy, and no issues were found.

Values, standards and rules — The way of doing things according to an accepted principle.

a. Regular, mindful care of my skin aligns with my values of health and self-care, allowing me to stay aware without constant checking.
b. Trusting in professional evaluations reflects my commitment to making informed health choices.
c. Following a routine of self-care and annual check-ups respects my values of proactive health management.

Authorities — A person, institution or organization that is perceived as important.

a. Medical professionals emphasize that annual skin check-ups are effective for catching significant issues in time.
b. Health authorities recommend balanced awareness of skin changes, not constant monitoring, which supports my approach.
c. Dermatologists acknowledge that most skin changes are benign and don't lead to serious health issues.

Hearsay and news — Information that you got from other people, substantiated or not.

a. Friends and family have shared that minor changes in skin are normal and nothing to worry about.
b. I've read articles discussing how most skin changes are natural and not indicators of serious health concerns.
c. Health magazines often highlight that skin health can be maintained without over-monitoring, which resonates with my own experience.

Anything else — Anything that does not fit well in the previous categories

a. Consistent care and awareness give me confidence in my health without needing to constantly check.
b. My routine offers a natural rhythm of care and observation that supports my well-being.
c. Having trusted professionals involved reassures me that my skin health is being effectively monitored.

Form 5.2. Case of Alex (Vignette 1.11)
Potential Reasons Behind a Contrasting Conclusion

Contrasting Conclusion
"My reality is grounded in true experiences and genuine connections"

Abstract facts and ideas — Things that you know or believe to be true in general.

a. Shared experiences and perceptions with others affirm a common reality, as we interpret and respond to the same events together
b. Genuine connections and emotions create a foundation for reality that goes beyond thoughts or theories.
c. A sense of reality and consistency is reinforced by common, universal human experiences and the world we all live in.

Personal experience — Your own personal experience, past or present

a. My experiences with friends and family feel real and meaningful, rooted in authentic connection.
b. Moments of joy, sadness, or excitement that I've felt with others are clear memories that shape my life and affirm a sense of reality.
c. Activities I enjoy, such as work, hobbies, or being in nature, make me feel genuinely engaged and present.

Values, standards and rules — The way of doing things according to an accepted principle.

a. I value being connected to the people in my life and feeling grounded in reality.
b. Experiencing life fully, including the highs and lows, aligns with my belief in living authentically.
c. I believe that genuine emotions and interactions are central to understanding who I am and where I fit in the world.

Authorities — A person, institution or organization that is perceived as important.

a. Philosophers and scientists acknowledge the shared human experience as a foundation for understanding reality.
b. Psychological research supports the notion that consistent experiences and memories affirm personal reality.
c. Experts agree that grounding oneself in daily experiences, routine, and relationships contributes to mental and emotional well-being.

Hearsay and news — Information that you got from other people, substantiated or not.

a. I've heard others talk about the importance of staying grounded in meaningful relationships and routines to stay connected with reality.
b. Friends have described feeling most "real" in the company of loved ones, and I resonate with that.
c. Articles and media often emphasize the stability that shared human experiences provide in understanding reality.

Anything else — Anything that does not fit well in the previous categories

a. The feeling of connection I have with others strengthens my sense of reality, showing me that I am part of something meaningful and tangible.
b. Observing life's consistency—like the change of seasons and daily routines—reinforces my understanding of reality.
c. The genuine sense of presence I feel during meaningful activities tells me that my experiences are real and significant.

Form 5.2. Case of Lily (Vignette 1.12)
Potential Reasons Behind a Contrasting Conclusion

Contrasting Conclusion
"My love for Ben is real, and our relationship is a genuine connection."

Abstract facts and ideas — Things that you know or believe to be true in general.

a. Genuine feelings often develop through shared experiences and a consistent sense of care and companionship.
b. Love is often expressed in the steady, everyday ways people support and understand each other
c. Strong relationships are often marked by mutual respect, trust, and a sense of partnership.

Personal experience — Your own personal experience, past or present

a. When I'm able to just enjoy being with Ben, I feel a sense of warmth and closeness that feels real.
b. There are many times when Ben's kindness and humor make me feel connected to him in a way that is natural and genuine.
c. I often feel a calm affection for Ben when we're spending time together, especially during moments when I'm fully present.

Values, standards and rules — The way of doing things according to an accepted principle.

a. I value honesty and self-awareness, and I recognize that I have genuine care and affection for Ben even if my doubts sometimes make it hard to trust those feelings.
b. In a relationship, I believe that being patient with myself and my partner creates room for a real, lasting connection.
c. I hold the view that a meaningful relationship is one where both people can be themselves, and Ben's steady support reminds me that I'm valued as I am.

Authorities — A person, institution or organization that is perceived as important.

a. Relationship experts often say that genuine love is a steady presence, something that's especially noticeable during times when I'm able to relax and appreciate what I have with Ben.
b. Experts often describe enduring love as steady and resilient, characterized by a sense of belonging and shared purpose.
c. Studies highlight that long-term love is often built on shared trust and stability, which I feel with Ben when I'm able to focus on our connection.

Hearsay and news — Information that you got from other people, substantiated or not.

a. Friends and family have commented on how they see me happy in my relationship with Ben.
b. People I know who are in strong relationships talk about the importance of shared respect and warmth, which I do experience with Ben.
c. I heard that the strongest relationships are those where you can truly relax and be yourself, something I feel with Ben when I'm not focused on questioning.

Anything else — Anything that does not fit well in the previous categories

a. When I imagine a future without Ben, it feels incomplete, as though something essential would be missing from my life.
b. There are times I feel completely at home with Ben, which suggests a closeness that doesn't disappear, even if I sometimes struggle to see it.
c. In the moments when I'm not questioning, I feel a sense of peace and belonging with Ben that's difficult to imagine with anyone else.

Form 5.2. Case of Lucas (Vignette 1.13)
Potential Reasons Behind a Contrasting Conclusion

Contrasting Conclusion *"My identity is secure and aligned with who I want to be."*

Abstract facts and ideas — Things that you know or believe to be true in general.

a. Authentic identity is often grounded in long-standing values and characteristics that don't easily shift due to external factors.
b. True personality and identity tend to remain stable, even when influenced by people, media, or changing circumstances.
c. Genetics and core characteristics establish a foundation for appearance and personality that doesn't change dramatically over short periods.

Personal experience — Your own personal experience, past or present

a. When I'm relaxed and just going about my day, I feel like myself—comfortable, familiar, and secure in my identity.
b. In times when I'm fully engaged with close friends or family, I experience a natural, effortless sense of who I am.
c. I've noticed that, even when spending time with different people or in new settings, my core traits and preferences remain the same.

Values, standards and rules — The way of doing things according to an accepted principle.

a. I value self-awareness and trust that I have a solid understanding of who I am and what I stand for.
b. Integrity is important to me, and I strive to remain true to my values, which reinforces my identity.
c. I see my personal growth as a reflection of my values, meaning that any change aligns with the core of who I am.

Authorities — A person, institution or organization that is perceived as important.

a. Psychological research suggests that identity and personality are generally stable over time, grounded in consistent patterns.
b. Experts in personal development emphasize that core identity is unlikely to shift simply from daily experiences or exposure to media.
c. Mental health professionals affirm that identity is inherently resilient and does not undergo sudden changes due to everyday interactions or influences.

Hearsay and news — Information that you got from other people, substantiated or not.

a. Friends have commented that people's true selves don't easily change—they believe that real personality remains stable.
b. I've read stories of people who, even in changing situations, find they remain true to their selves.
c. People I know have talked about how personality is something that deepens over time but doesn't fundamentally change.

Anything else — Anything that does not fit well in the previous categories

a. Knowing oneself includes recognizing that identity doesn't change dramatically without significant life events.
b. When I think about my future, I'm able to imagine myself continuing to grow in a way that's aligned with who I already am.
c. The things I care about and the qualities I admire in myself have stayed consistent, reinforcing that my identity is stable and secure.

Form 5.2. Case of Abigail (Vignette 1.14)
Potential Reasons Behind a Contrasting Conclusion

Contrasting Conclusion *"My progress is real, and I am capable of continuing to improve."* *"I have OCD and I am able to understand it.."*

Abstract facts and ideas — Things that you know or believe to be true in general.

a. Genuine progress often comes from sustained effort and applying strategies that work over time.
b. Recovery is a process, and periods of calm often reflect the hard work of managing symptoms effectively.
c. OCD is a defined mental health condition with specific patterns and symptoms.

Personal experience — Your own personal experience, past or present

a. I've experienced real changes in my symptoms since starting therapy.
b. The relief I've felt from applying OCD-specific techniques confirms my diagnosis.
c. My experiences with obsessions and compulsions align with what I've learned about OCD.

Values, standards and rules — The way of doing things according to an accepted principle.

a. Self-awareness and honesty have helped me understand and tackle my symptoms.
b. I value clarity, and understanding my diagnosis helps me take constructive steps forward.
c. I believe in learning about myself, and this understanding empowers me to manage my condition.

Authorities — A person, institution or organization that is perceived as important.

a. Experts emphasize that OCD can improve significantly with the right treatment and ongoing management.
b. Research supports the idea that behavioral and cognitive strategies can lead to lasting progress.
c. My therapist has confirmed my diagnosis, which is based on recognized patterns of OCD.

Hearsay and news — Information that you got from other people, substantiated or not.

a. Friends who have dealt with OCD have shared that progress feels fragile at first but becomes more stable over time
b. Online forums often describe recovery as a series of steps forward and back, with overall improvement in the long term.
c. Personal accounts of OCD in books and media often describe patterns that resonate with my own struggles.

Anything else — Anything that does not fit well in the previous categories

a. No two individuals experience OCD in exactly the same way, as each of us has our own unique story.
b. The improvements I've noticed in my daily routines are proof that progress is both real and tangible.
c. Progress is rarely linear; even relapses or shifts in symptoms can be meaningful parts of the recovery journey.

Form 5.2. Case of Oliver (Vignette 1.15)
Potential Reasons Behind a Contrasting Conclusion

Contrasting Conclusion *"Letting go of unnecessary items is a wise and thoughtful choice."*

Abstract facts and ideas — Things that you know or believe to be true in general.

a. Letting go of items can create space for a more organized and functional environment.
b. Items that no longer serve a purpose often take up unnecessary space and energy.
c. Many possessions are never used or serve no purpose.

Personal experience — Your own personal experience, past or present

a. I have enjoyed being in uncluttered space in the past.
b. I've found that certain things I worried about discarding could be replaced quickly and affordably.
c. Many things I've kept thinking they might be useful have sat untouched for years.

Values, standards and rules — The way of doing things according to an accepted principle.

a. I value simplicity and believe in prioritizing what truly enriches my life.
b. Letting go of what I don't need reflects respect for my space.
c. Prioritizing quality over quantity is a valuable principle.

Authorities — A person, institution or organization that is perceived as important.

a. Experts in organization and mental health emphasize the benefits of decluttering for emotional well-being.
b. Sustainability advocates promote donating and repurposing items to reduce waste and benefit others.
c. Books and research on minimalism show that focusing on essentials leads to greater happiness and productivity.

Hearsay and news — Information that you got from other people, substantiated or not.

a. Friends have shared how decluttering helped them feel freer and less burdened.
b. I've heard stories of people transforming their lives after letting go of clutter.
c. Articles often highlight how simplifying one's environment can lead to a better quality of life.

Anything else — Anything that does not fit well in the previous categories

a. Letting go of items aligns with my desire to create a space where I feel at peace.
b. Decluttering allows me to rediscover the joy and utility of the items I choose to keep.
c. Releasing unnecessary things creates room for opportunities and experiences in life that truly matter.

Form 5.5. An Alternative for Jack (Vignette 1.1)
"I am a peaceful person that is in control of himself"

I've always seen myself as someone who values peace and tries to keep things balanced. It's not that I'm perfect, but I've come to understand that my actions reflect a deep desire to approach life calmly and with care. Whether it's working on a design project or enjoying time outdoors, I try to be intentional about the choices I make. Sometimes I do get irritated, but I can step back and handle situations thoughtfully, rather than reacting impulsively. These choices are not random—they come from a place of wanting to live in a way that's true to my character.

On most days, my routine feels like a rhythm that keeps me grounded. I can recall countless mornings spent walking in the park, feeling the cool air and listening to the sound of leaves rustling in the trees. These walks are more than just a break—they're reminders of the calmness I try to bring into my life, even when I'm dealing with stress or pressure. Of course, not every day is easy, but I've learned to rely on my ability to take a breath, step back, and regain my balance. My work, too, is steady and focused. The hours spent designing, reviewing details, and refining projects give me a sense of control and satisfaction, helping me appreciate the way I approach challenges.

I see this same commitment in how I interact with others. Once, a friend came to me feeling really anxious about a decision they had to make. We sat down together, and I listened without judgment, just helping them feel heard. I'm not always able to fix things for people, and sometimes I feel unsure, but being there for my friends feels right. My friends and family often tell me they appreciate the calm I bring to conversations, especially during difficult moments.

I remember reading an article about how character is built over time through consistent actions. This idea speaks to me because it reflects how I try to live my life. I may not always have the perfect response, but I do my best to act with kindness and patience. I remember seeing an interview with a psychologist who said that people who value self-control tend to practice it in multiple areas of their lives. That feels true to me. Whether I'm working on a project, connecting with friends, or facing a challenge, I bring the same focus and respect for others.

My role as a graphic designer is another space where I see my peaceful and composed nature reflected. The process of designing can be demanding, but it requires a level of focus and self-control that aligns with my personality. When I'm designing, there's no rush—it's about making deliberate choices, adjusting, refining, and watching the project come together with patience and care. This calm and thoughtful approach to my work mirrors how I strive to handle all aspects of my life, reinforcing my sense of being a peaceful person in control of myself.

There's a balance in how I live that reassures me. A documentary I watched once explored how people's true nature reveals itself through their everyday actions. That thought stayed with me because it resonates with the choices I make. I've never been impulsive or rushed into a big decision without thinking it through. The way I treat people, with kindness and respect, reflects how I want to live. I'm not immune to stress, but I trust that I can stay steady, even when things feel overwhelming.

Even in moments of stress, I've found ways to keep a level head. Just last month, a deadline at work started to pile up, and instead of panicking, I broke the project into smaller tasks, tackling each one with focus. This steady approach allows me to stay grounded, trusting that I can handle whatever comes next. It's this kind of approach—taking things step by step—that allows me to stay in control and not get overwhelmed. I don't need to rush through things; I'm comfortable taking my time, making sure everything falls into place.

I came across a news feature once that emphasized how long-term behavior is a strong predictor of future actions. It's a reassuring thought because when I look back at my life, I see the consistency. This foundation I've built is something I can trust, knowing it reflects who I am. I don't claim to be perfect, but I know that my intentions—whether in my work, relationships, or personal time—are always centered around balance. The decisions I've made in the past show me that I can trust myself to continue acting in the same way.

Form 5.5. An Alternative Narrative for Rachel (Vignette 1.2)
"I have healthy and natural feelings towards children"

My role as an educator is driven by a deep-seated commitment to care, nurture, and protect the children I work with. Every day, I am reminded of the joy and fulfillment that comes from helping children grow, learn, and develop. The laughter, curiosity, and trust they bring into the classroom are a testament to the genuine and healthy bond I share with them. Parents frequently express their gratitude for the safe and encouraging environment I create, and my colleagues have consistently praised my patience, empathy, and ability to connect with my students. These affirmations reinforce that my feelings toward children are rooted in compassion and a commitment to their well-being.

The warmth and care I show align entirely with the values and standards of my profession. Ethical teaching guidelines emphasize the importance of empathy, trust, and creating a supportive environment for children. My actions, whether it's offering a comforting word, encouraging a student to try something new, or celebrating their achievements, reflect these principles. Studies have shown that effective teaching relies on building healthy, appropriate relationships with students, and this is something I strive to embody every day. The positive feedback I've received from colleagues and parents reminds me that my role is defined by these professional and ethical values.

I have seen how my commitment to nurturing children helps them thrive. Moments like watching a shy child gain confidence in their abilities or seeing a group of students come together to solve a problem reaffirm my purpose as a teacher. These experiences remind me that the emotional rewards I feel from helping children are not only healthy but are essential to the impact I have in their lives. They reflect the joy that comes from making a difference, not just academically but emotionally and socially.

My personal experiences further confirm the healthy and natural nature of my feelings. I have consistently maintained professional boundaries while offering support and encouragement to my students. The children in my care respond to me with trust and affection, showing that they feel secure and valued in my presence. These interactions are a reflection of my genuine desire to help them grow, learn, and feel safe in their environment.

Friends, colleagues, and even parents have commented on my ability to connect with children in a meaningful and appropriate way. I've often heard from parents that their children feel excited to come to my classroom because they feel understood and cared for. These moments are not only affirmations of my teaching abilities but also serve as reminders that my feelings and instincts are naturally aligned with my role.

I also understand that intrusive doubts are a hallmark of OCD, not a reflection of reality. The very nature of these doubts—a focus on questioning my values and instincts—demonstrates how far removed they are from who I truly am. The persistence of these doubts does not make them true; rather, they reveal my deep commitment to doing what is right and ensuring the safety and well-being of my students.

Decluttering my mind from these intrusive doubts allows me to focus on the joy and purpose of my work. The trust and affection I see in the children I teach affirm that my actions and intentions are entirely healthy and nurturing. My ability to create a positive and safe learning environment is proof of my commitment to their well-being. In prioritizing their needs and maintaining clear professional boundaries, I demonstrate not only my capability as a teacher but also the integrity and care that define my relationships with them.

By staying true to the values I hold dear—empathy, responsibility, and protection—I continue to fulfill my role in a way that supports the children's growth and development. These actions, grounded in my professional and personal principles, are the clearest evidence that my feelings and instincts are aligned with the healthy and positive role I play in their lives.

Form 5.5. An Alternative Narrative for John (Vignette 1.3)
"I am a faithful person who truly believes in God."

Every day, my faith guides me like a moral compass, directing my actions and decisions. It's in the quiet moments of prayer, in my daily routine, and in the choices I make. When I wake up in the morning and begin my day, I follow the path that God has set for me. Whether I'm at work, with family, or in prayer, I carry my faith with me. I know that being committed to prayer, worship, and service to others is a sign of my genuine belief. Even if I have days where I feel less focused, my faith is still there, grounding me through it all. My actions reflect my dedication to living by God's word.

Faith has always provided direction and meaning in my life. I remember many times when I felt deeply connected to God, especially during prayer and worship. I've experienced His presence in moments of quiet reflection, during worship, and even in the simple everyday tasks where I offer gratitude. There are times when my mind wanders, or I don't feel that intense connection, but I still trust that my faith is steady. It's in those moments that I know my faith is real. Whenever I've faced difficulties, I've turned to God for strength. My faith has always been my anchor, providing peace and comfort during even the most challenging times. I've relied on it consistently, and it has never failed me.

Living a life guided by faith is something I value deeply. My spiritual growth is a priority, and I take conscious steps to strengthen my relationship with God. Faith isn't just something I talk about—it's the foundation of my values and decisions. I might not have all the answers, but I know I'm doing my best to stay true to what I believe. My choices are shaped by my belief in God's teachings. I actively seek to deepen that connection by dedicating time to prayer, reading scripture, and reflecting on how I can better align my life with God's will. My commitment to these practices isn't out of obligation but a deep desire to remain close to God and to honor Him in every aspect of my life.

My spiritual mentors and leaders have always supported me in this journey. Their encouragement reminds me that my faith is genuine. They've emphasized the importance of my commitment to prayer and worship, reaffirming that this dedication is a sign of true belief. The scriptures themselves reinforce that living according to God's word is evidence of strong faith, and I strive to follow that path every day. Faith might not always feel the same, but it's something I've chosen to dedicate myself to, regardless of the ups and downs. My faith isn't something that wavers, because my connection to God is more than just a feeling—it's a lived experience. I make an active effort to stay connected to Him, knowing that this relationship gives my life purpose and strength.

It's not just spiritual leaders who see this in me—my family and friends have often spoken of my devotion. They've mentioned how they see me as someone deeply connected to God, and their words reflect the truth I feel in my heart. People close to me, including friends, family, and members of my church, often describe me as a spiritual role model. Their confidence in my faith is reassuring, and it mirrors what I know to be true about myself. It's comforting to know that others see my efforts to live faithfully, even if I'm not always as perfect as I'd like to be. These observations from those I care about reinforce that my faith isn't something hidden or fleeting—it is visible and recognized by those around me.

I've heard many stories and testimonies from others about how faith shapes their lives, and it always resonates with me. Religious programs I watch often feature people who live lives of devotion and commitment, just like mine. These stories remind me that my own faith journey is a testament to my belief in God. My life is centered around faith, and I take comfort in knowing that I am walking the same path as others who are deeply committed to their beliefs. The examples of other faithful people inspire me and remind me that I, too, am firmly planted in my belief in God, living a life of devotion.

My faith isn't just a part of my life—it is the core of who I am. It is reflected in my actions, choices, and relationships with others. My commitment to kindness, compassion, and integrity stems directly from my belief in God's teachings Sometimes I make mistakes or miss the mark, but I try to keep growing and improving, guided by my faith. I find fulfillment in living this way, knowing that my actions align with my faith. Whether I'm praying, helping others, or simply reflecting on the blessings in my life, my devotion to God provides meaning and purpose. Each day, I grow closer to Him, and each day, I reaffirm that I am a faithful person who truly believes in God. My relationship with God fills me with peace, and this faith shapes how I view the world, how I treat others, and how I make decisions. It's a fundamental part of who I am, and it strengthens me in everything I do.

My faith is what gives me clarity. It provides me with hope and the knowledge that I am never alone. God is always present in my life, guiding me through each season, and reminding me that through Him, I can overcome any obstacle. I find that my faith only grows stronger with time, and the more I engage with my spiritual practices, the deeper my connection to God becomes. My belief isn't just a fleeting feeling—it's a lifelong commitment that continues to enrich and guide every part of my life.

Form 5.5. An Alternative Narrative for Laura (Vignette 1.4)
"I am an honest and ethical person."

Honesty has always been important to me, though I know it doesn't mean being perfect. I try my best to act with integrity in both my work and personal life, even if I don't always get it right. When I make a mistake, I feel responsible for addressing it, and I try to make amends when I can. It's not easy, but I believe that handling errors honestly is part of what makes someone ethical. I don't need to be flawless to know that honesty matters deeply to me.

At work, I take pride in being reliable and transparent. My colleagues and clients trust me because I put effort into being fair and clear in my communication. While I've made mistakes, like forgetting to credit a teammate or occasionally missing a detail, I've always worked to correct them and learn from them. Over time, I've built a reputation for being conscientious, and I see that reflected in the trust others place in me. That trust reminds me that my actions, on the whole, align with my values.

I value fairness and try to make choices that reflect that, even when it's difficult. I don't always get it perfect, and I sometimes second-guess myself, but I know that my intentions are in the right place. Upholding my values has required effort and self-reflection, and while I sometimes struggle, I see those challenges as part of growing into the person I want to be. Ethics isn't about never faltering—it's about striving to do the right thing when it counts.

In my personal life, I think about the people who know me well—my friends, family, and colleagues. They trust me and often come to me for advice, which I take as a sign that they see me as dependable and honest. I've had conversations with friends where they've pointed out how much they appreciate my care in handling tricky situations. Those comments encourage me to keep prioritizing integrity, even when I feel uncertain.

I've been lucky to have mentors and coworkers who emphasize the importance of ethical decision-making. They've given me positive feedback about my approach, and that helps me stay grounded in my values. I know that being honest doesn't mean being perfect, and that reassurance lets me focus on how I handle situations rather than worrying about every small mistake. My effort to stay accountable, even in tough moments, shows me that I'm living according to the principles that matter most to me.

Of course, there have been moments when I could have taken the easier path and ignored an issue, but I've tried to address those situations directly. Whether it's owning up to an oversight at work or resolving a disagreement in my personal life, I've made an effort to choose transparency, even when it's uncomfortable. These experiences remind me that being ethical isn't always easy, but it's worth it to stay true to myself.

When I reflect on my actions and values, I know that honesty is at the core of how I try to live. While I'll never be perfect, I believe that my overall commitment to doing the right thing defines me more than any individual mistake. Every choice is an opportunity to grow, and knowing that I'm guided by a sense of fairness and integrity gives me confidence.

Form 5.5. An Alternative Narrative for Ethan (Vignette 1.5)
"I am thorough and attentive in my actions, ensuring that things are in order."
"The things around me are functioning as expected and are reliable."

Each day, with intentional and reasonable care, I can trust that my actions are sufficient to ensure a safe and reliable environment. Most appliances and systems I use are designed to work consistently and safely, with basic precautions in place. Manufacturers invest significant effort into creating safeguards, and this makes me feel confident that the items I use daily are dependable when handled appropriately. These safeguards, combined with occasional checks, are enough to keep things running smoothly.

I've noticed through experience that my belongings and appliances tend to work as expected over time. When I follow a simple routine to check things, they remain secure, allowing me to feel reassured in my efforts. Once I ensure something is in order—like locking a door or turning off a stove—it stays that way, enabling me to trust my initial actions. It's encouraging to reflect on how these small, reasonable habits are effective in maintaining a well-functioning home.

My approach to care and safety reflects a balanced sense of responsibility. I value attentiveness without overextending effort, which aligns with my principles of living thoughtfully and managing my environment efficiently. When I check things once and move on, I feel prepared, knowing that I've upheld my commitment to being thorough while avoiding unnecessary repetition. This standard of balance provides reassurance that my actions are both practical and reliable.

Experts and safety guidelines reinforce this approach, emphasizing that following basic instructions and occasional checks are enough to maintain safety. For example, industry standards highlight that periodic maintenance—rather than constant monitoring—is sufficient to ensure functionality. These guidelines support my belief that my habits are in line with what is needed for a secure and well-maintained space.

Hearing from friends and family also reinforces my sense of trust in my surroundings. They often share how they rely on their routines to manage their homes effectively without excessive worry. Their experiences remind me that most things function reliably when used correctly, and it's reassuring to know that I'm not alone in this perspective. Trusting in these shared principles helps me feel connected and supported in my approach to care and safety.

My ability to balance attentiveness with trust in the systems around me creates a sense of stability in my daily life. Knowing that small, thoughtful actions are enough allows me to shift my focus to other meaningful aspects of my day. The peace of mind that comes from this balance gives me confidence in my routines and in the reliability of my home. By embracing this trust, I create an environment where I can thrive without unnecessary concern.

This thoughtful approach brings a sense of security and self-assurance. Through reasonable care, I maintain a well-functioning space that reflects my values and supports my daily life. Trusting in the reliability of my actions and surroundings opens the door to greater peace, allowing me to move forward with clarity and focus.

Form 5.5. An Alternative Narrative for Sophie (Vignette 1.6)

"My environment and the products I use are safe, supporting the well-being of myself and others."

Each day, I can feel confident in the safe, healthy environment I've created for myself and others. My home is a place I can truly relax, knowing that the products I use are designed with health and safety in mind. Household products go through rigorous testing to meet strict health standards, especially for daily use. This allows me to trust that these products are built not only for convenience but for safety and cleanliness, reducing dust, bacteria, and other unwanted particles. Normal cleanliness is the foundation of health in my home, supporting my well-being every day.

I've been using a variety of household products for years, and they've consistently helped me maintain a welcoming, healthy environment. With my simple, effective routines, my space feels fresh and organized. I can see how this contributes to my health; a clean space feels brighter and supports my energy. Friends and family often comment on how comfortable and pleasant it feels here, and I'm glad to know they feel safe in my space, too. My routines bring us all peace of mind, knowing that we're in a place that promotes well-being. It's encouraging to see that others enjoy this environment as much as I do, which reinforces my belief that my space is safe and well-cared for.

For me, maintaining a clean environment is more than a habit—it's a reflection of the care I value deeply. My approach is simple yet effective, allowing me to support a healthy home without excessive effort. Basic cleaning is both practical and calming, giving me a safe, orderly space to unwind and recharge. By following standard cleaning guidelines, I'm confident I'm supporting a healthy environment that benefits everyone. This balanced, responsible approach gives me reassurance and helps me stay grounded. Knowing I don't need to overdo things to have a clean, healthy home makes my routine feel sustainable and balanced.

Experts also reinforce that the products I use are safe and effective when used as directed. Health agencies and environmental authorities ensure that consumer products meet rigorous standards, adding an extra layer of security to my choices. Scientific studies show that responsible, regular cleaning with these products poses minimal risks while offering real benefits for health. Guidelines from trusted sources, like health organizations, back up my choices, which reinforces my belief that I'm creating a truly safe environment. This information reassures me that my home is a safe, well-maintained space that protects my health.

I also feel encouraged by the experiences of others who share a similar approach to home care. Family and friends have described how their own routines help keep them healthy and comfortable, which reassures me that I'm making good choices. I often read articles and hear news reports that emphasize the importance of maintaining a clean home for health benefits. They remind me that a clean space supports both physical well-being and mental clarity, making it easier to relax and feel at peace. Stories I hear from others show me that a moderate, balanced approach keeps us all safe and healthy, aligning with what I believe about a well-cared-for space.

Overall, my home routines contribute to a healthy, balanced environment that supports my well-being. My space feels vibrant and clean, a source of calm and health that I can rely on. Knowing that my environment and the products I use are designed to be safe and effective makes me feel secure, and my commitment to maintaining this environment supports both my well-being and that of anyone who visits my home. Knowing that I've created an environment free from harmful risks and full of benefits brings me confidence and peace of mind. I feel reassured and at ease, knowing that my approach protects and supports both my well-being and that of anyone who visits my home.

Form 5.5. An Alternative Narrative for Matthew (Vignette 1.7)

"Things are placed well enough, done right, and adequately complete for their purpose."

As an architect, I've come to appreciate the value of tasks meeting clear, defined requirements. When I work on a project, I know there's a specific endpoint based on the goals of the design. Once I've verified my work to meet these standards, I trust that it's ready and doesn't need more adjustments. I find satisfaction in seeing a plan come together as intended, knowing it achieves what it's supposed to. My training emphasized that good design is functional and aligns with practical goals, and I've learned that meeting these standards signals a task is complete and reliable.

In my home, I also like things to feel orderly, but I understand that arrangements serve their purpose as long as they're generally in place. When I arrange books on my shelf or items on my desk, I know they meet my goal of creating a comfortable, organized space. I've noticed that once I set things up in a way that feels functional, they stay that way without needing constant adjustments. Friends and family seem at ease in my space, which reassures me that it's well-suited for daily life and gatherings. I feel comfortable knowing my initial arrangements support the function and flow of my home.

At work, I see that a completed project meets its purpose without needing extra checks once it's aligned with project goals. When I've double-checked my drafts and reviewed the necessary details, I trust that the design is ready to move forward. My training has taught me that precision and attention to detail achieve reliable results without needing endless revisits. My colleagues and clients are consistently satisfied with my work, and their feedback reflects that my initial efforts are thorough and effective. It's clear that a well-done task supports the project's goals as is, and that gives me confidence in my process.

I value clarity and efficiency, and I find that both are achieved when I trust my own process. This clarity allows me to focus on each task as needed, understanding that once I meet its requirements, it's effectively complete. I notice my colleagues approach work similarly, moving forward once they've met project requirements, which reinforces my own trust in my work. I see that a balanced approach makes a difference, allowing me to keep up with my workload without feeling the need to revisit completed tasks.

This approach gives me peace of mind. My attention to initial arrangements provides me with a functional, satisfying environment, and I feel reassured knowing my work and surroundings meet my needs and goals fully. I know that my attention to detail has served me well over time, producing results that align with the expectations I set for myself and with the demands of the task. I feel confident that my process is strong, allowing me to see each project and each task as successfully completed, with a sense of purpose and balance that I find rewarding.

Form 5.5. An Alternative Narrative for Olivia (Vignette 1.8)

"My body performs its natural functions effectively."
"I am in control of my attention and can direct my focus as I choose."

I can trust that my body and mind are designed to function effectively on their own. Each day, my body performs its natural functions smoothly, allowing me to go about my routines with confidence. My breathing, blinking, and other bodily processes happen automatically, without needing my direction. I can appreciate this harmony, which lets me focus on what truly matters in my life. My mind is naturally capable of shifting its attention where it's needed, and I can rely on that adaptability to help me stay engaged in the present moment.

I recall many moments in my life when my body handled everything seamlessly, from breathing to moving, even when I was deeply focused on something else. This memory reassures me that my body is inherently trustworthy, carrying out its tasks without me needing to direct it. At work, I can trust that my attention will follow the task at hand, and if a sensation or thought arises, it can pass on its own, allowing me to stay connected to what I'm doing. This ability to let go of monitoring feels empowering, and I know my mind can regulate itself, guiding my focus to adapt to each situation. My mind has always been resilient, guiding my attention naturally to what's most important in each moment. When I'm engaged in conversation or absorbed in a project, my mind shifts seamlessly, allowing me to respond thoughtfully and meaningfully. Knowing that my mind is resilient gives me a foundation of security, one I can rely on as I move through the day.

In my daily life, I can follow a practical approach to maintaining a healthy environment and body, knowing that these things are designed to be safe and effective without constant vigilance. I use household products and follow daily routines that support my well-being. This balanced approach is enough to create a safe and positive environment, one that allows me to live fully without needing to monitor every detail.

When I'm with friends, I can focus on the people I care about, trusting that my body will take care of its functions naturally. I can enjoy meals and social gatherings without feeling the need to monitor my sensations, allowing myself to be present and connected. Focusing on our conversations and shared moments brings a sense of calm. By letting go of my internal focus, I open up to the joy of these interactions, strengthening my bonds with the people I care about. Friends and family have shared their trust in their bodies, which reminds me that it's safe to allow my body to do its work without interference. This brings a sense of ease to social moments, helping me connect meaningfully with others.

Professionals I trust—health experts, psychologists, and mindfulness teachers—emphasize that the body and mind are equipped to self-regulate. Health experts remind us that the body's essential functions don't require constant monitoring, and that the mind's focus adapts naturally to life's demands. This guidance reassures me that I don't need to keep checking; I can rely on the natural systems designed to keep me safe and well. This approach supports a steady foundation, helping me trust that both my mind and body can function reliably in any situation.

In moments of quiet reflection, I can take comfort in knowing that life's small distractions and natural shifts in focus are enough to keep my body's functions on course. I see how little adjustments in my environment, or simple moments of engagement, show me that my mind naturally moves from one thing to the next, allowing me to engage with my surroundings fully. This confidence in my mind's natural flow lets me appreciate each moment more fully, without needing to monitor or control what happens within me.

Ultimately, my body and mind's natural and autonomous functioning is the status quo—a reliable and inherent part of who I am. There's nothing fundamentally wrong with me that prevents me from relying on these natural processes. I feel reassured knowing that my body and mind are aligned, always ready to support me, allowing me to move forward with trust and peace. I feel secure knowing that the natural functioning of my body and mind is steadfast. It's a core part of who I am, supporting me day by day, so I can live fully and move forward with peace.

Form 5.5. An Alternative Narrative for Henry (Vignette 1.9)

"My sexuality aligns with my heterosexual identity, and I am authentically connected to who I truly am."

As I reflect on my life, I find reassurance in the pattern of feelings and relationships that have always felt authentic to me. My connection with my girlfriend isn't just comfortable—it's meaningful and fulfilling in a way that feels deeply aligned with who I am. This relationship has brought me happiness and stability, reinforcing my sense of self and allowing me to experience love that feels genuine. I can't imagine feeling this same way in any other kind of relationship, as my attraction to women has been a steady, integral part of my identity.

Looking back on my relationships and connections, I can see a clear pattern. Throughout my life, my feelings of attraction toward women have been consistent and true to my experiences. This doesn't fluctuate for me; it's a foundation I can trust, a part of myself that feels certain and solid. Even though doubts sometimes arise, they don't change what I experience day to day. Spending time with my girlfriend reminds me of the closeness and compatibility we share, feelings that resonate on a deep level. I value the moments we spend together, and my connection with her is a reflection of the person I truly am.

Friends who know me well have often commented on the happiness they see in my relationship. It's comforting to know they recognize the fulfillment I find in this connection and support my understanding of myself. Hearing others' stories about the certainty they feel in their orientation reminds me that orientation is a stable part of identity, grounded in authentic experiences. Those around me see my connection with my girlfriend as genuine and supportive, which reinforces my own sense of stability in my relationship and my identity.

In speaking with people I trust, I'm reminded that knowing oneself often comes from a pattern of lived experiences, moments, and relationships that resonate on a genuine level. These conversations emphasize that orientation isn't something that shifts without reason; it's often rooted in lasting connections and patterns of attraction. I can feel reassured knowing that my life experiences and the connection I share with my girlfriend align with my values of honesty and integrity, further grounding my identity.

Reading stories from people who feel secure in their orientation helps me see that doubts, while sometimes present, don't need to define reality. Psychologists and experts in sexuality often highlight that one's orientation is usually reflected through a lifetime of steady attraction and relationships that feel meaningful. Experts note that consistent attractions and emotionally significant relationships often reinforce a person's authentic orientation, and I feel this consistency in my own life. For me, there's a natural stability in knowing that my relationships, feelings, and experiences all align in a way that is authentic and true.

There is a sense of comfort in knowing that the life I have chosen reflects my genuine self. When I imagine my future, it's with my girlfriend by my side, in a relationship that continues to feel real and deeply fulfilling. I know my values, my desires, and my understanding of myself align with this reality. As I think about the path my life has taken, I see a continuity that aligns naturally with my identity, confirming that my experiences are meaningful and true to who I am. My life, my connections, and the stability I feel in my relationship reassure me that I am grounded in my true self, confident in who I am and the path I have chosen.

Form 5.5. An Alternative Narrative for Mia (Vignette 1.10)
"My skin is healthy, and I am aware of its natural changes."

I know that by practicing a balanced routine, I am caring for my skin in a way that aligns with what professionals recommend. I protect my skin by applying sunscreen and following a routine that keeps it healthy. I trust that this care is enough to help me stay aware of any genuine changes without the need for constant checking. When I look in the mirror, I can appreciate that my skin is resilient and benefits from the care I put into it daily. I understand that changes in skin appearance, like freckles or moles are natural, arising as part of living a full life.

Over time, I've noticed that my body, including my skin, has a natural rhythm and stability. I see how my skin changes subtly with the seasons or after being outdoors, which reminds me of the normal shifts that happen naturally. These changes are just part of living fully and embracing all that life has to offer.

My approach to self-care allows me to appreciate these natural patterns without needing to examine every detail.

When I see my doctor for annual check-ups, I feel reassured by their expertise. In the past, every concern I raised has been met with careful evaluation and, ultimately, reassurance. This shows me that I can trust both my own observations and the expertise of professionals who are dedicated to my health. My doctor's guidance reflects a routine of self-care, where my regular appointments and mindful attention to my skin form a reliable rhythm. This approach aligns with my values and reinforces my confidence in my health.

I understand that skin health is largely stable, and I know that changes in skin don't suddenly emerge overnight. When I see minor changes, I can recognize them as natural parts of living. I've heard from friends, family, and health sources that these small variations are a common part of life. Knowing this, I feel empowered to let minor changes come and go without needing to scrutinize them. By embracing this balance, I can enjoy my life more fully, trusting that my healthy skin reflects the care I put into it.

I trust that my annual check-ups provide a solid foundation for my health. I value the professional expertise that assures me I'm taking the right steps, and that my level of care is aligned with what my body truly needs. I've read that dermatologists and health professionals don't recommend over-monitoring, as it creates unnecessary worry. Instead, I see how periodic, routine check-ups give me confidence that I am on the right track. Knowing that my doctor is there to support me provides peace of mind.

When I think of my future, I imagine continuing to care for myself in ways that feel balanced and realistic. I am reassured by my consistent efforts and the professionals who provide guidance along the way. My routine doesn't require constant scrutiny; instead, it promotes a gentle, steady awareness that enhances my life rather than taking from it. With this confidence, I can trust that I am caring for my skin in ways that truly matter, allowing me to enjoy each day with the assurance that I am supporting my health in a meaningful way.

Form 5.5. An Alternative Narrative for Alex (Vignette 1.11)
"My reality is grounded in true experiences and genuine connections."

Each morning, I wake up to familiar surroundings—my bed, the soft morning light filtering in, and the sounds of the world coming to life outside. These daily patterns provide a steady rhythm that roots me in something real and lasting. The continuity of these experiences reinforces my connection to the world around me, as well as my sense of being part of something meaningful. I see my routines as grounding rituals, small reminders that my life is made up of moments that feel purposeful and consistent.

At work, I see the impact of my actions and the purpose behind my efforts. Every line of code, every project we complete as a team, reflects my genuine skills and contributes to something valuable. In the structure of my work, the collaboration with my team, and the satisfaction of completing tasks, I find clear and tangible evidence that my reality is built on meaningful relationships and purposeful efforts. Working alongside my colleagues, sharing ideas, and seeing our projects come to life further assures me that my world is based on real interactions, personal growth, and shared goals. These everyday moments confirm the authenticity of my experiences and strengthen my sense of belonging to a shared reality.

When I spend time with friends, our conversations and shared laughter deepen the connections we've built over years. Every shared memory we've made—whether at gatherings, trips, or simply talking over coffee—feels vivid and true. My friendships are more than fleeting moments; they're rooted in years of mutual support, shared experiences, and personal growth. In these moments, I am reminded that our bonds carry a unique history that couldn't be replicated. These connections feel solid, grounded in something genuine and real. Through my relationships, I feel an undeniable link to the world, one that reaffirms my place within it.

In my hobbies—whether taking a walk in nature, reading a favorite book, or practicing a skill I enjoy— I find myself fully present and engaged. Each small detail, every interaction with the world around me, feels vivid and rewarding. The sights, sounds, and textures of these experiences offer a rich, sensory reality that confirms my place within a complex, vibrant world. The colors of a sunset, the feel of leaves crunching beneath my feet, and the comfort of familiar surroundings reflect a stable, shared reality that I participate in fully. Knowing that my senses connect me to a broader world makes my experiences feel real and fulfilling.

I've also come to understand that human experiences are central to the sense of reality we all share. The connections we build, the memories we create, and the consistent patterns in our lives are all part of this shared world. My life is full of routines, relationships, and places that reflect an enduring and grounded reality. In this world, I can trust that my place is defined by real relationships, tangible experiences, and a sense of purpose that connects me to something larger than myself.

Finally, I recognize that my curiosity and questions about the world stem from a desire to understand, rather than any lack of connection to it. In my personal values, I place high importance on clarity and truth, knowing that my search for meaning drives me to look for authenticity in my surroundings and relationships. This curiosity is a testament to my active engagement with reality, rather than a sign of doubt. With this awareness, I can embrace my experiences and relationships as meaningful parts of my life. I know that my reality is rooted in a world full of genuine interactions, real connections, and moments that shape who I am.

Form 5.5. An Alternative Narrative for Lily (Vignette 1.12)
"My love for Ben is real, and our relationship is a genuine connection."

In the moments when I allow myself to simply be with Ben, a natural warmth fills me. There's a quiet affection and a sense of ease that surfaces when we're together—whether we're laughing, sharing stories, or even just sitting in comfortable silence. These moments aren't forced; they feel like a natural part of our connection, grounded in something genuine. Ben's kindness and steady presence remind me that love often shines through in these everyday ways. I see his consistent support and care as reflections of a relationship that's real.

Reflecting on our time together, I see countless examples of how Ben's thoughtfulness and encouragement create a sense of belonging. When I'm fully present with him, I feel appreciated, understood, and safe. It's in these moments that I realize how deep my affection for him goes and how genuinely connected we are. He's become someone I can rely on in both small and significant ways. The respect and trust we've built over time ground me in the knowledge that my love for him is real, growing through the quiet moments that make up our everyday lives.

I know that love isn't always about feeling "in love" every second; it's often shown in the stability and security we build together. Lasting love, as I've heard from friends and experts, is about sharing mutual respect, kindness, and a sense of home with each other. When I'm with Ben, I see these qualities reflected in our interactions. Our relationship isn't about fleeting highs, but rather the steady companionship and trust I feel when I'm with him. I've come to understand that my true feelings for him show up in the stability and comfort we share, even in the moments that feel ordinary.

Friends and family have commented on the happiness they see in me when I'm with Ben, reminding me of the deep, lasting connection we share. When I look at people I know who are in strong relationships, I see that they're built on mutual respect and a sense of home with one another. Ben and I have this, too. He accepts me as I am, and I feel valued and free to be myself with him, which deepens our connection.

When I think about a future without Ben, it feels incomplete. There's a sense that something essential would be missing—a piece that has grown into an important part of who I am. Even when doubts cloud my mind, my feelings for Ben remain steady and true. I realize that in the moments when I'm not questioning, I feel a peaceful certainty about him that's difficult to imagine with anyone else. Our relationship is built on respect, trust, and shared moments of genuine affection, creating a sense of belonging that feels real and lasting.

Form 5.5. An Alternative Narrative for Lucas (Vignette 1.13)
"My identity is secure and aligned with who I want to be."

My identity has been shaped by years of experiences, values, and relationships. My core qualities, beliefs, and personality are the result of countless moments and choices that make me who I am, and real identity doesn't shift suddenly or without reason. Whether I'm with family, friends, or by myself, my values and characteristics feel familiar and consistent.

Identity is built on foundational values that don't simply disappear. Even as I grow or learn new things, the qualities I admire most in myself—like resilience, curiosity, and loyalty—remain a core part of who I am. These qualities aren't easily influenced by daily interactions, media, or conversations; they are intrinsic to me and don't change unless I choose to evolve in a specific direction. When I look back at photos from a few months or even years ago, I recognize myself as the same person I am today. While there may be minor changes, the essential parts of me have remained stable.

Experts in psychology and personal development suggest that a secure identity resists quick or superficial changes. Identity is something formed over time, inherently resilient and unshaken by ordinary influences or shifts in appearance. Friends I trust tell me that true personality deepens over time but doesn't fundamentally change. Hearing this reassures me that the things I value and the qualities I admire in myself are stable, reinforcing that my identity is not something fragile.

I often feel the strength of my true self when I'm fully present and connected in my relationships or engaged in something meaningful. Friends and family comment on the way I've stayed true to myself over the years, and these qualities they recognize in me have remained consistent, even as life brings new experiences. Friends who know me well see these qualities in me, and the things I care about have stayed steady, no matter the changes around me. These enduring traits are what make me feel secure and confident in who I am.

When I think about my future, I can imagine myself continuing to grow in ways that align with who I already am. I feel a natural continuity, a progression that feels true to my values. Even in unfamiliar situations, I find myself guided by my own principles, experiencing new things without losing my sense of self. I know that my identity, based on experiences, values, and personal growth, is secure and genuine.

Form 5.5. An Alternative Narrative for Abigail (Vignette 1.14)
"My progress is real, and I am capable of continuing to improve."
"I have OCD, and I am able to understand it."

I've lived with OCD for years, and managing it hasn't been easy, but I've made meaningful progress. The kind of endless rituals and overwhelming doubts that used to dominate my life have loosened their grip. My ability to resist compulsions and navigate obsessions shows that the strategies I've learned and applied in therapy are working. This isn't an accident—progress comes from sustained effort and applying techniques that are proven to help. The calm and reduced symptoms I'm experiencing aren't a prelude to something worse; they reflect the hard work I've done to improve.

When I reflect on my journey, I see proof of this progress. There was a time when I couldn't go an hour without checking, cleaning, or seeking reassurance. Now, I can recognize obsessive thoughts for what they are without acting on them, and I've reclaimed so much time and energy that used to be consumed by OCD. These changes remind me that recovery is a process—it's not linear, but every step forward matters. The relief I feel from using the tools I've learned confirms that my diagnosis is accurate and that my efforts are paying off.

I've come to understand OCD as a well-defined condition. The patterns I've experienced—obsessions followed by compulsions and the cycle of doubt—align perfectly with the criteria for OCD. My therapist has guided me through techniques that specifically target OCD, and they've worked. The changes I've noticed aren't just in my mind; they're evident in my behavior, my routines, and my ability to handle triggers that used to overwhelm me.

Self-awareness has been a cornerstone of my progress. I value honesty and clarity, and these values have helped me understand my experiences and move forward. By reflecting on my symptoms and how they've evolved, I've been able to build a stronger sense of control over my mental health. This clarity empowers me to take constructive steps, even when doubts arise.

I've also found reassurance in what I've learned from others. Experts emphasize that OCD is a condition that can improve significantly with the right treatment, and this has been true in my case. Friends who've experienced OCD have shared how progress can feel fragile but becomes more stable with time, which aligns with my own journey. Personal accounts and research highlight that recovery is rarely straightforward—it's a process of ups and downs—but each step builds toward long-term improvement.

Even in moments of doubt, I can see the evidence of my progress. The ability to let go of compulsions and to reclaim my time are all tangible signs of the strides I've made. Progress isn't always dramatic; sometimes, it's in the small changes that accumulate over time. Even if I face setbacks or new challenges, these moments don't erase the progress I've achieved—they're part of the journey.

My identity isn't tied to OCD, but my ability to understand and manage it is a reflection of my resilience. I know that I'm capable of continuing to improve because I've already proven to myself that change is possible. My progress is real, my understanding of OCD is clear, and I have the tools to navigate whatever comes next.

Form 5.5. An Alternative Narrative for Oliver (Vignette 1.15)
"Letting Go of Unnecessary Items Is a Wise and Thoughtful Choice"

Each day I make the decision to release items I no longer need, I find clarity and peace. Letting go of unnecessary possessions doesn't mean I'm losing anything important—it means I'm making room for what truly matters. When I clear away clutter, I can focus on the things that bring me joy, creativity, and a sense of purpose. My space begins to feel more like a home and less like a storage room, and I'm reminded of how much I value simplicity and order in my life.

When I look at the items I've chosen to let go of, I see how much lighter my environment feels. I remember a time when I finally donated a box of clothes I hadn't worn in years. At first, I hesitated, but once they were gone, I didn't miss them. In fact, I felt relieved, knowing they could serve someone else. That experience taught me that holding onto things "just in case" often creates more anxiety than letting go. It also showed me that what I truly value isn't tied to the objects themselves, but to the space and freedom their absence creates.

Clearing clutter allows me to appreciate the items I decide to keep. When I removed old stacks of magazines from my desk, I found space to work on my writing again. It felt like reclaiming a part of myself. My possessions are not my identity—they are tools that either support me or distract me. By choosing wisely, I can create an environment that reflects the person I want to be.

Each time I donate items to someone who needs them more, I feel like I'm contributing to a larger purpose. I don't have to hold onto every object to be responsible or prepared. Sometimes, the most responsible choice is letting something go so it can be useful elsewhere. Not every item needs to be recycled or repurposed perfectly, but doing what I can feels meaningful and aligns with my values of sustainability and kindness.

Letting go is also an act of trust—in myself and in the future. I've realized that I don't have to hold onto everything out of fear of regret. Most of the things I've worried about discarding in the past have turned out to be unnecessary, and if I ever do need something again, I trust that I'll find a solution. The idea of releasing items isn't about loss—it's about making thoughtful choices that support the life I want to lead. With every item I release, I'm creating space for the experiences, relationships, and opportunities that truly matter.

By focusing on one area at a time, I've started to see the transformation I longed for. Clearing my apartment has made it a place where I can think clearly, work productively, and feel proud of my surroundings. I've even found joy in the process of rediscovery—finding items I love that were buried under clutter, and recognizing that they shine brighter when they aren't competing with unnecessary things.

I see now that letting go doesn't mean losing—it means gaining control over my space, my time, and my energy. My home is becoming a place where I feel comfortable, organized, and free to live without the weight of unnecessary possessions. I'm learning that the things I choose to keep are enough to support me, and that simplicity is a gift I can give myself every day. Releasing the excess is not only wise but liberating, and it brings me closer to the life I truly want.

Resources

I-CBT Online

ICBT Online is a comprehensive resource dedicated to Inference-Based Cognitive-Behavioral Therapy (I-CBT), a specialized approach for treating OCD and related disorders. The platform offers information about the therapy model, practical self-help tools, and professional development opportunities, serving as a valuable hub for individuals, therapists, and researchers. Additionally, it features a directory of professionals providing I-CBT, simplifying the process of connecting with qualified therapists for this treatment. Designed to empower users with effective strategies, ICBT Online supports the application and growth of I-CBT for managing OCD and related conditions

Contact Information:
Website: https://icbt.online/
Contact Page: https://icbt.online/contact/

International OCD Foundation

The International OCD Foundation (IOCDF) is a nonprofit organization dedicated to helping individuals affected by OCD and related disorders lead full and productive lives. The foundation aims to increase access to effective treatment through research and training, foster a supportive community for those affected, and combat the stigma surrounding mental health issues. The IOCDF offers resources such as educational materials, support groups, and professional training programs to support individuals with OCD and their families

Contact Information:
Mailing Address: PO Box 961029, Boston, MA 02196
Phone: (617) 973-5801
Website: https://iocdf.org/

OCD-UK

OCD-UK is a national charity in the United Kingdom, run by and for individuals with lived experience of OCD. The organization is dedicated to supporting those affected by OCD through education, advocacy, and the promotion of recovery-focused services. OCD-UK provides a range of resources, including educational materials, support groups, and online discussion forums, to foster a supportive community and enhance public understanding of OCD. OCD-UK is committed to improving access to effective treatment, raising awareness, and challenging the stigma associated with OCD, empowering individuals to lead full and productive lives.

Contact Information:
Website: https://www.ocduk.org/
Phone: 01332 588112
Email: support@ocduk.org

OCD Action

OCD Action is a UK-based charity dedicated to supporting individuals affected by OCD and related conditions. The organization provides a range of services, including a confidential helpline, support groups, advocacy, and educational resources, aiming to increase awareness and understanding of OCD. OCD Action strives to ensure that those affected receive appropriate treatment and support, working towards a society where OCD is well understood and effectively treated.

Contact Information:
Website: https://ocdaction.org.uk/
Office Phone: 020 7253 5272
Office Email: info@ocdaction.org.uk
Helpline Phone: 0300 636 5478 (9am to 8pm)
Helpline Email: support@ocdaction.org.uk

OCD Ireland

OCD Ireland is a national organization dedicated to supporting individuals affected by OCD and related disorders. The organization provides resources such as educational materials, support groups, and information to assist individuals and their families in managing these conditions. OCD Ireland also works to reduce stigma and increase understanding through media engagement and educational talks at schools and universities.

Contact Information:
Website: https://ocdireland.org/
Email: information@ocdireland.org

The Anxiety and Depression Association of America

The Anxiety and Depression Association of America (ADAA) is an international nonprofit organization dedicated to the prevention, treatment, and cure of anxiety, depression, OCD, PTSD, and co-occurring disorders through education, practice, and research. Founded in 1979, ADAA aims to improve the quality of life for those affected by these conditions by promoting evidence-based treatments and fostering a supportive community. The organization offers resources such as educational materials, support groups, and professional training programs to support individuals with anxiety and depression and their families.

Contact Information:
Website: https://adaa.org/
Mailing Address: 8701 Georgia Avenue, Suite #412, Silver Spring, MD 20910
Phone: (240) 485-1001
Email: information@adaa.org

Association for Behavioral and Cognitive Therapies

The Association for Behavioral and Cognitive Therapies (ABCT) is a multidisciplinary organization committed to advancing scientific approaches to understanding and ameliorating human problems through behavioral, cognitive, and evidence-based principles. ABCT offers resources such as educational materials, support groups, and professional training programs to support individuals with behavioral and cognitive concerns and their families. The association also hosts an annual convention and publishes two journals—*Behavior Therapy* and *Cognitive and Behavioral Practice*—to disseminate research and promote best practices in the field.

Contact Information:
Website: https://www.abct.org/
Mailing Address: 305 7th Avenue, 16th Floor, New York, NY 10001
Phone: (212) 647-1890
Email: centraloffice@abct.org

The American Psychological Association

The American Psychological Association (APA) is the leading scientific and professional organization representing psychology in the United States, with over 157,000 members, including researchers, educators, clinicians, consultants, and students. Founded in 1892, the APA aims to advance the creation, communication, and application of psychological knowledge to benefit society and improve lives. The association provides resources such as educational materials, professional training programs, and publications to support individuals in the field of psychology and the broader community.

Contact Information:
Website: https://www.apa.org/
Mailing Address: 750 First Street, NE, Washington, DC 20002-4242
Phone: (800) 374-2721 or (202) 336-5500

The Canadian Association of Cognitive and Behavioural Therapies

The Canadian Association of Cognitive and Behavioural Therapies (CACBT) is a national organization dedicated to advancing the practice and science of cognitive behavioural therapy (CBT) in Canada. Established in 2010, CACBT focuses on training, advocacy, accreditation, and the dissemination of CBT knowledge. The association offers resources such as educational materials, professional development opportunities, and certification for qualified CBT practitioners. CACBT also maintains a directory of certified therapists, facilitating connections between individuals seeking evidence-based treatment and qualified professionals.

Contact Information:
Website: https://www.cacbt.ca/
Email: info@cacbt.ca

The Australian Association for Cognitive and Behaviour Therapy

The Australian Association for Cognitive and Behaviour Therapy (AACBT) is a multidisciplinary professional body dedicated to the practice, research, and training of evidence-based behavioral and cognitive therapies in Australia. Established in 1979, AACBT aims to improve the quality of these therapies by providing high-quality professional development opportunities, including workshops, webinars, and an annual national conference. The association fosters a community of practitioners and researchers committed to advancing cognitive and behavioral therapies and offers resources such as educational materials and events to support professionals in the field.

Contact Information:
Website: https://www.aacbt.org.au/
Mailing Address: PO Box 233, Northbridge, NSW 1560, Australia
Email: info@aacbt.org.au

The British Association for Behavioural and Cognitive Psychotherapies

The British Association for Behavioural and Cognitive Psychotherapies (BABCP) is the leading organization for Cognitive Behavioural Therapy (CBT) in the UK and Ireland. Established in 1972, BABCP is a multidisciplinary interest group dedicated to the practice, theory, and development of behavioral and cognitive psychotherapies. The association promotes high standards of CBT practice, supervision, and training, and supports its members through professional development opportunities and a vibrant community network. BABCP operates a respected voluntary register for accredited CBT practitioners, which is accredited by the Professional Standards Authority, ensuring public protection by upholding best practices.

Contact Information:
Website: https://www.babcp.com/
Mailing Address: Imperial House, Hornby Street, Bury, Lancashire, BL9 5BN, United Kingdom
Phone: +44 (0)161 705 4304
Email: babcp@babcp.com

About the Author

Dr. Frederick Aardema is a clinical psychologist, researcher, and professor in the Department of Psychiatry and Addiction at the University of Montreal. Dr. Aardema has dedicated nearly three decades advancing the understanding and treatment of Obsessive-Compulsive Disorder (OCD), pioneering innovative approaches to help individuals overcome the disorder.

As the co-creator of Inference-Based Cognitive Behavioral Therapy (I-CBT), he is at the forefront of its ongoing development, validation, and dissemination, providing individuals with OCD a novel and highly effective evidence-based treatment option. His research focuses on reasoning, imagination and feared-self perceptions in OCD, offering profound insights into how the disorder develops and persists.

In his role as director of the Obsessive-Compulsive Disorder Clinical Study Center at the Montreal Mental Health University Institute Research Center, Dr. Aardema leads cutting-edge clinical trials that compare I-CBT with other approaches, such as Exposure and Response Prevention (ERP). These studies consistently validate I-CBT as an innovative and highly effective treatment for OCD.

Dr. Aardema's extensive publications explore a wide range of topics related to OCD and its treatment, contributing significantly to the field's understanding of the disorder. His work is widely recognized, and he frequently presents at international conferences on the latest advancements in OCD treatment.

Beyond his research, Dr. Aardema is deeply committed to making I-CBT accessible worldwide through clinician training, online resources, and collaborative initiatives. His dedication to improving OCD treatment has empowered countless individuals to reclaim their lives and break free from the grip of obsessional doubt.

Made in United States
Troutdale, OR
12/14/2024

26503951R00197